ACHILLES TENDON D

A COMPREHENSIVE OVERVI
DIAGNOSIS AND TREATMEN ;

DJO PUBLICATIONS

A DJO Global, Inc. initiative
International Headquarters - London

www.DJOpublications.com

Project Manager: Francine Van Steenkiste
Cover Design: Simon Taylor
Compositor: DJO Publications (DJO Global, Inc.)
Secretary of the Achilles Tendon Study Group: Ruben Zwiers

First edition 2014

ISBN number: 978-0-9558873-4-5

Published by DJO Publications
1a Guildford Business Park
Guildford
Surrey
GU2 8XG
UK
www.DJOglobal.eu

Printed in the UK

ACHILLES TENDON Disorders
A COMPREHENSIVE OVERVIEW OF DIAGNOSIS AND TREATMENT

EDITORS:

Jón Karlsson
MD, PhD, Professor
Department of Orthopaedics
Sahlgrenska University Hospital
Sahlgrenska Academy
Gothenburg University
Gothenburg, Sweden

James D. F. Calder
MD, FRCS (Tr&Orth), FFSEM (UK)
Consultant Orthopeadic Surgeon
Fortius Clinic
Chelsea and Westminster Hospital
London, UK

C. Niek van Dijk
MD, PhD, Professor
Chief of Service
Orthopaedic Research Centre Amsterdam
Department of Orthopaedic Surgery
Academic Medical Center
University of Amsterdam
Amsterdam, The Netherlands

Nicola Maffulli
MD, MS, PhD, FRCP, FRCS(Orth), FFSEM
Professor of Musculoskeletal Disorders
Consultant Trauma and Orthopaedic Surgeon
School of Medicine and Surgery
University of Salerno
Salerno, Italy
Queen Mary University of London
Centre for Sports and Exercise Medicine
Mile End Hospital
London, UK

Hajo Thermann
MD, PhD, professor
Center for Knee & Foot Surgery / Sports Trauma
ATOS Clinic
Heidelberg, Germany

LIST OF CONTRIBUTORS

Paul W. Ackermann
MD, PhD, Associate Professor
Department of Orthopaedics and
Sports Medicine
Karolinska University Hospital
Karolinska Institutet
Stockholm, Sweden

Erica Arverud
MD
Integrative Orthopaedic Laboratory
Department of Molecular Medicine and Surgery
Karolinska Institutet
Stockholm, Sweden

Alp Bayramoğlu
MD, Professor
Department of Anatomy
Acibadem University School of Medicine
İstanbul, Turkey

James H. Beaty
MD
Department of Orthopaedic Surgery &
Biomechanical Engineering
Le Bonheur Children's Hospital
University of Tennessee-Campbell Clinic
Memphis, TN, USA

Christoph Becher
MD, PhD
Orthopaedic Department
Hanover Medical School
Hannover, Germany

Onur Bilge
MD, Assistant Professor
Department of Orthopaedics & Traumatology
Necmettin Erbakan University
Konya, Turkey

Murat Bozkurt
MD, Professor
Department of Orthopaedics and Traumatology
Atatürk Training and Research Hospital
Yıldırım Beyazıt University
Ankara, Turkey

Annelie Brorsson
PT, MSc
Capio Lundby Hospital
Institute of Clinical Sciences
Sahlgrenska Academy
Sahlgrenska University Hospital
University of Gothenburg
Gothenburg, Sweden

James D. F. Calder
MD, FRCS (Tr&Orth), FFSEM (UK)
Consultant Orthopeadic Surgeon
Fortius Clinic
Chelsea and Westminster Hospital
London, UK

Michael R. Carmont
MD
Orthopaedic Department
Princess Royal Hospital
Telford, UK

Angelo Del Buono
MD
Department of Orthopaedic and Trauma
Surgery Campus Biomedico
University of Rome
Rome, Italy

Vincenzo Denaro
MD
Department of Orthopaedic and Trauma
Surgery Campus Biomedico
University of Rome
Rome, Italy

Brian Donley
MD, Professor of Surgery
Cleveland Clinic Lerner College of Medicine
President Regional Hospitals & Family
Health Centers
Cleveland Clinic
Cleveland, OH, USA

Gürhan Dönmez
MD
Department of Sports Medicine
Hacettepe University School of Medicine
Ankara, Turkey

Mahmut N. Doral
MD, Professor
Department of Orthopaedics and Traumatology
Department of Sports Medicine
Hacettepe University School of Medicine
Ankara, Turkey

C. Niek van Dijk
MD, PhD, Professor
Chief of Service
Orthopaedic Research Centre Amsterdam
Department of Orthopaedic Surgery
Academic Medical Center
University of Amsterdam
Amsterdam, The Netherlands

LIST OF CONTRIBUTORS

Robin R. Elliot
MA (Oxon,) MB BS, FRCS (Tr & Orth)
Consultant Orthopaedic Surgeon
Basingstoke and North Hampshire Hospital
The Hampshire Clinic
Basingstoke, UK

Sven Feil
MA, Chief Scientific Department
Center for Knee & Foot Surgery / Sports Trauma
ATOS Clinic
Heidelberg, Germany

Ralph M. Fisher
Center for Knee & Foot Surgery / Sports Trauma
ATOS Clinic
Heidelberg, Germany

John P. Furia
MD
SUN Orthopedics and Sports Medicine
Evangelical Community Hospital
Lewisburg, PA, USA

Pau Golanó
MD, Professor
Laboratory of Arthroscopic and Surgical
Anatomy
Human Anatomy Unit
Department of Pathology and Experimental
Therapeutics
University of Barcelona
Department of Orthopaedic Surgery
University of Pittsburgh
Barcelona, Spain

Gazi Huri
MD, Fellow
Department of Orthopaedics Surgery
Division of Sports Medicine and Shoulder
Surgery
Johns Hopkins University
Baltimore, MD, USA

Bernard C. S. Lee
MD
Consultant Orthopaedic Surgeon
Jurong Healthcare (Alexandra Hospital)
Singapore

Jón Karlsson
MD, PhD, Professor
Department of Orthopaedics
Sahlgrenska University Hospital
Sahlgrenska Academy
Gothenburg University
Gothenburg, Sweden

Defne Kaya
PT, PhD, Associate Professor
Department of Sports Medicine
Hacettepe University School of Medicine
Ankara, Turkey

Derek M. Kelly
MD, Associate Professor
University of Tennessee-Campbell Clinic
Department of Orthopaedic Surgery &
Biomechanical Engineering Le Bonheur
Children's Hospital
Memphis, TN, US

John G. Kennedy
MD, FRCS (Orth)
Hospital for Special Surgery
New York, NY, US

Gino M.M.J. Kerkhoffs
MD, PhD, Professor
Orthopaedic Research Centre Amsterdam
Department of Orthopaedic Surgery
Academic Medical Center
University of Amsterdam
Amsterdam, The Netherlands

Feza Korkusuz
MD, Professor
Department of Sports Medicine
Hacettepe University School of Medicine
Ankara, Turkey

Umile G. Longo
MD, PhD
Department of Orthopaedic and Trauma
Surgery
Campus Biomedico University
Rome, Italy

Nicola Maffulli
MD, MS, PhD, FRCP, FRCS(Orth), FFSEM
Professor of Musculoskeletal Disorders
Consultant Trauma and Orthopaedic Surgeon
School of Medicine and Surgery
University of Salerno
Salerno, Italy
Queen Mary University of London
Centre for Sports and Exercise Medicine
Mile End Hospital
London, UK

Peter Malliaras
PT, PhD
Centre for Sports and Exercise Medicine
Queen Mary University of London
Mile End Hospital
London, UK

LIST OF CONTRIBUTORS

Sean Matuszak
MD
Troy Orthopaedic Associates
Troy, MI, USA

Katerina Nilsson Helander
MD, PhD
Department of Orthopaedic Surgery
Kungsbacka Hospital
Tölövägen, Sweden

Nicklas Olsson
MD, PhD
Department of Orthopaedics
Sahlgrenska University Hospital
Sahlgrenska Academy
Gothenburg University
Gothenburg, Sweden

Christopher J. Pearce
FRCS (Tr&Orth), MFSEM (UK)
Consultant Orthopaedic Surgeon
Jurong Healthcare (Alexandra Hospital)
Singapore

Jan D. Rompe
MD, Professor
Orthopeadic Surgery
Ortho Trauma Evaluation Center
Mainz, Germany

Jeffrey R. Sawyer
MD, Professor
Department of Orthopaedic Surgery &
Biomechanical Engineering
University of Tennessee-Campbell Clinic
Pediatric Orthopaedics and Spinal Deformity
Le Bonheur Children's Hospital
Memphis, TN, USA

Karin Grävare Silbernagel
PT, ATC, PhD Assistant Professor
Department of Physical Therapy
Samson College of Health Professions
University of the Sciences
Philadelphia, PA, USA

Niall A. Smyth
MD
Hospital for Special Surgery
New York, NY, US

Maayke N. van Sterkenburg
MD, PhD
Department of Surgery
Zaans Medical Center
Zaandam, The Netherlands

Hajo Thermann
MD, PhD, professor
Center for Knee & Foot Surgery / Sports Trauma
ATOS Clinic
Heidelberg, Germany

Johannes L. Tol
MD, PhD
Sports Medicine Department
Aspetar; Qatar Orthopaedic and Sports
Medicine Hospital
Doha, Qatar

Egemen Turhan
MD, Associate Professor
Department of Orthopaedics & Traumatology
Hacettepe University School of Medicine
Ankara, Turkey

Jordi Vega
MD
Foot and Ankle Unit
Etzelclinic Pfäffikon
Zurich, Switzerland

William C. Warner
MD, Professor
Department of Orthopaedic Surgery &
Biomechanical Engineering
Le Bonheur Children's Hospital
University of Tennessee-Campbell Clinic
Memphis, TN, USA

Johannes I. Wiegerinck
MD, PhD–Fellow
Orthopaedic Research Centre Amsterdam
Department of Orthopaedic Surgery
Academic Medical Center
University of Amsterdam
Amsterdam, The Netherlands

W. James White
MBBS, BSc, MRCS
North West Thames Deanery
London, UK

Ruben Zwiers
MSc, PhD-fellow
Orthopaedic Research Centre Amsterdam
Department of Orthopaedic Surgery
Academic Medical Center
University of Amsterdam
Amsterdam, The Netherlands

CONTENTS

PREFACE

After the series of three consensus books *Achilles Rendon Rupture* (2008), *Achilles Tendinopathy* (2010) and *Disorders of the Achilles Tendon Insertion* (2012), we are proud to present you with the fourth production in the line of consensus books on Achilles Tendon Pathology.

Within this book we bring together the previous three editions, updated and supplemented with new chapters. Therefore, this production will provide an overview of the current concepts of all Achilles-related problems, both acute injuries and chronic disorders, based on the best available evidence and expert opinions. The production of this book was made possible by DJO Publications.

The Achilles Tendon Study Group (ATSG) was founded to promote the research and scientific study of injuries to the Achilles tendon. In collaboration with world leaders in this field, ATSG has reviewed the available literature to provide a balanced consensus on the scope of Achilles tendon disorders.

Although the Achilles tendon is the thickest and strongest tendon in the human body, it remains susceptible to injury. Achilles tendon disorders are relatively common in the physical active population. In this book, we distinguished acute and chronic disorders: Achilles tendon ruptures and Achilles tendinopathies. The Achilles tendinopathies are divided into mid-portion and insertional problems, of which the insertional disorders are divided into pathology of the tendon itself (insertional tendinopathy) and the surrounding tissue (retrocalcaneal bursitis). All of these pathologies are extensively addressed in this book.

The focus of this fourth book is mainly on the available treatments and the basis on which they are founded, diagnostics, the outcome measures available to standardize future clinical studies, and future treatment. Surgical techniques are extensively described and a comprehensive overview of the outcomes, based on the best available evidence, is provided. Furthermore, general issues like anatomy, epidemiology, and the aetiology of Achilles tendon disorders are addressed, as well as current insights in the field of biomechanics, sport resumption and Achilles problems in the paediatric population.

Some chapters may be open to debate, as their content may be based on limited clinical evidence. These chapters were nonetheless included to promote debate and force discussion in order to emphasize the present state of affairs and promote future studies of controversial subjects.

The Editors

"They certainly give very strange names to diseases."

Plato

Chapter 1

Terminology for Achilles Tendon Disorders

Johannes I. Wiegerinck, Ruben Zwiers, Jón Karlsson, Nicola Maffulli, C. Niek van Dijk

Take Home Message

• *Uniform and clear terminology based on the combination of anatomic location, symptoms, clinical findings and pathological changes is necessary for proper research, diagnosis and treatment.*

• *Haglund's disease, Haglund's syndrome, Haglund's deformity, pump bump and tendinitis are confusing, inadequate terms that should therefore not be used.*

• *Restraint is advocated regarding the adoption of new terms or the modification of a pre-existing terminology solely on personal interpretation or preference.*

Introduction

The Achilles heel of Achilles tendon problems may very well be the terminology of Achilles tendon pathology. The terminology, description and nomenclature of the tendon itself and its surrounding structures has changed continuously ever since the Dutch surgeon Philip Verheyen changed 'tendo magnus of Hippocrates' to 'Achilles tendon' in 1693 [11]. From the beginning of the twentieth century, many terms have been used to describe the structures and pathology around the Achilles tendon insertion[1,2,5,7,12,15,18,19,22,23,30]. For there is no agreement regarding the definition or description of the pathology, and over the years various terms have been added to describe the same pathological process[2,5,7,12,18,19,22,30]: 'Haglund', for example, is a much used eponym for pathologies around the Achilles tendon insertion. However, there are numerous pathologies related to Haglund: Haglund's syndrome, Haglund's deformity, Haglund's disease, Haglund's triad. All describe pathology in the foot, most describe different pathologies and some, however, describe the same pathologies[2,5,7,12,18,19,22,30]. The multiplicity of terms has led to substantial confusion, not only over Haglund' definitions but also over other pathologies around the tendon[1,2,5,8-10,12,15,17,19,23,30].

Many have tried to systematically categorise Achilles tendon pathology[4,14,20,21,25]. In 1976, Perugia and co-workers introduced a new terminology on inflammatory problems of the Achilles tendon[20,21]. It took until 1992 to divide the definitions of Achilles 'tendinitis' into insertional and non-insertional[4]. Confused by the aforementioned Haglund terms, Sella and co-workers proposed new definitions for Haglund's disease, Haglund's syndrome and Haglund's deformity[25]. Despite the proposal, many continued using Haglund terms interchangeably[3,9,10,13,16,24]. In that same year, Maffulli and co-workers suggested changing the (still confusing) terminology concerning overuse tendon conditions[14]. Among others, Maffulli and co-workers proposed naming the clinical syndrome of pain, swelling and impaired performance 'tendinopathy'[14]. Despite all efforts, the terminology has remained confusing[17,26-28]. This confusion leads to problems in the scientific literature and daily clinical practice[6,14,27,28]. Influenced by previous work, van Dijk and co-workers proposed a structured terminology to provide neutral, descriptive, uniform and clear definitions of Achilles tendon pathology to be used in both the scientific literature and daily clinical practice[29]. The terminology is based on the combination of anatomic location, symptoms, clinical findings and pathological changes[29]. In addition, van Dijk and co-workers proposed departing from previous confusing terms, such as Haglund's disease, Haglund's syndrome, Haglund's deformity, pump bump and tendinitis[29]. The following definitions of Achilles tendon disorders, based on the aforementioned terminology, will be used throughout this publication (Table 1).

Terminology

Mid-portion Achilles tendinopathy

Achilles tendinopathy is a clinical syndrome characterized by a combination of pain, swelling and impaired performance. The swelling can be diffuse or localized. Typically, the nodular swelling is located at 2–7 cm from the insertion onto the calcaneus. This part of the tendon has also been described as the "main body of the Achilles tendon." This entity involves isolated pathology of the tendon proper and includes - but is not limited to - the histopathological diagnosis of tendinosis. Tendinosis implies the histopathological diagnosis of tendon degeneration without clinical or histological signs of intratendinous inflammation, and it is not necessarily symptomatic. However, it should be kept in mind that, although the histological term 'tendinosis' is also widely used, the essential lesion of tendinopathy is not, *strictu sensu*, of a degenerative nature: it has the features of a failed healing response, in which the tendon attempts to heal but, for some reason - including, possibly, continuous inappropriate mechanical stimuli - the healing process appears non-finalized [29].

Achilles paratendinopathy

Paratendinopathy is defined by acute or chronic inflammation and/or degeneration of the thin membrane around the Achilles tendon. Exercise-induced pain and local swelling around the tendon's mid-portion are the most important symptoms. Histopathologically, acute paratendinopathy is characterized by edema and hyperaemia of the paratenon, with infiltration of inflammatory cells, possibly with the production of a fibrinous exudate that fills the space between the tendon sheath and the tendon, causing palpable crepitations on physical examination. In chronic Achilles paratendinopathy, exercise-induced pain is the major symptom, while crepitations and swelling are less pronounced. Histopathologically, the paratenon becomes thickened as a result of fibrinous exudate, the prominent and widespread proliferation of (myo)fibroblasts, the formation of new connective tissue and adhesions between the tendon, paratenon, and crural fascia [29].

Insertional Achilles tendinopathy

Insertional Achilles tendinopathy is located at the insertion of the Achilles tendon onto the calcaneus, possibly with the formation of bone spurs and calcifications in the tendon proper at the insertion site. In case of calcifications or spurs - proven by imaging - this condition is termed 'calcified insertional Achilles tendinopathy'. Patients complain of pain, stiffness and - sometimes - a solid swelling. On physical examination, the tendon insertion (at the mid-portion of the posterior aspect of the calcaneus) is painful. A swelling may be visible and a bony spur may be palpable. Histopathologically, there is ossification of entheseal fibrocartilage and sometimes small tendon tears occur at the tendon-bone junction [29].

Retrocalcaneal bursitis

An inflammation of the bursa in the recess between the anterior inferior side of the Achilles tendon and the postero-superior aspect of the calcaneus (retrocalcaneal recess) results in a visible and painful soft tissue swelling, medial and lateral to the Achilles tendon at the level of the postero-superior part of the calcaneus. Frequently, a postero-superior calcaneal prominence can be identified on plain radiographs. Histopathologically, the fibro-cartilaginous bursal walls show degeneration and/or calcification, with hypertrophy of the synovial infoldings and accumulation of fluid in the bursa itself. Alternatively, the bursa may be primarily inflamed or an infectious bursitis might be caused by an inflammatory arthropathyt [29].

Superficial calcaneal bursitis

This is an inflammation of the bursa located between the Achilles tendon and the skin resulting in a visible, painful, solid swelling and discoloration of the skin. It is most often located at the postero-lateral aspect of the calcaneus. It is frequently associated with shoes with a rigid posterior portion. The Achilles tendon, however, is usually not involved. Histopathologically, the subcutaneous bursa is an adventitious bursa, which is acquired after birth and develops in response to friction. It is lined by hypertrophic synovial tissue and fluid. A superficial calcaneal bursitis can be further specified by its location, i.e., posterior, postero-lateral or postero-medial[29].

Non-insertional Achilles tendinopathy consists of mid-portion Achilles tendinopathy and paratendinopathy – these entities often co-exist. Retro-calcaneal bursitis is frequently seen in combination with an insertional Achilles tendon. Other combinations are possible, but occur less frequently[29].

	Term	Anatomic Location	Symptoms	Clinical Findings	Histopathology
Insertional Achilles Tendon Disorders	**Insertional Achilles Tendinopathy**	Insertion of the Achilles tendon onto the calcaneus, most often with the formation of bone spurs and calcifications in the tendon proper at the insertion site.	Pain, stiffness, sometimes a (solid) swelling.	Painful tendon insertion at the mid-portion of the posterior aspect of the calcaneus; swelling may be visible and a bony spur may be palpable.	Ossification of entheseal fibrocartilage and sometimes small tendon tears occurring at the tendon-bone junction.
	Retrocalcaneal Bursitis	Bursa in the recess between the anterior inferior side of the Achilles tendon and the postero-superior aspect of the calcaneus (retrocalcaneal recess).	Painful swelling superior to calcaneus.	Painful soft tissue swelling, medial and lateral to the Achilles tendon at the level of the postero-superior calcaneus.	Fibro-cartilaginous bursal walls show degeneration and/or calcification, with hypertrophy of the synovial infoldings and accumulation of fluid in the bursa. Alternatively, the bursa may be primarily involved by inflammatory or infectious bursitis due to an inflammatory arthropathy.
	Superficial Calcaneal Bursitis	Bursa located between the calcaneal prominence or the Achilles tendon and the skin.	Visible, painful, solid swelling of the postero-lateral calcaneus (often associated with shoes with a rigid posterior portion).	Visible, painful, solid swelling and discoloration of the skin. Most often located at postero-lateral calcaneus; sometimes posterior or postero-medial.	Acquired adventitious bursa, developing in response to friction. When inflamed, lined by hypertrophic synovial tissue and fluid.
Non-insertional Achilles Tendon Disorders	**Mid-portion Achilles Tendinopathy**	2-7 cm from the insertion onto the calcaneus.	A combination of pain, swelling and impaired performance.	Diffuse or localized swelling.	Includes, but is not limited to, the histopathological diagnosis of tendinosis: implies histopathological diagnosis of tendon degeneration without clinical or histological signs of intratendinous inflammation (not necessarily symptomatic).
	Paratendinopathy *Acute*	Around the mid-portion Achilles tendon.	Oedema and hyperaemia.	Palpable crepitations, swelling.	Oedema and hyperaemia of the paratenon, with infiltration of inflammatory cells, possibly with the production of a fibrinous exudate that fills the space between the tendon sheath and tendon.
	Paratendinopathy *Chronic*	Around the mid-portion Achilles tendon.	Exercise-induced pain.	Crepitations and swelling less pronounced.	Paratenon thickened as a result of fibrinous exudate, prominent and widespread proliferation of (myo) fibroblasts, formation of new connective tissue and adhesions between the tendon, paratenon and crural fascia.

Table 1. Terminology for Achilles tendon disorders, including the anatomic location, symptoms, clinical findings histopathology [29].

Term/ Imaging	Plain Radiography	Ultrasound	CT	MRI
Insertional Achilles Tendon Disorders				
Insertional Achilles Tendinopathy	May show ossification or a bone spur at the tendon's insertion; possible deviation of soft tissue contours.	Calcaneal bony abnormalities.	Bone formation at insertion. CT scan is indicated mainly for pre-operative planning. It shows the exact location and size of the calcifications and spurs.	Bone formation and/ or on STIR (short tau inversion recovery) hyperintense signal at tendon insertion.
Retrocalcaneal Bursitis	A postero-superior calcaneal prominence can be identified; radio-opacity of the retrocalcaneal recess; possible deviation of soft tissue contours.	Fluid in the retrocalcaneal area/bursa (hyperechoic).	–	Hyperintense signal in retrocalcaneal recess on T2 weighed images.
Superficial Calcaneal Bursitis	Possible deviation of soft tissue contours.	Fluid between the skin and the Achilles tendon.	–	Hyperintense signal between Achilles tendon and subcutaneous tissue on T2 weighed images.
Non-insertional Achilles Tendon Disorders				
Mid-portion Achilles Tendinopathy	Deviation of soft tissue contours is usually present. In rare cases calcifications can be found.	Tendon larger than normal in both its cross-sectional area and anterior posterior diameter. Hypoechoic areas within the tendon; disruption of fibrillar pattern; increase in tendon vascularity (Echo-Doppler), mainly in the ventral peritendinous area.	In case (massive) calcifications are seen on plain radiography. CT imaging can be helpful in pre-operative planning, showing the exact size and location of the calcifications.	Fat-saturated T1 or T2 images: fusiform expansion, central enhancement consistent with intratendinous neovascularisation.
Paratendinopathy *Acute*	–	Normal Achilles tendon with circumferential hypoechogenic halo.	–	Peripheral enhancement on fat-saturated T1 or on T2 images.
Paratendinopathy *Chronic*	–	Thickened hypoechoic paratenon with poorly defined borders may show as a sign of peritendinous adhesions; increase in tendon vascularity (Echo-Doppler), mainly in the ventral peritendinous area.	–	–

Table 2. Radiologic findings in Achilles tendon disorders [29].

Conclusion

Uniform and clear terminology is necessary for proper research, diagnosis and treatment. The terminology described by van Dijk and co-workers will be used throughout this publication. The following terms are specifically not used as they are confusing and inaccurate: Haglund's disease, Haglund's syndrome, Haglund's deformity, pump bump and tendinitis[29]. We advise scientists and physicians to use one, broadly accepted terminology in their daily practice. Restraint is advocated regarding the adoption of new terms or the modification of a pre-existing terminology solely on personal interpretation or preference.

References

1. Albert E. Achillodynie. Wiener Medizinische Presse 1839;2:41-3.
2. Biyani A, Jones DA. Results of excision of calcaneal prominence. Acta Orthop Belg 1993;59:45-9.
3. Brunner J, Anderson J, O'Malley M, Bohne W, Deland J, Kennedy J. Physician and patient-based outcomes following surgical resection of Haglund's deformity. Acta Orthop Belg 2005 Dec;71:718-23.
4. Clain MR, Baxter DE. Achilles tendinitis. Foot Ankle 1992 Oct;13:482-7.
5. Dickinson PH, Coutts MB, Woodward EP, Handler D. Tendo Achillis bursitis. Report of twenty-one cases. J Bone Joint Surg Am 1966 Jan;48:77-81.
6. Fry HJH. Overuse syndrome, alias tenosynovitis/tendinitis: the terminological hoax. Plast Recons Surg 1986;78:414-7.
7. Haglund P. Beitrag zur Klinik der Achillessehne. Zeitschr Orthop Chir 1928;49-58.
8. Harris CA, Peduto AJ. Achilles tendon imaging. Australas Radiol 2006 Dec;50:513-25.
9. Jerosch J, Nasef NM. Endoscopic calcaneoplasty - rationale, surgical technique, and early results: a preliminary report. Knee Surg Sports Traumatol Arthrosc 2003 May;11:190-5.
10. Jerosch J, Schunck J, Sokkar SH. Endoscopic calcaneoplasty (ECP) as a surgical treatment of Haglund's syndrome. Knee Surg Sports Traumatol Arthrosc 2007 Jul;15:927-34.
11. Kirkup J. Mythology and history. In: Helal B, Wilson D, editors. The Foot. Churchill Livingstone; 1988. p. 1-8.
12. Le TA, Joseph PM. Common exostectomies of the rearfoot. Clin Podiatr Med Surg 1991 Jul;8:601-23.
13. Leitze Z, Sella EJ, Aversa JM. Endoscopic decompression of the retrocalcaneal space. J Bone Joint Surg Am 2003 Aug;85-A:1488-96.
14. Maffulli N, Khan KM, Puddu G. Overuse tendon conditions: time to change a confusing terminology. Arthroscopy 1998 Nov;14:840-3.
15. Nielson AL. Diagnostic and therapeutic point in retrocalcanean bursitis. J Am Med Assoc 1921;77:463.
16. Ortmann FW, McBryde AM. Endoscopic bony and soft-tissue decompression of the retrocalcaneal space for the treatment of Haglund deformity and retrocalcaneal bursitis. Foot Ankle Int 2007 Feb;28:149-53.
17. Paavola M, Jarvinen TA. Paratendinopathy. Foot Ankle Clin 2005 Jun;10:279-92.
18. Painter C.F. Inflammation of the post-calcaneal bursa associated with exostosis. J Bone Joint Surg Am 1898;s1-11:169-80.
19. Pavlov H, Heneghan MA, Hersh A, Goldman AB, Vigorita V. The Haglund syndrome: initial and differential diagnosis. Radiology 1982 Jul;144:83-8.
20. Perugia L, Ippolitio E, Postacchini F. A new approach to the pathology, clinical features and treatment of stress tendinopathy of the Achilles tendon. Ital J Orthop Traumatol 1976 Apr;2:5-21.
21. Puddu G, Ippolito E, Postacchini F. A classification of Achilles tendon disease. Am J Sports Med 1976 Jul;4:145-50.
22. Reinherz RP, Smith BA, Henning KE. Understanding the pathologic Haglund's deformity. J Foot Surg 1990 Sep;29:432-5.
23. Rössler. Zur Kenntniss der Achillodynie. Deutsch Ztschr f Chir 1895;52:274-91.
24. Schunck J, Jerosch J. Operative treatment of Haglund's syndrome. Basics, indications, procedures, surgical techniques, results and problems. Foot Ankle Surg 2005;11:123-30.
25. Sella EJ, Caminear DS, McLarney EA. Haglund's syndrome. J Foot Ankle Surg 1998 Mar;37:110-4.
26. Sorosky B, Press J, Plastaras C, Rittenberg J. The practical management of Achilles tendinopathy. Clin J Sport Med 2004 Jan;14:40-4.
27. van Dijk CN, Jakobsen BW, ackney R. ISAKOS/ESSKA STANDARD TERMINOLOGY, DEFINITIONS, CLASSIFICAchilles tendonION AND SCORING SYSTEMS FOR ARTHROSCOPY. 2007. http://www.esska.org/upload/PDF/Standard_Terminology.pdf.
Ref Type: Online Source
28. van Dijk CN. The future is in our hands. Knee Surg Sports Traumatol Arthrosc 2010 Aug;18:1003-4.
29. van Dijk CN, van Sterkenburg MN, Wiegerinck JI, Karlsson J, Maffulli N. Terminology for Achilles tendon related disorders. Knee Surg Sports Traumatol Arthrosc 2011 May;19(5):835-41
30. Vega MR, Cavolo DJ, Green RM, Cohen RS. Haglund's deformity. J Am Podiatry Assoc 1984 Mar;74:129-35.

"Anatomy is to physiology as geography is to history; it describes the theatre of events."

Jean Francois Fernel

Chapter 2

Anatomy of the Achilles Tendon

Mahmut N. Doral, Pau Golanó, Gürhan Dönmez, Jordi Vega, Murat Bozkurt, Gazi Huri, Alp Bayramoğlu, Egemen Turhan

Take Home Message

- *The anatomy of the Achilles tendon is complex. The tendon originates from three separate muscles and inserts at the calcaneus; therefore, it is involved in the motion of three joints: the knee, the ankle and the sub-talar joints.*

- *The calcaneal insertion of the Achilles tendon is not at a single point.*

- *The Achilles tendon lacks a synovial sheath. Instead, it has a paratenon, which is a thin layer of fibrovascular tissue. The main blood supply to the mid-portion of the tendon is provided through the paratenon.*

- *Knowledge of the anatomical variations of the sural nerve is extremely important for performing both percutaneous and open Achilles tendon surgery.*

Introduction

It is hypothesized that the Achilles tendon developed two million years ago, enabling humans to run much faster. Besides the fact that the Achilles tendon played a key role in the evolution of human running, it is known as the strongest tendon in the human body. In addition, the Achilles tendon is also one of the longest tendons in the human body (Figure 1). On the other hand, this tendon is most prone to injury, especially in active individuals[14]. During running, jumping and skipping, the tendon has to withstand a load of up to twelve times body weight [10,13.] It is the conjoint tendon of the gastrocnemius and soleus muscles (triceps surae), and may have a small contribution from the plantaris muscle.

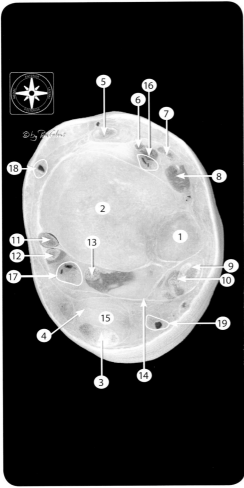

1   Lateral malleolus
2   Tibia
3   Achilles tendon
4   Plantaris tendon
5   Tibialis anterior tendon
6   Extensor hallucis longus tendon
7   Extensor digitorum longus tendon
8   Peroneus tertius tendon
9   Peroneus longus tendon
10 Peroneus brevis tendon
11 Tibialis posterior tendon
12 Flexor digitorum longus tendon
13 Flexor hallucis tendon
    (musculo-tendinous)
14 Deep sural/crural fascia
15 Kager's fat pad
16 Anterior neurovascular bundle
    (deep peroneal nerve and anterior
    tibial artery and veins)
17 Posterior neurovascular bundle
    (posterior tibial nerve and
    posterior tibial artery and veins)
18 Saphenous nerve and great
    saphenous vein
19 Sural nerve and small saphenous
    vein

Figure 1. Transversal section at the level of the tibiofibular syndesmosis showing the difference in size of the Achilles tendon with other tendons.

The mean length of the Achilles tendon is approximately 15 cm and ranges from 11 to 26 cm. The width of the tendon depends on the location. The mean width at origin is 6.8 cm (range 4.5-8.6 cm) and the tendon gradually becomes thinner towards the midsection, were the tendon width is 1.8 cm (1.2-2.6 cm). More distally, it becomes more rounded until approximately 4 cm above the calcaneus before expanding in the shape of a delta (Figure 2 and Figure 3). At the insertion to the midpoint of the posterior surface of the calcaneus, the mean width is 3.4 cm (2.0-4.8 cm) [1].

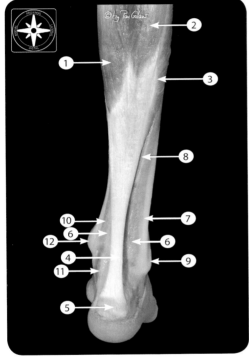

1   Medial head of the gastrocnemius muscle

2   Lateral head of the gastrocnemius muscle

3   Soleus muscle

4   Achilles tendon

5   Calcaneal insertion of the Achilles tendon

6   Deep sural/crural fascia

7   Peroneal tendons

8   Postero-lateral inter-muscular septum (cut)

9   Lateral malleolus

10 Tibialis posterior and flexor digitorum tendon

11 Posterior neurovascular bundle

12 Medial malleolus

Figure 2. Posterior view of the Achilles tendon.

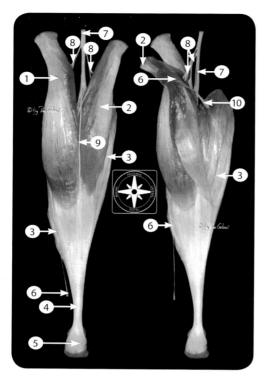

1 Medial head of the gastrocnemius muscle

2 Lateral head of the gastrocnemius muscle

3 Soleus muscle

4 Achilles tendon

5 Calcaneal insertion of the Achilles tendon

6 Plantaris muscle

7 Tibial nerve

8 Motor branches to the heads of the gastrocnemius

9 Medial cutaneous sural nerve

10 Motor branch to the soleus muscle

Figure 3. Triceps surae and its components. Posterior view.

Histology

Tenoblasts and tenocytes account for 90-95% of the cellular elements of tendons, while the remaining 5-10% consists of chondrocytes, vascular cells, synovial cells and smooth muscle cells.

Like other fibrous connective tissues, the Achilles tendon is composed primarily of type I collagen (65% to 80%) and elastin. Elastin accounts for approximately 2% of the dry mass of tendons[13,16]. Elastic fibres within the tendon may contribute to the shock-absorbing capacity of the tendon and may also play a role in the maintenance of the collagen crimp pattern. Although elastin is able to undergo a strain up to 200% of its unloaded length, increasing the proportion of elastin would reduce the efficiency of force dissipation from muscle to bone[13].

The collagen fibres are tightly packed in parallel bundles containing nerve, blood and lymphatic vessels, forming fascicles[16]. The fascicles are surrounded by endotenon and group together to form the macroscopic tendon.

The tendon is surrounded by endotenon, which in turn is enveloped by epitenon. The paratenon, a layer of thin, areolar tissue, is wrapped around the epitenon[1,19]. The paratenon and epitenon are separated by a thin layer of fluid to reduce friction during tendon motion. The mean distance between the confluence of the fascia cruris and paratenon from the postero-superior calcaneal tubercle is 37.3 mm (range 17-58 mm)[3].

Tendons are stiff and resilient, with high tensile strength: they can be stretched up to 4% before damage occurs. At rest, a tendon has an undulating configuration due to the crimping of the collagen fibrils. This undulating configuration disappears when it is stretched by more than 2%[8]. The tendon is able to regain its normal undulating appearance if the strain exerted on it is less than 4%. At strain levels greater than 8%, macroscopic rupture is produced by tensile failure.

The Achilles tendon fibres are not strictly aligned vertically, instead displaying a variable degree of spiralling. Due to this rotation, the gastrocnemius tendinous fibres insert into the postero-lateral, and the soleus tendinous fibres insert into the postero-medial aspect of the calcaneus. The extent of this rotation is determined by the position of fusion between the two muscles, with a more distal fusion resulting in more rotation. The spiralization of the fibres of the tendon produces an area of concentrated stress and confers a mechanical advantage [1,19] (Figure 4).

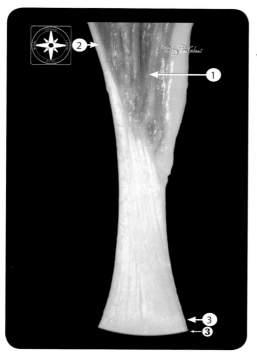

1   Soleus muscle

2   Tendinous fibres of the lateral head of the gastrocnemius muscle

Figure 4. Anterior view of the Achilles tendon showing the rotation fibres. Due to this rotation, the Gastrocnemius tendinous fibres attach in the postero-lateral aspect of the calcaneus, while the soleus tendinous fibres attach in the postero-medial aspect of the calcaneus.

Muscle Origins

The relative contribution of the soleus muscle and gastrocnemius muscle to the Achilles tendon is variable. Due to the changing orientation of the tendon fibres, the exact degree of contribution is difficult to determine.

Gastrocnemius

The gastrocnemius is the most superficial muscle of the dorsal aspect of the leg, and gives the calf its characteristic bulge. It is a fusiform muscle formed by two heads - medial and lateral - each separately crossing the knee joint (Figure 3). The muscle heads fuse in a single muscle belly located at the posterior superficial compartment of the leg [7]. The lateral and medial heads of gastrocnemius arise from the back of the femur just above the lateral and medial femoral condyles, respectively [10]. Contributions to the two muscle heads may be found from the posterior knee joint capsule, particularly at the lateral aspect of the popliteal ligament [21]. Compared with the lateral head, the medial head is broader and longer, and extends more distally in the calf (Figure 3). The gastrocnemius muscle usually contains a larger proportion of fast-twitch (Type II) muscle fibres, which enable it to produce explosive and rapid movement [7].

Soleus

The soleus lies deep in the gastrocnemius and it is a broad, multipennate muscle. The soleus muscle is wider than the gastrocnemius, and its muscle fibres extend more distally than those of the gastrocnemius. It originates from the oblique line (soleal line) and the middle third of the medial border of the tibia, from a fibrous arch between the fibula and the tibia and from the posterior surface of the head of the fibula. The soleus fuses with the gastrocnemius and forms the deepest portion of the Achilles tendon. The tendinous portion of the soleus is usually the largest tendinous part contributing to the Achilles tendon, and is the main plantar flexor [16] (Figure 3 and Figure 5). It acts only on the ankle joint and can be palpated on either side of the gastrocnemius when the subject stands on tiptoes [8]. The soleus consists primarily of type I slow twitch muscle fibres. Muscle fibre hypotrophy of the soleus occurs more rapidly than that of the gastrocnemius, making the soleus muscle a more sensitive indicator of hypotrophy as a result of injury or denervation [7].

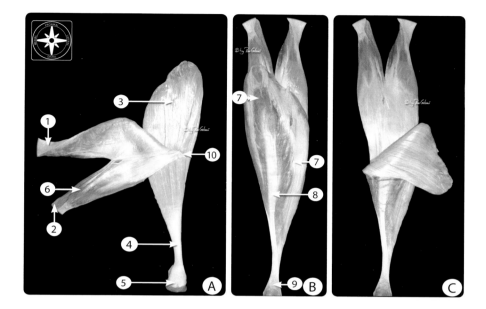

1. Medial head of the gastrocnemius muscle
2. Lateral head of the gastrocnemius muscle
3. Soleus muscle
4. Achilles tendon
5. Calcaneal insertion of the Achilles tendon
6. Plantaris muscle
7. Intramuscular aponeurosis
8. Median septum
9. Retrocalcaneal bursa

Figure 5. Triceps surae and its components. A. Posterior view. The Gastrocnemius muscle was rejected from its normal location. B. Anterior view showing the anterior surface of the soleus muscle. C. Anterior view. The soleus muscle was rejected from its normal location.

Plantaris

The plantaris muscle is located between the gastrocnemius and soleus muscles. It is a small, thin, vestigial muscle, originating from the popliteal surface of the femur with its tendon running distally between the gastrocnemius and soleus muscles. The plantaris tendon has its origin close to the lateral head, runs an oblique course between the gastrocnemius and the soleus, and usually inserts in the medial aspect of the calcaneus anterior to the Achilles tendon. The muscle belly is 5 to 10 cm in length, with a long tendon that extends distally between

17

the gastrocnemius and the soleus (Figure 1, Figure 3 and Figure 6). According to Sarrafians' atlas of foot and ankle anatomy, 4% of plantaris tendons insert on the medial border of the Achilles tendon, 1-16 cm above its insertion into the calcaneus. Occasionally, the tendon is lost in the laciniate ligament or in the fascia of the leg. It is absent in up to 8% of individuals, and may be preferred for augmentation or a graft source [16,19].

The gastrocnemius, soleus and plantaris muscles act as ankle flexors, while the gastrocnemius is also a knee flexor. The main function of the gastrocnemius muscle is the propulsion of the body forward during gait, whereas the soleus is a postural muscle that also acts as a peripheral vascular pump [6]. The soleus muscle is also a stabilizer of the foot during standing.

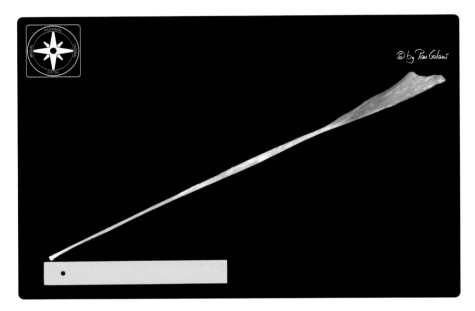

Figure 6. Plantaris muscle overview.

Calcaneal insertion

The Achilles tendon starts at the musculo-tendinous junction of the gastrocnemius and the soleus in the middle of the calf. The tendon is flattened at its junction with the gastrocnemius to become rounded until approximately 4 cm proximal to the insertion [16]. At this level, it flattens and then expands and becomes cartilaginous, to insert into a rough area on the middle of the inferior part of the posterior surface of the calcaneus (Figure 1, Figure 2 and Figure 3).

It should be mentioned that the calcaneal insertion of the Achilles tendon is not at a single point. The Achilles tendon has three insertions: (1) osseous to the tuberosity of the calcaneus, (2) fascial around the calcaneus and into the plantar fascia, and (3) into the skin via the plantar fat pad and its intricate system of fibrovascular septae [10,11,18]. The calcaneal insertion of the Achilles tendon is highly specialized and has been described as an 'enthesis organ', designed to aid stress dissipation from the tendon to its bony attachment [2,17]. The enthesis organ is formed by the osteotendinous junction between the Achilles tendon and the calcaneus.

Deep, and just proximal to the insertion, the retrocalcaneal bursa is located between the tuberosity on the posterior surface of the calcaneus and the Achilles tendon (Figure 7). It protects the distal Achilles tendon from frictional wear against the calcaneus. It has an anterior bursal wall composed of fibro cartilage and a thin posterior wall which blends with the thin epitenon of the Achilles tendon. Less common are an adventitious bursa superficial to the Achilles tendon and a subcalcaneal bursa between the inferior surface of the calcaneus and the origin of the plantar aponeurosis.

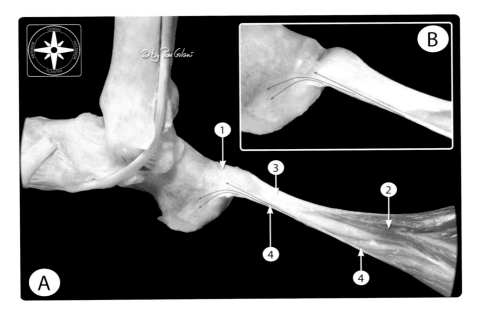

1   *Retrocalcaneal bursa*

2   *Soleus muscle*

3   *Achilles tendon (anterior surface)*

4   *Plantaris muscle and its insertion*

Figure 7. Calcaneal insertion of the Achilles tendon. Medial view. The Achilles tendon was retracted from its normal location.
A. Retrocalcaneal bursa.
B. Retrocalcaneal bursa opened.

The shape of the insertion into the calcaneus has previously been described as a wide, deltoid-shaped attachment, with the Achilles tendon becoming broad prior to its insertion[16]. However, a more recent anatomical study suggests a crescent-shaped insertion with medial and lateral extensions[12]. The medial extensions were more prominent than the lateral side, with maximum extensions of 9.1 mm and 5.5 mm medially and laterally, respectively[12]. This has important implications for surgery in this region, since care needs to be taken to avoid sacrificing healthy Achilles tendon. The posterior one-third of the calcaneus is rough and concavo-convex. The convexity is transverse and supports the Kager's fat pad which is the fibroadipose tissue between the Achilles tendon and the ankle joint. Kager's fat pad is a mass of adipose tissue located within Kager's triangle. This triangle is surrounded by the Achilles tendon posteriorly, the flexor hallucis longus anterio-medially, and the superior cortex of the calcaneus inferiorly. Although it predominantly serves as a variable space-filler, it has been reported to have biomechanical importance. Kager's fat pad protrudes into the retrocalcaneal bursa during plantarflexion (Achilles tendon contraction) and retracts during ankle dorsiflexion. The protrusion into the bursa during plantarflexion is thought to reduce the development of negative pressure in the bursa and perhaps reduce Achilles tendon kinking under loading. The Kager's fat pad provides sub-tendinous lubrication, promoting low wear and suggesting that the fat pad may provide protection to the tendon. Additionally, its neural and vascular supplies promise to provide sensory function as well as being significant for the blood supply of the Achilles tendon.

Innervation

Tendons are thought to receive their sensory innervation from overlying superficial nerves or from adjacent deep nerves [15]. The Achilles tendon derives its innervation from the nerves of the attaching muscles and cutaneous nerves, in particular the sural nerve with a smaller supply from the tibial nerve[15]. The sural nerve is formed by branches from the tibial and common peroneal nerves. In the proximal calf, after its formation, the sural nerve lies at the lateral border of the Achilles tendon. The sural nerve crosses its lateral border at about half the length of the Achilles tendon. Cadaveric dissections with computer-assisted modelling in the sagittal and transverse plane have revealed that on average the sural nerve crossed the Achilles tendon at 11 cm proximal to the calcaneal tuberosity, and at 3.5 cm distal to the gastrosoleus musculo-tendinous junction [5] (Figure 8). In this area, the nerve is especially vulnerable to iatrogenic injury during surgery [1], especially minimally-invasive surgery [5]. Anatomical variations of the sural nerve are common.

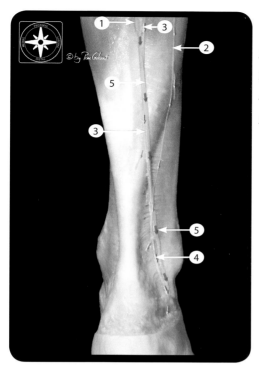

1   *Fascial sural/crural perforation*
2   *Lateral cutaneous sural nerve*
3   *Medial cutaneous sural nerve*
4   *Sural nerve*
5   *Small saphenous nerve*

Figure 8. Sural nerve anatomy. Posterior view.

Vascularization

The blood supply of tendons is provided by three sources: (1) the musculo-tendinous junction, (2) vessels in the surrounding connective tissue, and (3) the osteotendinous junction. Historically, the Achilles tendon has been known to be poorly vascularized and it was once considered to be avascular because of its pale colour and lack of visible blood vessels [4,20]. However, the posterior tibial artery was found to supply the majority of the Achilles tendon, – mainly the peritendinous tissues. The peroneal artery, probably through anastomoses with the posterior tibial artery, makes small contributions, whereas the anterior tibial artery appears not to be involved. The vascularization can also be classified in three sections, with the midsection supplied by the peroneal artery, and both the proximal and distal sections supplied by the posterior tibial artery. The mid-portion of the Achilles tendon has the lowest vascularity in the Achilles tendon [16]. This relatively poor vascularization might explain the frequent incidence of pathology at this site [4,9].

The Achilles tendon has no true synovial sheath; it is surrounded by a paratenon, a double-layered sheath composed of an inner, visceral layer, and an outer, parietal layer [29]. The main blood supply to the middle portion of the tendon is by way of the paratenon [13] (Figure 9). The small blood vessels in the paratenon run transversely toward the tendon and branch several times before running parallel to the long axis of the tendon. Whilst the paratenon is known to be a highly vascular tissue, disagreement exists as to whether the vessels are uniformly distributed throughout its length or whether they provide a higher blood flow at the site of insertion.

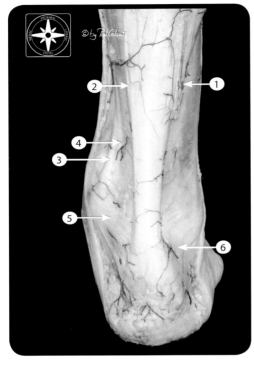

1   *Sural nerve and small saphenous vein*

2   *Plantaris tendon*

3   *Tibialis posterior tendon*

4   *Flexor digitorum longus tendon*

5   *Flexor retinaculum*

6   *Extensor retinaculum*

Figure 9. The blood supply of the Achilles tendon. The arteries were filled with black latex.

References

1. Apaydin N, Bozkurt M, Loukas M, Vefali H, Tubbs RS, Esmer AF. Relationships of the sural nerve with the calcaneal tendon: an anatomical study with surgical and clinical implications. Surg Radiol Anat. 2009;31(10):775-80.

2. Benjamin M, Toumi H, Ralphs JR, Bydder G, Best TM, Milz S. Where tendons and ligaments meet bone: attachment sites ('entheses') in relation to exercise and/or mechanical load. J Anat. 2006;208(4):471-90.

3. Carmont MR, Highland AM, Rochester JR, Paling EM, Davies MB. An anatomical and radiological study of the fascia cruris and paratenon of the Achilles tendon. Foot Ankle Surg. 2011;17(3):186-92.

4. Chen TM, Rozen WM, Pan WR, Ashton MW, Richardson MD, Taylor GI. The arterial anatomy of the Achilles tendon: Anatomical study and clinical implications. Clin Anat. 2009;22(3):377-85.

5. Citak M, Knobloch K, Albrecht K, Krettek C, Hufner T. Anatomy of the sural nerve in a computer-assisted model: implications for surgical minimal-invasive Achilles tendon repair. Br J Sports Med. 2007;41(7):456-8.

6. Cohen JC. Anatomy and biomechanical aspects of the gastrocsoleus complex. Foot Ankle Clin. 2009;14(4):617-26.

7. Del Buono A, Chan O, Maffulli N. Achilles tendon: functional anatomy and novel emerging models of imaging classification. Int Orthop. 2013;37(4):715-21.

8. Doral MN, Alam M, Bozkurt M, Turhan E, Atay OA, Dönmez G, Maffulli N. Functional anatomy of the Achilles tendon. Knee Surg Sports Traumatol Arthrosc. 2010;18(5):638-43.

9. Doral MN, Bozkurt M, Turhan E, Ayvaz M, Atay ÖA, Üzümcügil A, Leblebicioğlu G, Kaya D, Aydoğ T. Percutaneous suturing of the ruptured Achilles tendon with endoscopic control. Arch Orthop Trauma Surg. 2009;129 (8): 1093-101.

10. Hernández-Díaz C, Saavedra MÁ, Navarro-Zarza JE, Canoso JJ, Villaseñor-Ovies P, Vargas A, Kalish RA. Clinical anatomy of the ankle and foot. Reumatol Clin. 2012;8 Suppl 2:46-52.

11. Kachlik D, Baca V, Cepelik M, Hajek P, Mandys V, Musil V. Clinical anatomy of the calcaneal tuberosity. Ann Anat. 2008;190(3):284-91.

12. Lohrer H, Arentz S, Nauck T, Dorn-Lange NV, Konerding MA. The Achilles tendon insertion is crescent-shaped: an in vitro anatomic investigation. Clin Orthop Relat Res. 2008;466(9):2230-7.

13. Maffulli N. Rupture of the Achilles tendon. J Bone Joint Surg Am. 1999;81(7):1019-36.

14. Malvankar S, Khan WS. Evolution of the Achilles tendon: the athlete's Achilles heel? Foot (Edinb). 2011;21(4):193-7.

15. O'Brien M. Functional anatomy and physiology of tendons. Clin Sports Med. 1992;11(3):505-20.

16. O'Brien M. The anatomy of the Achilles tendon. Foot Ankle Clin. 2005;10(2):225-38.

17. Shaw HM, Vázquez OT, McGonagle D, Bydder G, Santer RM, Benjamin M. Development of the human Achilles tendon enthesis organ. J Anat. 2008;213(6):718-24.

18. Standring S. Gray's Anatomy: The Anatomical Basis of Clinical Practice. 39th Ed. Philadelphia: Elsevier Churchill Livingstone; 2005. pp.1499-500.

19. Theobald P, Bydder G, Dent C, Nokes L, Pugh N, Benjamin M. The functional anatomy of Kager's fat pad in relation to retrocalcaneal problems and other hindfoot disorders. J Anat. 2006;208(1):91-7.

20. Watanabe Y, Moriya H, Takahashi K, Yamagata M, Sonoda M, Shimada Y, Tamaki T. Functional anatomy of the posterolateral structures of the knee. Arthroscopy. 1993;9(1):57-62.

21. Snow SW, Bohne WH, DiCarlo E, Chang VK. Anatomy of the Achilles tendon and plantar fascia in relation to the calcaneus in various age groups. Foot Ankle Int. 1995;16(7):418-21.

"Not everything that counts can be counted and not everything that can be counted counts."

William Bruce Cameron

Chapter 3

Epidemiology of Achilles Tendon Disorders

Bernard C.S. Lee, Christopher J. Pearce, James D.F. Calder

Take Home Message

• *The incidence of Achilles tendon disorders is rising.*

• *There is a strong association with sporting activities, mostly recreational sports.*

• *Little epidemiological data is available from rural populations or developing countries.*

Introduction

Disorders of the Achilles tendon are commonly seen in general practice as well as in hospital settings. The incidence of these conditions appears to be rising, at least in the developed world [33,34,37,41,42,48,49]. Current efforts to quantify the incidence of each disease entity are limited by the fact that most epidemiological papers study a small sample population with the attendant problem of selection bias. In addition, studies investigating the incidence of Achilles tendon ruptures largely review surgical data for surgically-treated patients, while the data concerning Achilles tendinopathy mostly come from surveys at sporting events, sports clubs or small databases. In particular, milder cases of Achilles tendinopathy may not even be recorded if the patient never consults a doctor. The majority of the available literature on the epidemiology of Achilles tendon problems has come from developed countries, and hence the strong association with sporting activities. Little is known about their incidence in rural life or developing countries, where a more physical occupational lifestyle may potentially affect the overall incidence of these problems.

All is not lost, however, as was aptly put by the epidemiologist John M Cowden – "Consistency is more important than accuracy." This chapter will examine the available evidence for the incidence of, and epidemiological factors that contribute to, problems of the Achilles tendon within the limitations mentioned above. The epidemiology of Achilles tendon ruptures as well as insertional and non-insertional Achilles tendinopathies will be included. Based on the currently available epidemiological studies, it is apparent that although there is a distinction made between the different locations of tendon pathology, many of the epidemiological factors are common to all conditions. There will inevitably be some overlap between epidemiological and aetiological contributors, which are commonly classified as 'intrinsic' and 'extrinsic' factors, and the latter will be expanded upon further in Chapter 4 – Aetiology of Achilles Tendon Disorders.

Incidence

The incidence of Achilles tendinopathy and ruptures is increasing, especially in the developed world. This has been attributed to an increase in sporting activity both in the young and especially in older populations, as well as a general increase in the duration and intensity of training [23, 36, 52].

Much of the currently available epidemiological data are from Scandinavia. Based on these studies, the annual incidence of Achilles tendon ruptures has been rising, with a peak as high as 37.3 per 100,000 population [33, 34, 41, 42, 48]. Other studies from Scotland and Canada have also shown a similar increase, although of a smaller magnitude [37, 49] (Table 1).

Study	Study Population	Study Period	Incidence per 100,000 at the Start of the Study Period	Incidence per 100,000 at the End of the Study Period
Leppilahti 1996 [33]	Oulu, Finland	1979-1994	2	18
Moller 1996 [41]	Malmo, Sweden	1987-1991	–	13.3
Levi 1997 [34]	Copenhagen, Denmark	1978-1995	–	13.4
Houshian 1998 [19]	Esbjerg, Denmark	1984-1996	18.2	37.3
Maffulli 1999 [37]	Scotland	1981-1994	4.7	6
Suchak 2005 [49]	Edmonton, Canada	1998-2002	5.5	9.9
Sode 2007 [48]	Funen, Denmark	1991-2002	22.1	32.6
Nyyssönen 2008 [42]	Finland	1987-1999	8.3	14.8

Table 1. Increasing annual incidence of Achilles tendon ruptures.

The incidence of Achilles tendinopathy in the general population is harder to ascertain. Based on epidemiological data from a cohort of 57,725 patients in a Dutch primary care setting, this was reported as 1.85/1000 of GP-registered patients. However, in patients aged 21 to 60 years, the rate was 2.35 per 1,000 [9]. The incidence may well be higher due to the inherent study limitations discussed earlier.

Intrinsic Factors

Age

Studies have consistently reported a peak incidence of Achilles tendon rupture in the 30-39 age group, with the peak incidence in men being several years earlier than that in women [33, 37, 49].

	Overall Peak Incidence Age/Years	**Peak Incidence in Men/Years**	**Peak Incidence in Women/Years**
Leppilahti 1996 [33]	30-39	Not reported	Not reported
Houshian 1998 [19]	30-49	Not reported	Not reported
Maffulli 1999 [37]	30-39	30-39	>80
Suchak 2005 [49]	30-39	30-39	40-49
Nyyssonnen 2008 [42]	30-45	41.7	44.4

Table 2. Summary of peak incidence of Achilles tendon ruptures with respect to age.

Some reports describe a bimodal distribution, corresponding to younger athletes and older non-athletic individuals [19, 37, 41], while others found no such bimodal distribution [42, 49]. This is likely due to the overlap between the older patients with sports-related ruptures and the peak of the non-sports-related ruptures, which does not show up as a second peak in the age distribution. Several authors have reported that the majority of sports-related Achilles tendon ruptures occur between the ages of 30 and 49 years, while the peak in non-sports-related ruptures was between the ages of 50 and 59 years [19, 33]. Indeed, Leppilahti and co-workers [33] as well as Houshian and co-workers [19] showed that the peaks in incidence were different when sports-related and non-sports-related ruptures were studied separately. However, due to the high incidence of sports-related injuries (81%), they found no bimodal distribution in the overall incidence.

Histological studies have shown that the incidence of degenerative tendinopathy increases with age. Kannus and co-workers found that while only 30% of tendons from young, previously-healthy cadavers (mean age 38 years) had histological evidence of degenerative tendinopathy, almost half of the older cadavers (mean age 66 years) had degenerative tendinopathy [25]. They concluded that degenerative changes were more common in people older than 35 years of age, and as a result patients older than 35 had a higher risk of spontaneous rupture than younger patients.

These findings may show a clinical correlation with two studies involving badminton players in Sweden. Young, elite badminton players (aged 16 to 34 years) showed no correlation between age and symptomatic Achilles tendino-pathy [11]. In contrast, the incidence of symptomatic Achilles tendinopathy in middle-aged competitive badminton players (aged 35 to 57 years) was significantly higher in the older players within that range [12].

Biomechanics

Multiple studies have looked at the biomechanical factors contributing to Achilles tendinopathy. These include the gastrocnemius-soleus complex, the tibio-talar joint and the sub-talar joint.

Decreased peak dorsiflexion velocity and gastrocnemius-soleus insufficiency with decreased plantar flexion strength have been shown to be associated with Achilles tendinopathy [5, 16, 38, 45]. One study suggested that lower eccentric torques of the gastrocnemius-soleus were associated with tendinopathy, while there was no relation to concentric torque [16].

The effect of ankle dorsiflexion range of motion is less clear. Mahieu and co-workers found that military cadets with increased dorsiflexion excursion were at greater risk of developing overuse tendinopathy [38]. In contrast, Kvist and co-workers [31] found that decreased ankle dorsiflexion with the knee in extension was a predisposing cause of tendinopathy. The former may be due to larger excursion distances, while the latter may be due to a tight gastrocnemius.

Increased eversion displacement of the sub-talar joint during mid-stance and 'functional overpronation' in runners has also been found to be associated with non-insertional tendinopath [5]. Ryan and co-workers found trends towards Achilles tendinopathy with greater overall frontal plane ankle joint motion [45]. However, Kvist and co-workers also found that limited total passive sub-talar motion and ankle dorsiflexion (with the knee in extension) was found in 58% and 70% of patients with non-insertional tendinopathy and insertional tendinopathy respectively [31]. More recently, Waldecker and co-workers [50] did not find any association between hindfoot valgus and Achilles tendinopathy. In fact, in their study of 1,394 feet in patients with various orthopaedic complaints and who were not active in sports, it was found that 78.3% of patients with Achilles tendinopathy had varus hindfoot malalignment [50].

The contribution of sub-talar mobility to Achilles tendinopathy is thus not clear, and other factors such as a tight gastrocnemius may be the greater driving force towards tendinopathy.

Co-morbidities

Achilles tendinopathy has been associated with various other disease processes, such as inflammatory arthropathies, gout, familial hyperlipidaemia, sarcoidosis and diffuse idiopathic skeletal hyperostosis.

Diabetes mellitus has been shown to be a predisposing factor [3, 18]. Batista and co-workers showed that in diabetic patients with no prior history of diabetic foot morbidity, 89% had disorganized tendon fibres and 76% had intratendinous calcifications on ultrasonography [3]. They also found a trend between the duration of diabetes disease as well as age and the degree of tendon disorganization. They did not, however, find any correlation between glycosylated haemoglobin levels and tendon alterations.

Inflammatory conditions have long been associated with Achilles pathology. Gout was found to be present in 14.3% of ruptured tendons in one study [4]. The presence of rheumatoid arthritis was also shown to increase the chance of sustaining an Achilles tendon rupture (odds ratio: 1.9) [46]. The correlation between systemic lupus erythematous with associated Jaccoud's arthropathy and steroid use has also recently been highlighted as a predisposing factor for spontaneous Achilles tendon ruptures [1].

Achilles tendinopathy has also been significantly correlated with hypertension, most likely as a result of the end organ's effect on microvascularity [18]. Other causes include seronegative arthropathies and their associated enthesitis, as well as what we now know are much rarer conditions such as xanthomas of the Achilles tendon.

The association of obesity with Achilles tendon disorders has also been well studied [11,12]. Data from surveys of running events and competitive badminton players have shown no association between BMI and an increased incidence of Achilles tendon problems [11, 12, 39]. However, these data are limited by the fact that the number of participants with a high BMI playing competitive sports is small. In contrast, Holmes and co-workers showed a positive correlation between obesity and Achilles tendinopathy in patients seen in the clinic setting [18]. At the same time, Seeger and co-workers showed that the odds ratio for Achilles tendon ruptures with obesity based on insurance claims within a health insured cohort was 2 [46].

Certainly, a previous history of local symptoms has been associated with Achilles tendon ruptures in 15-21% of cases [4, 10, 21].

Deformity

It is common belief that a postero-superior calcaneal prominence (sometimes referred to as Haglund's deformity) is associated with insertional Achilles tendinopathy [17]. In a group of patients not active in sports, the prevalence of a postero-superior calcaneal prominence in subjects with Achilles tendinopathy was 39.2% [50]. However, a retrospective review published in the same year found that the presence of a postero-superior calcaneal prominence was not indicative of insertional tendinopathy, with the deformity being present in many asymptomatic patients [24]. In their study, they also found that 73% had intratendinous calcifications, leading them to conclude that the excision of the postero-superior calcaneal prominence may not always be necessary in the management of these conditions.

Ethnicity and blood group

The contribution of ethnicity and, therefore, a presumed genetic predisposition to the development of Achilles tendon problems is highly likely. However, it is also important to rule out or control for cultural and socio-economic factors that may also contribute to the observed difference in incidence. As previously stated, there are few studies available that describe the incidence of Achilles tendon problems in the developing world; consequently, most of the available literature regarding ethnicity is from the US military, where comparisons have been made between black and white service members. Based on these studies, the risk of Achilles tendon rupture has been quoted at between 3.6 to 13 times greater in service members of black ethnicity [8, 43, 51]. Taking into account that 64.9% of injuries in black service members were Achilles tendon ruptures while only 34% of injuries in non-black service members were ruptures, there was still an increased risk (RR 1.82) in black basketball players compared to non-black service members [8]. There is little other information available about the epidemiology of Achilles tendon problems in other ethnic groups.

The ABO blood group distribution of patients with a rupture of the Achilles tendon and of patients with chronic tendo Achillis tendinopathy differed from the controls in a study by Kujala and co-workers with the O and A blood groups being predominant in these conditions [29].

Gender

Most epidemiological studies report a higher incidence of tendon ruptures in males than females. The odds ratio for being male was as high as 3 in two studies [34, 46].

	Study Population	**Male : Female**
Leppilahti 1996 [33]	Oulu, Finland	5.5 : 1
Levi 1997 [34]	Copenhagen	3 : 1
Houshian 1998 [19]	Esbjerg, Denmark	3 : 1
Maffulli 1999 [37]	Scotland	1.55 : 1

Table 3. Ratios of Achilles tendon rupture incidences between men and women.

It has been described that men sustain Achilles tendon ruptures on average two to three years younger than women [42]. These differences in incidence may be due to differences between sporting levels between men and women, and not necessarily because of intrinsic differences between the sexes.

In two separate studies involving young (age 16-34 years) and middle-aged (age 35-57) elite, competitive badminton players, there was no difference in the sex distribution between patients with and without symptomatic Achilles tendinopathy [11, 12]. Another study from Dunedin, New Zealand, showed that although 73% of Achilles tendon ruptures occurred in males, in patients up to the age of 50 years there were equal numbers of Achilles tendon ruptures in males and females [15]. They found that netball was the most common cause of ruptures, thus possibly accounting for the high incidence in females.

It may thus be possible that the differences in the incidence of Achilles tendon problems are due to factors other than gender, such as sporting and occupational activities.

Extrinsic factors

Activity

Achilles tendinopathy and ruptures have been strongly associated with increased sporting activity. In the publications from Scandinavia, the incidence of sports-related ruptures is as high as 81%, with up to 89% of sports-related ruptures due to involvement in ball games [19, 31, 33]. Achilles tendon ruptures are associated with sports that involve jumping or sudden and abrupt movements, as it is usually an eccentric load that causes the injury. These include badminton, volleyball, basketball, netball and football [8, 14, 19, 41, 42]. Indeed, daily physical activities may affect incidence rates, with Nyyssonen and co-workers showing geographical variation within Finland whereby the incidence of Achilles tendon ruptures is higher around the urban centres than in the rural areas [42].

	Study Population	Sports-Related Ruptures / %	Ruptures Related to Ball Games / %
Kvist 1994 [32]	Turku, Finland	75	–
Leppilahti 1996 [33]	Oulu, Finland	81	88
Houshian 1998 [19]	Esbjerg, Denmark	74.2	89
Gwynne-Jones 2011 [15]	Dunedin, New Zealand	78.5	61.4

Table 4. Incidence of sports-related Achilles tendon ruptures.

The incidence of Achilles tendon ruptures has also been shown to be high for sprinters (odds ratio 14.9) in male former elite athletes [30]. Veteran master track and field athletes have been shown to have an increased risk of Achilles tendon rupture (odds ratio 14.87) after the age of 45 compared to previously healthy controls [26].

The incidence of Achilles tendinopathy on the other hand, has been reported to be higher in individuals who start a new or unaccustomed activity, in runners and badminton players, and in sportsmen who increase their training load, change their shoes or change their usual running surfaces.

In a cohort of German patients who were not active in sports, the overall incidence of Achilles tendinopathy was 5.6%, of which 3.7% were insertional, 4% were non-insertional and 1.9% were combined insertional and non-insertional [50]. Meanwhile, 35% of patients seen in a Dutch GP practice for Achilles tendinopathy showed some sports involvement [9]. As with tendon ruptures, the incidence of sports-related Achilles tendinopathy has been reported to be higher than in the rest of the population, at up to 69% in a Swedish study [44].

New military recruits and officer cadets have been shown to have an incidence of Achilles tendinopathy of 6.8% to 14.5% [38, 40]. This is believed to be due to unaccustomed activity, although these studies were not done in comparison with a baseline incidence for the general population.

Amongst athletes, Achilles tendinopathy has been reported in 66% of joggers, 32% of tennis players and 24% of runners. These comprised non-insertional tendinopathy in 66%, insertional in 23% and myotendineal 8% [31].

The lifetime risk of Achilles tendinopathy in former elite male distance runners is between 52% and 56.6% [27, 55,] while 34% of middle-distance runners have also been reported to have had Achilles tendon problems at some point [16]. The incidence of Achilles tendinopathy before the age of 45 has also been shown to be high for middle- and long-distance runners (adjusted odds ratio of 31.2) when compared with controls [30].

In a study of elite runners (aged mean 42 years) who run an average of 65.2 km per week, overuse injuries were shown to be 7-times more frequent than acute injuries, with Achilles tendinopathy being the most predominant injury and Achilles tendon ruptures being rare [27]. Non-insertional tendinopathy was twice as common as insertional tendinopathy in these athletes.

From these studies, it is evident that Achilles tendinopathy is a common overuse injury in runners. An epidemiological survey of participants in a 16 km race showed 'Achillodynia' to be the most common single chronic overuse injury, comprising 4.6% of running injuries in the 12 months preceding the race [39]. A separate study of club runners found an annual incidence of Achilles tendon problems of 7% to 9% [35].

The cumulative running load has been correlated with the incidence of Achilles tendinopathy. Marti and co-workers found that Achilles tendinopathy was significantly and positively correlated with age, weekly mileage and previous jogging injury [39]. Likewise, Haglund-Akerlind and co-workers found that patients with Achilles tendinopathy had longer exposure time, with significantly more years of training, and significantly longer distances per week than those without tendinopathy [16]. Indeed, the risk of developing Achilles tendinopathy in elite runners with more than 10 years' experience has been shown to be higher (RR 1.6) [27]. Overtraining was found to be the most common cause of overuse Achilles tendinopathy in runners (75.2%) [5].

Running surfaces have also been implicated in the development of Achilles tendinopathy. Knobloch and co-workers found that in elite runners, running on asphalt, decreased the non-insertional tendinopathy risk (RR 0.47), while running on sand increased the relative risk tenfold (RR 10) [27]. In contrast, however, Marti and co-workers found that in patients surveyed at a 16 km race, the usual running surface was not associated with increased injuries [39].

The contribution of the type of running shoes worn is harder to study. Although we might expect that the incidence of Achilles tendinopathy to be higher in runners with cheap (and, therefore, presumably poorer quality) shoes, Marti and co-workers found that cheap shoes did not increase the incidence of Achilles tendinopathy. On the contrary, they found that expensive running shoes were associated with more running injuries, although this may simply mean that patients with running injuries tend to prefer expensive shoes [39].

The incidence of Achilles tendon problems in badminton players has also been studied. In a group of elite and recreational badminton players, 10.5% of overuse injuries were Achilles tendon-related [22]. In young, elite badminton players (age 16-34), 32% reported having had disabling Achilles tendon problems during the previous five years. Of these, 57% were non-insertional. Symptomatic individuals were also found to have had higher weekly training loads [11]. In older, competitive badminton players (age 35-57) the incidence of Achilles tendon pain in the previous five years was 44%. The affected individuals were found to be significantly older. In contrast with the study on younger players, however, there was no relationship found between symptoms of pain and the amount of training or years of playing badminton [12]. It is questionable, however, whether some older individuals with disabling symptoms had stopped competitive badminton, and hence were self-excluded from the study population.

Climate

The incidence of Achilles tendinopathy and ruptures in relation to climate and seasonal changes has been investigated. Infantry recruits were found to have a statistically higher incidence of Achilles tendinopathy in the winter months at 9.4% compared to a 3.6% incidence in the summer [40]. They attributed 94% of the cases to paratendinitis, and this was postulated to be due to a fall in the temperature of the Achilles paratenon, resulting in decreased lubrication and increased friction.

There was no such seasonality found in other epidemiological studies looking at the incidence of Achilles tendon ruptures [37, 42, 49]. One study showed more ruptures in the spring, although there were no significant differences by season [49].

Drugs

The use of certain drugs has been implicated in the development of Achilles tendon ruptures. Achilles tendinopathy has been significantly correlated with hormone replacement therapy and oral contraceptives [18].

The role of corticosteroids in the development of Achilles tendon ruptures has also been studied. Previous steroid injections have been reported in 7% of patients [4]. A separate study found that the risk of rupture was increased with local steroid injections (odds ratio 2.2) [46]. The same study found a smaller magnitude but still an increased risk with oral corticosteroid (odds ratio 1.4).

The use of fluoroquinolones is associated with an increase in the risk of Achilles tendon rupture and tendinopathy. A World Health Organization (WHO) survey in Australia found that fluoroquinolone use was associated with 112 cases of Achilles tendon-related problems up until 2002. Of these, 30 were tendon ruptures and 90% (100 cases) were associated with Ciprofloxacin use (World Health Organization. Pharmaceutical Newsletter) [2]. Clinically, the risk has also been shown to be dose-dependent, and ciprofloxacin has been shown in laboratory studies to decrease proteoglycan synthesis and increase matrix-degrading proteolytic activity [53]. The use of fluoroquinolones has been reported to triple the risk of Achilles tendon rupture (age- and sex-standardized incidence ratio of 3.1) [48]. However, a separate study showed that when compared to the controls, the elevation in Achilles tendon rupture risk with fluoroquinolones (odds ratio 1.2) was similar in magnitude to that associated with oral corticosteroids (odds ratio 1.4) and non-fluoroquinolone antibiotics (OR 1.2). In line with the earlier laboratory study (Williams 2000), a stronger association was found with higher cumulative fluoroquinolone dosing (OR 1.5) [46]. Fluoroquinolone antibiotics, including ciprofloxacin, have long been associated with the development of tendinopathies [6, 7, 13, 20, 28, 47, 53, 54].

Women taking the oral contraceptive pill and post-menopausal women on hormone replacement therapy also appear to have a higher incidence of tendo Achillis tendinopathy than national controls [18].

Conclusion

The incidence of Achilles tendon disorders is rising notably in developed countries, where most of the epidemiological data comes from. The increasing incidence is likely due to changes in lifestyle and sporting activities in these urban communities, and less likely due to factors such as gender. While age plays an important part in the development of degenerative tendinopathy, the contribution of sporting activities greatly increases the incidence of Achilles tendinopathy and rupture beyond the baseline incidence for spontaneous rupture or degenerative tendons. Sports such as badminton are popular in the Scandinavian countries, perhaps resulting in a high incidence of Achilles tendon ruptures there. Unfortunately, we do not have data from other major badminton-playing countries, such as China, with which to correlate these findings. With jogging and running becoming more popular globally, we should expect to see an even greater increase in the incidence of Achilles tendinopathy.

The contribution of biomechanical abnormalities and deformities to the increased risk of Achilles tendon problems needs to be better studied and understood so that we can prophylactically manage high-risk athletes with appropriate orthotics and strengthening programmes.

With a greater understanding of associated medical conditions and pharmacotherapy, we can also better advise our active population on the kinds of sports they are safe to participate in, especially in the developed countries where health and fitness is becoming more important.

Finally, the effect of ethnicity and global geographical differences, with their intrinsic cultural, occupational, socio-economic as well as climate differences, requires further study. It has been shown that even within a country, there are geographical differences in the incidence rates between rural and urban areas [42]. There is also very little data from developing countries and the tropics.

A better understanding of the contribution of all of these factors will not only aid in the understanding of Achilles tendon disorders as a global problem, but also aid in identifying high-risk groups. Until then, we will continue to advise our athletes and patients based on what little we already know: "The man who insists on seeing with perfect clearness before he decides, never decides." – Henri-Frederic Amiel (philosopher, 1821-1881).

References

1. Alves EM, Macieira JC, Borba E, Chiuchetta FA,Santiago MB. Spontaneous tendon rupture in systemic lupus erythematosus: association with Jaccoud's arthropathy. Lupus. 2010;19(3):247-54.

2. Australian Adverse Drug Reactions Bulletin 21:15, Dec 2002. Available from URL: http://www.health.gov.au

3. Batista F, Nery C, Pinzur M, Monteiro AC, de Souza EF, Felippe FH, Alcantara MC,Campos RS. Achilles tendinopathy in diabetes mellitus. Foot Ankle Int. 2008;29(5):498-501.

4. Beskin JL, Sanders RA, Hunter SC, Hughston JC. Surgical repair of Achilles tendon ruptures. Am J Sports Med. 1987 ;15(1):1-8

5. Clement DB, Taunton JE, Smart GW. Achilles tendinitis and peritendinitis: etiology and treatment. Am J Sports Med. 1984;12(3):179-84.

6. Corps AN, Curry VA, Harrall RL, Dutt D, Hazleman BL, Riley GP. Ciprofloxacin reduces the stimulation of prostaglandin E(2) output by interleukin-1beta in human tendon-derived cells. Rheumatology (Oxford). 2003;42(11):1306-10.

7. Corps AN, Harrall RL, Curry VA, Fenwick SA, Hazleman BL, Riley GP. Ciprofloxacin enhances the stimulation of matrix metalloproteinase 3 expression by interleukin-1beta in human tendon-derived cells. A potential mechanism of fluoroquinolone-induced tendinopathy. Arthritis Rheum. 2002;46(11):3034-40.

8. Davis JJ, Mason KT, Clark DA. Achilles tendon ruptures stratified by age, race, and cause of injury among active duty U.S. Military members. Mil Med. 1999;164(12):872-3.

9. de Jonge S, van den Berg C, de Vos RJ, van der Heide HJ, Weir A, Verhaar JA, Bierma-Zeinstra SM, Tol JL. Incidence of midportion Achilles tendinopathy in the general population. Br J Sports Med. 2011;45(13):1026-8.

10. Fahlstrom M, Bjornstig U, Lorentzon R. Acute Achilles tendon rupture in badminton players. Am J Sports Med. 1998;26(3):467-70.

11. Fahlstrom M, Lorentzon R, Alfredson H. Painful conditions in the Achilles tendon region in elite badminton players. Am J Sports Med. 2002;30(1):51-4.

12. Fahlstrom M, Lorentzon R, Alfredson H. Painful conditions in the Achilles tendon region: a common problem in middle-aged competitive badminton players. Knee Surg Sports Traumatol Arthrosc. 2002;10(1):57-60.

13. Fleisch F, Hartmann K, Kuhn M. Fluoroquinolone-induced tendinopathy: also occurring with levofloxacin. Infection. 2000;28(4):256-7.

14. Flood L, Harrison JE. Epidemiology of basketball and netball injuries that resulted in hospital admission in Australia, 2000-2004. Med J Aust. 2009 19;190(2):87-90.

15. Gwynne-Jones DP, Sims M, Handcock D. Epidemiology and outcomes of acute Achilles tendon rupture with operative or nonoperative treatment using an identical functional bracing protocol. Foot Ankle Int. 2011;32(4):337-43.

16. Haglund-Akerlind Y, Eriksson E. Range of motion, muscle torque and training habits in runners with and without Achilles tendon problems. Knee Surg Sports Traumatol Arthrosc. 1993;1(3-4):195-9.

17. Haglund P. Bietrag zur klink der achillessehne. Z. Orthop.Chir. 1928 49 49-58.

18. Holmes GB, Lin J. Etiologic factors associated with symptomatic Achilles tendinopathy. Foot Ankle Int. 2006;27(11):952-9.

19. Houshian S, Tscherning T, Riegels-Nielsen P. The epidemiology of Achilles tendon rupture in a Danish county. Injury. 1998;29(9):651-4.

20. Huston KA. Achilles tendinitis and tendon rupture due to fluoroquinolone antibiotics. N Engl J Med. 1994 15;331(11):748.

21. Inglis AE, Sculco TP. Surgical repair of ruptures of the tendo Achillis. Clin Orthop Relat Res. 1981;(156):160-9.

22. Jorgensen U, Winge S. Injuries in badminton. Sports Med. 1990;10(1):59-64.

23/ Kader D, Saxena A, Movin T, Maffulli N. Achilles tendinopathy: some aspects of basic science and clinical management. Br J Sports Med. 2002;36(4):239-49.

24. Kang S, Thordarson DB, Charlton TP. Insertional Achilles tendinitis and Haglund's deformity. Foot Ankle Int. 2012;33(6):487-91.

25. Kannus P, Jozsa L. Histopathological changes preceding spontaneous rupture of a tendon. A controlled study of 891 patients. J Bone Joint Surg Am. 1991;73(10):1507-25.

26. Kettunen JA, Kujala UM, Kaprio J, Sarna S. Health of master track and field athletes: a 16-year follow-up study. Clin J Sport Med. 2006;16(2):142-8.

27. Knobloch K, Yoon U, Vogt PM. Acute and overuse injuries correlated to hours of training in master running athletes. Foot Ankle Int. 2008;29(7):671-6.

28. Koeger AC, Bellaiche L, Roger B. Magnetic resonance imaging in fluoroquinolone induced tendinopathy. J Rheumatol. 1997;24(5):1015-7.

29. Kujala UM, Jarvinen M, Natri A, Lehto M, Nelimarkka O, Hurme M, Virta L, Finne J. ABO blood groups and musculoskeletal injuries. Injury. 1992 23(2):131-3.

30. Kujala UM, Sarna S, Kaprio J. Cumulative incidence of Achilles tendon rupture and tendinopathy in male former elite athletes. Clin J Sport Med. 2005;15(3):133-5.

31. Kvist M. Achilles tendon injuries in athletes. Ann Chir Gynaecol. 1991 80(2):188-201.

32. Kvist M. Achilles tendon injuries in athletes. Sports Med. 1994;18(3):173-201.

33. Leppilahti J, Puranen J, Orava S. Incidence of Achilles tendon rupture. Acta Orthop Scand. 1996;67(3):277-9.

34. Levi N. The incidence of Achilles tendon rupture in Copenhagen. Injury. 1997;28(4):311-3.

35. Lysholm J, Wiklander J. Injuries in runners. Am J Sports Med. 1987 Mar-;15(2):168-71.

36. Maffulli N, Sharma P, Luscombe KL. Achilles tendinopathy: aetiology and management. Journal of the Royal Society of Medicine. 2004;97(10):472-6.

37. Maffulli N, Waterston SW, Squair J, Reaper J, Douglas AS. Changing incidence of Achilles tendon rupture in Scotland: a 15-year study. Clin J Sport Med. 1999;9(3):157-60.

38. Mahieu NN, Witvrouw E, Stevens V, Van Tiggelen D, Roget P. Intrinsic risk factors for the development of Achilles tendon overuse injury: a prospective study. Am J Sports Med. 2006;34(2):226-35.

39. Marti B, Vader JP, Minder CE, Abelin T. On the epidemiology of running injuries. The 1984 Bern Grand-Prix study. Am J Sports Med. 1988 ;16(3):285-94.

40. Milgrom C, Finestone A, Zin D, Mandel D, Novack V. Cold weather training: a risk factor for Achilles paratendinitis among recruits. Foot Ankle Int. 2003;24(5):398-401.

41. Moller A, Astron M, Westlin N. Increasing incidence of Achilles tendon rupture. Acta Orthop Scand. 1996;67(5):479-81.

42. Nyyssonen T, Luthje P, Kroger H. The increasing incidence and difference in sex distribution of Achilles tendon rupture in Finland in 1987-1999. Scand J Surg. 2008 97(3):272-5.

43. Owens B, Mountcastle S, White D. Racial differences in tendon rupture incidence. Int J Sports Med. 2007;28(7):617-20.

44. Rolf C, Movin T. Etiology, histopathology, and outcome of surgery in achillodynia. Foot Ankle Int. 1997;18(9):565-9.

45. Ryan M, Grau S, Krauss I, Maiwald C, Taunton J, Horstmann T. Kinematic analysis of runners with Achilles mid-portion tendinopathy. Foot Ankle Int. 2009;30(12):1190-5.

46. Seeger JD, West WA, Fife D, Noel GJ, Johnson LN, Walker AM. Achilles tendon rupture and its association with fluoroquinolone antibiotics and other potential risk factors in a managed care population. Pharmacoepidemiol Drug Saf. 2006;15(11):784-92.

47. Sendzik J, Shakibaei M, Schafer-Korting M,Stahlmann R. Fluoroquinolones cause changes in extracellular matrix, signalling proteins, metalloproteinases and caspase-3 in cultured human tendon cells. Toxicology. 2005 15;212(1):24-36.

48. Sode J, Obel N, Hallas J, Lassen A. Use of fluroquinolone and risk of Achilles tendon rupture: a population-based cohort study. Eur J Clin Pharmacol. 2007;63(5):499-503.

49. Suchak AA, Bostick G, Reid D, Blitz S, Jomha N. The incidence of Achilles tendon ruptures in Edmonton, Canada. Foot Ankle Int. 2005;26(11):932-6.

50. Waldecker U, Hofmann G, Drewitz S. Epidemiologic investigation of 1394 feet: coincidence of hindfoot malalignment and Achilles tendon disorders. Foot Ankle Surg. 2012;18(2):119-23.

51. White DW, Wenke JC, Mosely DS, Mountcastle SB, Basamania CJ. Incidence of major tendon ruptures and anterior cruciate ligament tears in US Army soldiers. Am J Sports Med. 2007;35(8):1308-14.

52. Wilder RP, Sethi S. Overuse injuries: tendinopathies, stress fractures, compartment syndrome, and shin splints. Clin Sports Med. 2004;23(1):55-81, vi.

53. Williams RJ, 3rd, Attia E, Wickiewicz TL, Hannafin JA. The effect of ciprofloxacin on tendon, paratenon, and capsular fibroblast metabolism. Am J Sports Med. 2000 ;28(3):364-9.

54. Zabraniecki L, Negrier I, Vergne P, Arnaud M, Bonnet C, Bertin P, Treves R. Fluoroquinolone induced tendinopathy: report of 6 cases. J Rheumatol. 1996;23(3):516-20.

55. Zafar MS, Mahmood A, Maffulli N. Basic science and clinical aspects of Achilles tendinopathy. Sports Med Arthrosc. 2009;17(3):190-7.

"I like the dreams of the future better than the history of the past."

Thomas Jefferson

Chapter 4

Aetiology of Achilles tendon disorders

Nicola Maffulli, Umile G. Longo, Angelo Del Buono, Vincenzo Denaro

Take Home Message

• *The aetiology of Achilles tendon pathology remains unclear, and many factors have been implicated.*

• *Proposed intrinsic factors include tendon vascularity, gastrocnemius-soleus dysfunction, gender, age, body weight and height, pes cavus and lateral ankle instability.*

• *Proposed extrinsic factors for Achilles tendinopathy include poor technique, previous injuries, changes in training patterns, footwear and environmental factors such as training on hard, and slippery or slanting surfaces.*

• *Achilles tendon injuries have been reported to occur more frequently in individuals with increased adiposity. Treatment also appears to have poorer outcomes among these individuals.*

• *Variants within the TNC, COL5A1, MMP3, GDF5 and CASP8 genes have been independently associated with the risk of Achilles tendon pathology. Changes in the composition of the extracellular matrix of the tendon are likely to be reflected in the biomechanical properties of this connective tissue.*

Introduction

Achilles tendon pathology is common. The exact aetiology of Achilles tendon injury is still unclear. The pathology of tendinopathy has been described as a degenerative or failed healing response. Neither of these descriptions fully explain the heterogeneity of presentation. A continuum of pathology has been proposed [16]. Genetic risk factors have been proposed, but not completely clarified [63].

Histology

Tendons mainly consist of collagen, non-collagenous proteins, glycosaminoglycans, cells and water [69, 70]. About 90–95% of the cellular elements of tendons are tenoblasts and tenocytes, aligned in rows between collagen fibre bundles [67]. Tenoblasts transform into mature tenocytes, and are highly metabolically immature, spindle-shaped cells, with numerous cytoplasmic organelles [77]. Tenocytes produce extracellular matrix (ECM) proteins [64-66]. Tenoblasts have variable shapes and sizes, and are arranged in long parallel chains [37]. The presence of an easily harvestable stem cell population within adult human tendons has been demonstrated [108]. These cells exhibit features such as clonogenicity, multi-potency and mesenchymal stem cells markers expression. The age-related variations in human tendon stem cells affect the number of isolated cells and their self-renewal potential, while multi-potency assays are not influenced by tendon ageing, even though cells from younger individuals expressed higher levels of osteogenic and adipogenic genes, while chondrogenic genes are highly expressed in cells from older individuals.

Collagen constitutes about 90% of tendons' protein, or approximately 70% of the dry weight of a tendon [45]. The collagen fibres are tightly packed in parallel bundles [51]. Type I collagen is the commonest – it forms 95% of tendon collagen and is held in parallel bundles by small proteoglycan molecules [75]. Elastin accounts for only about 2% of the dry mass of tendon [45] and can undergo up to 200% strain before failure.

Aging significantly decreases tendon glycosaminoglycans and increases collagen concentration [131]. Acute exercise increases type I collagen formation in peritendinous tissue [58].

M_2 macrophages reduce inflammation and resolve necrotic debris in the first phase, whereas they promote angiogenesis in the proliferative stage [93]. These findings are indicative of post-injury 'failed healing' as well as matrix disorganization, increased extracellular ground substance and separation between collagen fibres [61, 50]. All these detections may result in greater vulnerability to future mechanical strain [3].

Several patterns of degeneration have been described with microscopy, including hypoxic degeneration, hyaline degeneration, mucoid or myxoid degeneration, fibrinoid degeneration, lipoid degeneration, calcification, fibrocartilaginous and bony metaplasia. All can coexist, depending on the anatomical site and the nature of their causal insult. Therefore, tendinopathy can be considered the end result of a number of aetiological processes with a relatively narrow spectrum of histopathological features [76, 80, 81].

Aetiology

The aetiology of Achilles tendon pathology remains unclear, and many factors have been implicated. Proposed common intrinsic factors include tendon vascularity, gastrocnemius-soleus dysfunction, gender, age, body weight and height, pes cavus and lateral ankle instability [82]. However, in competing track and field athletes, no influence of age, gender, weight, height and impact profile on Achilles tendinopathy was found [68].

Excessive motion of the hindfoot in the frontal plane, especially a lateral heel strike with excessive compensatory pronation, is thought to cause a 'whipping action' on the Achilles tendon and predispose it to tendinopathy. Excessive loading of tendons during vigorous physical training is regarded as the main pathological stimulus for tendinopathy [60], possibly as a result of imbalance between muscle power and tendon elasticity. The Achilles tendon may respond to repetitive supra-physiological overload by either inflammation of its sheath or degeneration of its body, or a combination of both [42, 56].

It remains unclear whether different stresses induce different responses. Experimental evidence suggests that moderate exercise exerts a protective effect on the tendon structure while sudden discontinuation of physical activity has a negative effect on tendons, suggesting that after a period of sudden de-training (such as after an injury) physical activity should be restarted with caution and with appropriate rehabilitation programmes [24]. The active repair of fatigue damage must occur or tendons will weaken and eventually rupture. The repair mechanism is probably mediated by resident tenocytes, which continually monitor the ECM. Failure to adapt to recurrent excessive loads results in the release of cytokines, leading to further modulation of cell activity [60]. Tendon damage may even occur from stresses within physiological limits, as frequent cumulative microtrauma may not allow enough time for repair [112]. Microtrauma can also result from non-uniform stress within tendons, producing abnormal load concentrations and frictional forces between the fibrils with localized fibre damage [60].

Free radical damage occurring on reperfusion after ischaemia, hypoxia, hyperthermia and impaired tenocyte apoptosis have been linked to tendinopathy [7].

Such reactive oxygen species are continually produced during normal cell metabolism. The principal site for reactive oxygen species formation in non-stressed cells is the mitochondrial respiratory chain. This series of coupled redox reactions leads to the formation of ATP with molecular oxygen. Molecular oxygen is the ultimate electron acceptor and is being reduced to water. Under normal physiological conditions, approximately 1% of electron flux leaks from this reductive chain, resulting in the univalent reduction of molecular oxygen and the generation of O_2- [19, 23, 109].

Exercise stimulates immune responses [5, 40, 41, 136], with increased leucocyte numbers - in particular granulocytes - generated with bouts of moderate exercise. Exhaustive exercise in cross-country skiers produces neutrophil mobilization and increased reactive oxygen species generation on subsequent stimulation [136]. Enhanced phagocytic O_2- generation is found approximately 24 h after exhaustive exercise [31]. However, the extent to which granulocyte activity is consistently enhanced by exercise is contested [40]. Increased phagocyte activity probably does not contribute to elevated reactive oxygen species levels during short-term exercise, but may act as a secondary source of reactive oxygen species during recovery from heavy exercise [40].

During cyclical tendon loading, the period of maximum tensile load is associated with ischaemia, and relaxation with reperfusion. This restoration of normal tissue oxygenation may lead to enhanced oxy-free radical production [27, 31].

Classical ischaemia-reperfusion injury involves the conversion, within the ischaemic-reperfused tissues, of hypoxanthine/xanthine dehydrogenase to the O_2- generating oxidase Neutrophil; infiltration may also be a source of enhanced reactive oxygen species in reperfusion injury [23]. However, for the tendon, ischaemia is a constant feature of loading rather than a pathophysiological occurrence, and neutrophil infiltration is not a feature of tendinopathy [46, 76]. It is therefore unlikely that the classical mechanism of reperfusion-mediated O_2- generation will be encountered during normal tendon use. However, mitochondria may leak more electrons during reoxygenation. As degeneration develops, the tendon may be more prone to classical (xanthine/hypoxanthine oxidase-mediated) reperfusion injury. We suggest, therefore, that there is the potential for re-oxygenation resulting in a cycle of enhanced reactive oxygen species production, most probably at sub-lethal levels, within the non-degenerate tendon.

Of possible importance for tendinopathy, non-professional phagocytes such as tenocytes also possess the ability to specifically generate reactive oxygen species in response to biochemical and physical stimuli that might be encountered on wounding and subsequent healing. Human fibroblasts produce reactive oxygen species in response to the cytokines TNF-α and interleukin-1 as well as to growth factors [26, 34, 53, 91, 124]. Indeed, fibroblasts apparently possess the capacity to produce O_2-/H_2O_2 by an NADPH oxidase complex similar to that in 'professional' phagocytes [53, 91].

Considerable tissue damage can be generated through phagocyte overactivity, and exercise seems to enhance the potential for phagocytes to generate O_2-

when stimulated. Phagocytic activity involves the generation and release - to the phagosome - of O_2-, H_2O_2, HO, $^1O_2$, HOCl and minor quantities of NO [97, 107]. While this is a vital component of immune surveillance and healing, it also has the potential for collateral damage to 'normal' cells and tissues through extra cellular bursts of reactive oxygen species and reactive oxygen species leakage [107, 133, 134]. While non-exhaustive exercise does not produce any consistent findings of oxidative damage [40], the inflammatory response may contribute to over-training damage in muscle [130, 136].

In animal studies, the local administration of cytokines and inflammatory agents, such as prostaglandins, has resulted in tendinopathy [127]. Fluoroquinolones have also been implicated in the pathogenesis of tendinopathy. Ciprofloxacin causes enhanced interleukin-1β-mediated MMP3 release, inhibits tenocyte proliferation and reduces collagen and matrix synthesis.

Degenerative tendinopathy is the most common histological finding in spontaneous tendon ruptures. Tendon degeneration may lead to reduced tensile strength and a predisposition to rupture. Indeed, ruptured Achilles tendons have more advanced intratendinous changes than tendinopathic tendons [129]. In Achilles tendinopathy, changes in the expression of genes regulating cell-cell and cell-matrix interactions have been reported, with down-regulation of matrix metalloproteinase [3] (MMP3) mRNA [120]. Significantly higher levels of type I and type III collagen mRNAs have been reported in tendinopathic samples compared with normal samples. Imbalance in MMP activity in response to repeated injury or mechanical strain may result in tendinopathy [83-87].

Pain is the main symptom of Achilles tendinopathy, but the underlying mechanism causing pain is not fully understood. Traditionally, pain has been thought to arise through inflammation or via collagen fibre separation or disruption [81]. However, chronically painful Achilles tendons present no evidence of inflammation [73]. As tendinopathies are not inflammatory conditions, pain may originate from a combination of mechanical and biochemical causes [74].

Inflammation

In acute tendon injuries, different phases define the healing process [3]. An acute inflammatory state occurs in the first few days - generally three to seven - after the injury, with a prevalence of inflammatory cells such as monocytes and macrophages [3]. During this phase, haematoma, platelet activation and the invasion of cells form a granuloma, and cells migrate from the extrinsic peritendinous tissue (tendon sheath, periosteum, subcutaneous tissue and fascicles), the epitenon and the endotenon [104].

Successively, a 'proliferative phase' persists for roughly three weeks after the injury. Cells proliferate and differentiate, and migrated fibroblasts start producing collagen (mostly collagen type III). In this way, elastic deformation and mechanical signalling take part in the process. Collagen type I is increasingly produced in the tendon and its ECM, allowing repair callus to enlarge and the tendon's strength to increase and sustain considerable traction loads [33, 25]. Tenocytes are the main cell type, and collagen synthesis continues for the next five weeks until eight weeks after the initial injury [33]. The vascular endothelial growth factor (VEGF) release facilitates neovascularization and stimulates the formation of granulation tissue. In this stage, continuous, intermittent or activity-related pain occurs [25, 33].

In the remodelling phase, the maturation and remodelling of collagen result in better tissue organization and increasing cross-linking [49]. The callus transverse area progressively decreases, and mechanical tissue properties improve. Remodelling continues, taking up to a year to complete healing [49]. Nevertheless, tendon regeneration is never completely achieved; hypercellularity, altered collagen diameter and fibrils thinning result in the reduced biomechanical strength and resistance of the tendon [79].

Adiposity

Achilles tendon injuries have been reported to occur more frequently in individuals with increased adiposity. Treatment also appears to have poorer outcomes among these individuals. Four longitudinal cohorts, 14 cross-sectional studies, eight case-control studies and two interventional studies (28 in total) met the inclusion criteria in a systematic review [25], providing a total of 19,949 individuals. Forty-two subpopulations were identified, 18 of which showed elevated adiposity to be associated with tendon injury (43%). Sensitivity analyses indicated a clustering of positive findings among studies that included clinical patients (81% positive) and among case-control studies (77% positive). Adiposity is frequently associated with tendon injury. Some studies suggest that adiposity is a risk factor for tendon injury, although this association appears to vary depending on aspects of study design and measurement. Adiposity is of particular interest in tendon research because, unlike a number of other reported risk factors for tendon injury, it is preventable and modifiable [1, 2, 25].

Metalloproteases in tendinopathy of the Achilles tendon

The tendon matrix constantly remodels, with higher rates of turnover at sites exposed to high levels of strain. Matrix metalloproteases (MMPs), a family of zinc- and calcium-dependent endopeptidases active at a neutral pH, are involved in the remodelling of the ECM through their broad proteolytic capability [117]. The degradation of collagen in the tendon ECM is initiated by MMPs. Twenty-three human MMPs have been identified, with a wide range of extracellular sub-strates [118]. MMPs can be subdivided into four main groups: collagenases, which cleave native collagen types I, II and III; gelatinases, which cleave denatured collagens and type IV collagen; stromelysins, which degrade proteoglycans, fibronectin, casein, collagen types III, IV and V; and membrane-type MMPs. The activity of MMPs is inhibited reversibly by TIMPs in a non-covalent fashion in a 1:1 stoichiometry. There are four types of TIMPs: TIMP1, TIMP2, TIMP3 and TIMP4. The balance between the activities of MMPs and TIMPs regulates tendon remodelling, and an imbalance produces collagen disturbances in tendons.

MMP3 may play a major role in the regulation of tendon ECM degradation and tissue remodelling. An increased expression of MMP3 may be necessary for appropriate tissue remodelling and the prevention of tendinopathic changes [120]. The timing of MMP3 production is probably also critical in this process. MMP3 and TIMP1, TIMP2, TIMP3 and TIMP4 are downregulated in tendinopathic tendons [119]. Decreased MMP3 expression may, therefore, lead to tendinopathic changes in tendons. The expression of MMP2 can be upregulated in Achilles tendinopathy. Physical exercise can influence local MMP and TIMP activities in the human tendo Achillis with a pronounced increase in local levels of pro-MMP9 after exercise [120]. MMP9 may have a role in a potential inflammation reaction in the human tendo Achillis induced by intensive exercise. Also, exercise causes a rapid increase in serum MMP9, a probable result of increased leucocytes in the circulation [120].

MMPs and their inhibitors are crucial to ECM remodelling, and a balance exists between them in normal tendons. The alteration of MMP and TIMP expression from basal levels leads to the alteration of tendon homoeostasis. Tendinopathic tendons have an increased rate of matrix remodelling, leading to a mechanically less-stable tendon which is more susceptible to damage [47, 55, 81, 83-89].

Genetics

Variants within the *TNC, COL5A1, MMP3, GDF5* and *CASP8* genes have been independently associated with the risk of Achilles tendon pathology [78]. All polymorphisms which have been associated with Achilles tendinopathy to date encode for proteins that are either structural and/or regulatory in function. Additional genes encoding for ECM-specific proteinases and their inhibitors are, therefore, good candidates for further investigation. In addition to the MMP family of proteins, the ADAM (a disintegrin and metalloproteinase), ADAMTS (a disintegrin and metalloproteinase with thrombospondin motifs), and the TIMP (tissue inhibitor metalloproteinase) family of proteins are all involved in the regulation of the composition of the ECM of the tendon and other connective tissues. Changes in the composition of the ECM of the tendon are likely to be reflected in the biomechanical properties of this connective tissue [18].

COL1A1 (Collagen type I alpha 1 gene)

Collagen type I fibrils are a major constituent of the bone matrix and form strong parallel bundles of fibres in tendons and ligaments. The major two genes that regulate collagen production are the collagen Iα1 *(COLIA1)* and the collagen Iα2 *(COLIA2)* genes. *COLIA1* and *COLIA2* encode collagen Iα1 and collagen Iα2 polypeptides, respectively, which associate in a 2:1 ratio to form collagen type I [35]. The *COL1A1* gene (located on chromosome 17q21.33) contains a polymorphism in the region of intron 1 (rs1800012), a predicted binding site for the transcription factor Sp1 [90]. Posthumus and co-workers [102] showed no significant association in the allelic or genotype frequencies of the Sp1 binding site polymorphism in 126 patients with Achilles tendinopathy and 126 healthy Caucasian controls.

COL5A1 (Collagen type V alpha 1 gene)

Based on its known biological function and chromosome location, the *COL5A1* gene has been selected as specific candidate gene for Achilles tendon injuries. The *COL5A1* gene encodes for the α1 chain of type V collagen, which is a minor fibrillar collagen found in ligaments and tendons, as well as other tissues [32]. Type V collagen, which makes up approximately 10% of the collagen content in ligaments, intercalates into the core of type I collagen fibrils, where it is believed to be involved in the organization and regulation of type I collagen fibril diameters [98]. Furthermore, some investigators have reported an association of the ABO blood group with Achilles tendon injury [48] - the ABO blood group is determined by a single gene located on the end of the long arm of chromosome [9] (9q34), close to the chromosomal localization of the *COL5A1* gene and other genes that will be discussed further in this review. The *COL5A1* gene contains BstUI and DpnII restriction fragment length polymorphisms (RFLPs) within its 3'-untranslated region (UTR) [30]. Some studies investigated whether genetic variants within the *COL5A1* gene were associated with Achilles and quadriceps tendon injuries, anterior cruciate ligament (ACL) rupture and altered musculo-tendinous flexibility.

In particular, Mokone and co-workers [96] investigated whether the BstUI (rs12722, C to T *substitution*) and/or the DpnII (rs13946, C to T *substitution*) poly-morphisms were associated with Achilles tendon injuries in 111 Caucasian patients and 129 healthy Caucasian controls from a South African population. The main biological finding was a significant difference in the allele distribution of the three *COL5A1* BstUI RFLP alleles (A1, A2 and A3 derivating from two single nucleotide polymorphism substitutions: rs12722 and *rs55748801*) when control subjects were compared with the Achilles tendon injuries group. The frequencies of the A1 and A3 alleles were higher in the Achilles tendon injuries group (A1, 76.1% and A3, 5.9%) than in the control group (A1, 67.1% and A3, 3.1%), while the frequencies of the A2 allele (corresponding to the C allele of the rs12722 single nucleotide polymorphism substitution) was significantly higher in the control subjects (A2, 29.8%) than in the patients group (A2, 29.8%). Based on this statistical evidence, the authors concluded that individuals with the cytosine-cytosine genotype were, therefore, less likely to develop symptoms of tendon pathology[96]. Finally, there were no significant differences in the genotype frequencies of the *COL5A1* DpnII RFLP alleles between the control subjects and the Achilles tendon injuries group [96].

Moving from first evidence, September and co-workers [113] decided to study the association of the *COL5A1* gene and Achilles tendinopathy in two different populations: white South Africans and Australians [113]. The researchers selected seven genetic variants within the *COL5A1* gene: the already investigated rs12722 (BstUI RFLP) and rs13946 (DpnII RFLP), and five other variants (rs10858286, rs3196378, rs11103544, rs4504708 and rs3128575). The first two variants rs12722 and rs13946 had already been analysed in the South African population by Mokone and co-workers [96] and, as mentioned, the rs12722 was strongly associated with chronic Achilles tendinopathy in this study, while the rs13946 was not associated. Thus, the authors evaluated these two variants in a second case-control population study of subjects from Australia, while the other five variants were investigated in both the South African and the Australian population[113]. There was a highly significant difference in the genotype distribution of rs12722 between the Australian controls and the Australian Achilles tendon injuries group. Moreover, individuals with a cytosine-cytosine genotype had a significantly decreased risk of developing chronic Achilles tendinopathy than those with a T allele (thymine-guanine- or thymine- thymine) in both the Australian and South African groups. As for the South African population, there was no significant association of the marker rs13946 (DpnII RFLP) and tendinopathy disease in the Australian population[113].

A significant difference in the genotype distribution between the Australian controls and the Australian Achilles tendon injuries groups was noted for rs3196378, which spans a putative mRNA binding site. The AC genotype was significantly associated with the increased risk of developing Achilles tendon injuries in the Australian population. These data were not confirmed in the South African study. None of the differences in genotype distribution between the Australian controls and the tendon injuries groups for markers rs10858286, rs4504708 and rs3128575 were significant. For this reason, these markers were not analysed in the South African group. In conclusion, the relevant finding of this report was that the *COL5A1* BstUI RFLP is associated with Achilles tendinopathy in two independent populations.

Finally, Laguette and co-workers [57] investigated the relationship between the sequence of the *COL5A1* 3'-UTR and the mRNA stability, comparing patients with Achilles tendinopathy and asymptomatic controls.

The predominant forms were T-allele in patients with Achilles tendinopathy and C-allele in the controls. The authors reported a significantly increased mRNA stability for T-allele and proposed that it could be a molecular mechanism underlying musculoskeletal soft tissue injuries.

COL12A1 (Collagen type XII alpha 1 gene)

As with the *COL5A1* gene and the *COL1A1* gene, any other proteins involved in similar biological processes can be studied to test the association between the selected candidate gene and the Achilles tendon injuries and or anterior cruciate ligament rupture. For this reason, it was decided to investigate additional candidate genes such as the *COL12A1* and *COL14A1* genes [101, 114]. The types XII and XIV collagens belong to a family of non-fibrillar collagens and are associated with the surface of the collagen fibril as well as members of the fibril associated collagens with interrupted triple helices (FACITs) subfamily [122]. The type XII collagen is a homotrimer consisting of 3 α1 (XII) chains and is encoded by a single gene, *COL12A1*, mapped to chromosome 6q12–q13 [28]. Similar to the type V collagen, the type XII collagen is believed to regulate fibril diameter (fibrillogenesis) [9, 99, 139]. September and co-workers [114] investigated the association of two *COL12A1* single nucleotide polymorphisms (SNP rs970547 and SNP rs240736) with Achilles tendon injuries and reported no significant association in the selected group [114].

COL14A1 (Collagen type XIV alpha 1 gene)

Based on its known biological function, the *COL14A1* gene has been selected as a specific candidate gene for Achilles tendon injuries [114]. Unlike the fibrillar collagens, the type XIV collagen is associated with the surface of the collagen fibril and is a member of the FACITs subfamily [122]. The type XIV collagen is a homotrimeric molecule consisting of α1 (XIV) chains and encoded by a single gene, *COL14A1*, mapped to chromosome 8q23 [20, 110]. September and co-workers investigated two informative exonic SNPs of the *COL14A1* gene, the A to C transversion at position 90 of exon 14 (rs4870723) that causes a missense substitution of Asn to His at position 563, and the intronic SNP as well with a high heterozygosity of the A to T transversion at position 93 of intron 43 (rs1563392). The authors selected for this case-control study a total of 137 physically active, Caucasian, unrelated individuals with chronic Achilles tendinopathy and 44 with acute Achilles tendon rupture, while 131 physically active Caucasians without any history of clinical symptomatic Achilles tendon injuries were selected as controls [114]. There were no significant differences in the genotype or allele distribution of the *COL14A1* SNPs between any of the affected or control subjects, suggesting that the *COL14A1* gene is not associated with an increased risk of developing Achilles tendinopathy [114].

TNC (Tenascin C gene)

Some investigators have reported an association of the ABO blood group with Achilles tendon injury [48] - these findings suggest that either the ABO gene or a closely linked gene(s) may be associated with tendon injury. In addition, it has been reported that persons in blood group O are more susceptible to tendon injuries [44, 46, 48, 54]. The ABO blood group is determined by a single gene located on the end of the long arm of chromosome 9 (9q34), close to the chromosomal localization of the already discussed *COL5A1* and *TNC* gene, and closely linked to the ABO gene on chromosome 9q32-q34.3 [106]. The ECM glycoprotein tenascin-C is expressed in a variety of tissues, including tendons [72], and is encoded by the tenascin-C (*TNC*) or hexabrachion (*HXB*) genes. Tenascin-C binds other components of the ECM and cell receptors, and plays an important role in regulating cell-matrix interactions [43]. In normal adult tendons, it is expressed predominately in regions responsible for transmitting high levels of mechanical force, such as the myotendinous and osteotendinous junctions [13, 14, 39]. The *TNC* gene contains a guanine-thymine dinucleotide repeat polymorphism (a tandem repeat consisting of a repeated two–base pair sequence of varying lengths in different people) within intron [17]. The influence of this polymorphism on the expression of the gene or the biological function of tenascin-C is, to our knowledge, unknown. Mokone and co-workers [95] investigated the association of the guanine-thymine dinucleotide repeat polymorphism of the *TNC* gene with Achilles tendon injuries. The authors selected 114 physically active patients with symptomatic Achilles tendon injuries (72 chronic Achilles tendinopathies and 42 acute Achilles tendon ruptures) and 127 apparently healthy physically active white subjects without any history of symptoms as a control. Eighteen different alleles of the guanine-thymine dinucleotide repeat polymorphism in the *TNC* gene were identified within the two groups. There was a significant difference in the distribution of the alleles between the Achilles tendon injuries and control groups, with the alleles containing 12 and 14 guanine-thymine dinucleotide repeats being significantly more frequent in the Achilles tendon injuries group. The alleles containing 13 and 17 repeats were, on the other hand, significantly less frequent in the Achilles tendon injuries subjects. The alleles were grouped according to those that were significantly overrepresented, containing 12 or 14 guanine-thymine dinucleotide repeats (O), those that were significantly underrepresented, containing 13 or 17 repeats (U), and those that were evenly distributed (E). They were then paired by genotype and the genotype distributions were analysed between case and control. Those subjects with a genotype of UU or UE were significantly underrepresented in the Achilles tendon injuries group. With respect to the O alleles, those subjects who were either homozygous or heterozygous were overrepresented in the Achilles tendon injuries. The novel finding of this study was that the allele distributions of the guanine-thymine dinucleotide repeat polymorphism within the *TNC* gene were significantly different between the subjects presenting with symptoms of Achilles tendon injuries and the asymptomatic subjects. Alleles containing 12 and 14 guanine-thymine repeats were overrepresented in subjects with Achilles tendon injuries, while the alleles containing 13 and 17 repeats were underrepresented[95].

MMP3 (Matrix metallopeptidase 3 gene)

Besides the already discussed genes which encode for the ECM proteins, the genes which encode for any protein that regulates tendon and ligament biological processes - such as adaptation, healing and remodelling - are probably also associated with these injuries[15, 115]. Raleigh and co-workers[103] investigated the role of the MMPs proteins in the aetiology of tendinopathy. The MMPs have regulatory roles in maintaining ECM homeostasis. The MMPs are known to consist of over 20 distinct endopeptidases that can catalyse a broad spectrum of both ECM and non-ECM substrates[123]. One of the family, *MMP3*, can catalytically degrade multiple substrates, including: types II, IV, V, IX and X collagens, laminin, fibronectin, proteoglycan, decorin and aggrecan[10, 123]. The *MMP3* gene is located at the long arm of chromosome 11 (11q22.3), in a cluster together with five other *MMP* genes (*MMP-7* and *MMP*-10, -11, -12, -13)[126]. The promoter region of *MMP-3* is characterized by a 5A/6A promoter polymorphism at position -1171, in which one allele has six adenosines (6A) and the second has five adenosines (5A). It has been shown that the expression of the *MMP3* gene can be substantially altered by the 5A/6A promoter polymorphism[137], and this variant has been associated with a number of pathological states[8, 138]. Interestingly, reduced levels of *MMP3* mRNA[4, 38] and immunochemically detectable *MMP3* protein have been observed in resected Achilles tendinopathy tissue compared to control tissue [38]. Raleigh and co-workers [103] investigated the relationship between variants within the *MMP3* gene and Achilles tendinopathy or Achilles tendon rupture. One-hundred-and-fourteen Caucasian subjects diagnosed with Achilles tendon injuries were recruited (including 75 with chronic Achilles tendinopathy and 39 with partial or complete ruptures of the Achilles tendon). An additional 98 apparently healthy, unrelated, Caucasian subjects were recruited as controls. Three exonic SNPs were identified and selected for this case-control study. The rs679620 (E45K) and the rs602128 (D96D) in exon 2 and rs520540 (A362A) in exon 8 all had a high heterozygous frequency and, therefore, were considered potentially informative [103].

There were no significant differences in the genotypes and allele distributions of the selected SNPs between patients with Achilles tendon injuries and the control groups. Since differences have been detected in genotype distributions between subjects with chronic Achilles tendon or Achilles tendon ruptures [114], the Achilles tendon pathology group was sub-divided into 75 patients with chronic Achilles tendinopathy and 39 patients rupture sub-groups. There were significant differences in the distribution of the genotype and allele frequencies of the *MMP3* rs679620 SNP between the control and 75 patients with chronic Achilles tendinopathy. The guanine- guanine genotype was significantly more frequent in the chronic Achilles tendinopathy (37.3%; n=28) when compared to the control group (19.4%; n=19). The cytosine- cytosine genotype of SNP rs591058 was over-represented in the chronic Achilles tendinopathy (35.6%; n=26) compared with the controls (19.6%; n=19) and the adenine-adenine genotype of SNP rs650108 was over-represented in the chronic Achilles tendinopathy (9.5%; n=7) compared to the controls (2.1%; n=2). There were, however, no significant differences in the distribution of the genotype and allele frequencies of the three *MMP3* SNPs between the control and the 39 patients rupture sub-group. The authors evaluated the *MMP3* rs679620 G/A and *COL5A1* rs12722 C/T genotype pairs, together with their frequencies within the 75 patients with chronic Achilles tendinopathy and control groups, as well as their estimated risk (OR) and the risk order. The *MMP3* rs679620 A allele (adenine-adenine or adenine-guanine genotype) combined with the *COL5A1* rs12722 cytosine-cytosine genotype had the lowest risk for Achilles tendinopathy [103]. In conclusion, the authors reported the evidence that variation within the human *MMP3* gene is associated with Achilles tendinopathy. They also studied and discovered an interaction of the *MMP3* variant and the *COL5A1* gene variant to increase risk of Achilles tendinopathy. Further study and repetition of this work in other, larger population analysis must to be done to confirm these associations.

TGFB1 (Transforming growth factor beta 1 gene)

To study further candidate genes as possible predisposing factors to Achilles tendon pathology Posthumus and co-workers [100] selected a functional polymorphism of the *TGFB1* gene (the TGFB1 rs1800469 variant) and investigated is association with Achilles tendon pathology within an Australian and a South

African case-control cohort study. The TGF-b superfamily, which includes various growth/differentiation factors (GDFs), plays an essential role in tissue (including tendon) growth and homoeostasis. Two members of this family, TGF-b1 (an isoform of TGF-b) and *GDF-5*, have been shown to increase mechanical strength after gene transfection in experimentally injured animal Achilles tendons [11, 36, 105]. The *GDF-5* gene will be discussed further in this review, the TGF-b1 is released in response to a number of stimuli (including mechanical loading [71]) and is known to increase cell proliferation, migration and the synthesis of ECM. The gene coding for TGF-b1, *TGFB1*, is located on chromosome 19q13. The 5' UTR of the *TGFB1* gene contains a functional promoter single nucleotide polymorphism (SNP) (rs1800469, cytosine to thymine substitution) that has been associated with various multifactorial pathologies [52, 59, 62, 116, 121, 132, 140]. Moreover, retrospective regression analysis estimated the mean acid-activated TGF-b concentration to be approximately twice as high in the thymine-thymine genotype compared with the cytosine-cytosine genotype of the TGFB1 rs1800469 variant [29]. Posthumus and co-workers [100] enrolled subjects from the Australian cohort study [113], and in particular they selected 59 Caucasian patients, all of whom were diagnosed with chronic Achilles tendinopathy, and 142 healthy subjects as controls. Meanwhile, from the South African cohort study [95, 96], they selected 112 Caucasian subjects diagnosed with Achilles tendon pathology, and 96 healthy subjects as controls. The genotype and allele frequency of the *TGFB1* rs1800469 variant showed no significant differences between the Achilles tendon pathology and the control groups within the South African and Australian cohorts [100]. In conclusion, the study suggests that the *TGFB1* polymorphism rs1800469 is unlikely to be a predisposition factor for the Achilles tendon pathology disease, especially in subjects of European descent.

GDF-5 (Growth/differentiation factor-5 gene)

The specific role of *GDF-5* in the tendon is largely unknown [22, 28]. *GDF-5* is involved in the maintenance, development and repair of bones, cartilage and various other musculoskeletal soft tissues (including tendons) [22, 28, 92]. The gene-coding for *GDF-5*, is located on chromosome 20q11. Mutations in the *GDF5* gene are known to cause several inherited developmental disorders [6, 111, 128]. A possible role of *GDF-5* in tendon and ligament biology was first suggested by Wolfman and co-workers [135]. In this study, the ectopic administration of *GDF-5* resulted in the synthesis of new tendon tissue. The 5' UTR of the *GDF5* gene contains a functional promoter SNP (rs143383; thymine to cytosine substitution) that has been associated with multifactorial disorders, such as osteoarthritis [12] and congenital hip dysplasia [17], as well as phenotypic data such as height, hip axis length and fracture risk [17]. The function of this SNP has been reported by luciferase reported assays [94] and differential allelic expression analysis [21, 125]. The thymine allele of *GDF5* rs143383 was correlated with the reduced expression of the *GDF5* gene in a wide range of soft tissues [21, 125]. To further investigate the role of *GDF-5* in the tendon, Posthumus and co-workers [100] decided to determine whether the functional polymorphisms rs14338 of the *GDF5* gene were associated with Achilles tendon pathology in an Australian and a South

African case-control cohort study. Given the known functional effect of the selected SNP, the hypothesis was that the thymine-thymine genotype of the *GDF5* rs143383 variant increased the risk of Achilles tendon pathology. There were significant genotype differences between the Australian chronic Achilles tendinopathy and Australian control groups for the *GDF5* rs143383 variant. Although similar frequencies and trends were observed in the South African cohort, there were no significant genotype or allele differences. When the data from the Australian and the South African cohort were combined, both genotype and allele frequencies were significantly different between the case and control groups. Similar results were observed when individuals with a thymine-thymine genotype for the *GDF5* rs143383 variant were compared with individuals with a C allele (combined thymine-cytosine and cytosine-cytosine). Within the Australian cohort, the thymine-thymine genotype increased the susceptibility to Achilles tendinopathy by 2.24 times. Although there was a similar pattern in the South African cohort, the thymine-thymine genotype was not significantly over-represented in the Achilles tendinopathy. The thymine-thymine genotype remained significantly over-represented when both cohorts (Australian and South African) were analysed together. The main finding of this study was that the *GDF5* gene was associated with Achilles tendon pathology within the Australian population both independently and when combined with an additional South African population [100].

Conclusions

The aetiology of Achilles tendon pathology remains unclear, and many factors have been implicated. Proposed common intrinsic factors include tendon vascularity, gastrocnemius-soleus dysfunction, gender, age, body weight and height, pes cavus and lateral ankle instability. Extrinsic factors for Achilles tendinopathy include poor technique, previous injuries, changes in training patterns, footwear and environmental factors, such as training on hard, slippery or slanting surfaces. Variants in the *TNC, COL5A1, MMP3, GDF5* and *CASP8* genes have been independently associated with the risk of Achilles tendon pathology. Changes in the composition of the ECM of tendon are likely to be reflected in the biomechanical properties of this connective tissue.

References

1. Abate M, Oliva F, Schiavone C, Salini V. Achilles tendinopathy in amateur runners: role of adiposity (Tendinopathies and obesity). Muscles Ligaments Tendons J. 2012;2(1):44-48.
2. Abate M, Schiavone C, Salini V, Andia I. Occurrence of tendon pathologies in metabolic disorders. Rheumatology (Oxford). 2013;52(4):599-608.
3. Abate M, Silbernagel KG, Siljeholm C. Pathogenesis of tendinopathies: inflammation or degeneration? Arthritis Res Ther. 2009;11(3):235.
4. Alfredson H, Lorentzon M, Backman S, Backman A, Lerner UH. cDNA-arrays and real-time quantitative PCR techniques in the investigation of chronic Achilles tendinosis. J Orthop Res. 2003;21(6):970-975.
5. Aruoma I. Free radicals and antioxidant strategies in sports. J Nutr Biochem. 1994(5):370-381.
6. Basit S, Naqvi SK, Wasif N, Ali G, Ansar M, Ahmad W. A novel insertion mutation in the cartilage-derived morphogenetic protein-1 (CDMP1) gene underlies Grebe-type chondrodysplasia in a consanguineous Pakistani family. BMC Med Genet. 2008;9:102.
7. Bestwick CS, Maffulli N. Reactive oxygen species and tendinopathy: do they matter? Br J Sports Med. 2004;38:672-674.
8. Beyzade S, Zhang S, Wong YK, Day IN, Eriksson P, Ye S. Influences of matrix metalloproteinase-3 gene variation on extent of coronary atherosclerosis and risk of myocardial infarction. J Am Coll Cardiol. 2003;41(12):2130-2137.
9. Birk DE, Fitch JM, Babiarz JP, Doane KJ, Linsenmayer TF. Collagen fibrillogenesis in vitro: interaction of types I and V collagen regulates fibril diameter. J Cell Sci. 1990;95 (Pt 4):649-657.
10. Birkedal-Hansen H, Moore WG, Bodden MK, . Matrix metalloproteinases: a review. Crit Rev Oral Biol Med. 1993;4(2):197-250.
11. Bolt P, Clerk AN, Luu HH, . BMP-14 gene therapy increases tendon tensile strength in a rat model of Achilles tendon injury. J Bone Joint Surg Am. 2007;89(6):1315-1320.
12. Chapman K, Takahashi A, Meulenbelt I, . A meta-analysis of European and Asian cohorts reveals a global role of a functional SNP in the 5' UTR of GDF5 with osteoarthritis susceptibility. Hum Mol Genet. 2008;17(10):1497-1504.
13. Chiquet M, Fambrough DM. Chick myotendinous antigen. I. A monoclonal antibody as a marker for tendon and muscle morphogenesis. J Cell Biol. 1984;98(6):1926-1936.
14. Chiquet M, Fambrough DM. Chick myotendinous antigen. II. A novel extracellular glycoprotein complex consisting of large disulfide-linked subunits. J Cell Biol. 1984;98(6):1937-1946.
15. Collins M, Raleigh SM. Genetic risk factors for musculoskeletal soft tissue injuries. Med Sport Sci. 2009;54:136-149.
16. Cook JL, Purdam CR. Is tendon pathology a continuum? A pathology model to explain the clinical presentation of load-induced tendinopathy. Br J Sports Med. 2009;43(6):409-416.
17. Dai J, Shi D, Zhu P, . Association of a single nucleotide polymorphism in growth differentiate factor 5 with congenital dysplasia of the hip: a case-control study. Arthritis Res Ther. 2008;10(5):R126.
18. Del Buono A, Oliva F, Longo UG, . Metalloproteases and rotator cuff disease. J Shoulder Elbow Surg. 2012;21(2):200-208.
19. Dennery PA. Introduction to serial review on the role of oxidative stress in diabetes mellitus. Free Radic Biol Med. 2006 40:1-2.
20. Dublet B, van der Rest M. Type XIV collagen, a new homotrimeric molecule extracted from fetal bovine skin and tendon, with a triple helical disulfide-bonded domain homologous to type IX and type XII collagens. J Biol Chem. 1991;266(11):6853-6858.
21. Egli RJ, Southam L, Wilkins JM, . Functional analysis of the osteoarthritis susceptibility-associated GDF5 regulatory polymorphism. Arthritis Rheum. 2009;60(7):2055-2064.
22. Eliasson P, Fahlgren A, Aspenberg P. Mechanical load and BMP signaling during tendon repair: a role for follistatin? Clin Orthop Relat Res. 2008;466(7):1592-1597.
23. Flowers F, Zimmerman JJ. Reactive oxygen species in the cellular pathophysiology of shock. New Horizons. 1998;6:169-180.
24. Frizziero A, Fini M, Salamanna F, Veicsteinas A, Maffulli N, Marini M. Effect of training and sudden detraining on the patellar tendon and its enthesis in rats. BMC Musculoskelet Disord. 2011;12:20.
25. Gaida JE, Ashe MC, Bass SL, Cook JL. Is adiposity an under-recognized risk factor for tendinopathy? A systematic review. Arthritis Rheum. 2009;61(6):840-849.
26. Goldman R, Moshonov S, Zor U. Generation of reactive oxygen species in a human keratinocyte cell line: role of calcium. Arch Biochem Biophys. 1998;350:10-18.
27. Goodship AE, Birch HL, Wilson AM. The pathobiology and repair of tendon and ligament injury. Veterinary Clinics of North America: Equine Practice. 1994;10:323-348.

28. Gordon MK, Gerecke DR, Olsen BR. Type XII collagen: distinct extracellular matrix component discovered by cDNA cloning. Proc Natl Acad Sci USA. 1987;84(17):6040-6044.

29. Grainger DJ, Heathcote K, Chiano M, . Genetic control of the circulating concentration of transforming growth factor type beta1. Hum Mol Genet. 1999;8(1):93-97.

30. Greenspan DS, Pasquinelli AE. BstUI and DpnII RFLPs at the COL5A1 gene. Hum Mol Genet. 1994;3(2):385.

31. Hack V, Strobel G, Rau JP, Weicker H. The effect of maximal exercise on the activity of neutrophil granulocytes in highly trained athletes in a moderate training period. Eur J Appl Physiol. 1992;65:520-524.

32. Hildebrand KA, Frank CB, Hart DA. Gene intervention in ligament and tendon: current status, challenges, future directions. Gene Ther. 2004;11(4):368-378.

33. Hirai S, Takahashi N, Goto T, . Functional food targeting the regulation of obesity-induced inflammatory responses and pathologies. Mediators Inflamm. 2010:367838.

34. Hiran ST, Moulton PJ, Hancock JT. Detection of superoxide and NADPH oxidase in porcine articular chondrocytes. Free Rad Biol Med. 1997;23:736-743.

35. Hoffmann A, Gross G. Tendon and ligament engineering in the adult organism: mesenchymal stem cells and gene-therapeutic approaches. Int Orthop. 2007;31(6):791-797.

36. Hou Y, Mao Z, Wei X, . The roles of TGF-beta1 gene transfer on collagen formation during Achilles tendon healing. Biochem Biophys Res Commun. 2009;383(2):235-239.

37. Ippolito E, Natali PG, Postacchini F, Accinni L, De Martino C. Morphological, immunochemical, and biochemical study of rabbit Achilles tendon at various ages. J Bone Joint Surg Am. 1980;62(4):583-598.

38. Ireland D, Harrall R, Curry V, . Multiple changes in gene expression in chronic human Achilles tendinopathy. Matrix Biol. 2001;20(3):159-169.

39. Jarvinen TA, Jozsa L, Kannus P, . Mechanical loading regulates tenascin-C expression in the osteotendinous junction. J Cell Sci. 1999;112 Pt 18:3157-3166.

40. Ji LL. Antioxidants and oxidative stress in exercise. PSEBM. 2000;222:283-292.

41. Ji LL, Leeuwenburgh C, Leichtweis S, . Oxidative stress and aging. Role of exercise and its influences on antioxidant systems. Ann N Y Acad Sci. 1998;854:102-117.

42. Johnson KW, Zalavras C, Thordarson DB. Surgical management of insertional calcific Achilles tendinosis with a central tendon splitting approach. Foot Ankle Int. 2006;27(4):245-250.

43. Jones FS, Jones PL. The tenascin family of ECM glycoproteins: structure, function, and regulation during embryonic development and tissue remodeling. Dev Dyn. 2000;218(2):235-259.

44. Jozsa L, Balint JB, Kannus P, Reffy A, Barzo M. Distribution of blood groups in patients with tendon rupture. An analysis of 832 cases. J Bone Joint Surg Br. 1989;71(2):272-274.

45. Jozsa L, Kannus P. Human Tendon: anatomy, physiology and pathology. Human Kinetics. 1997.

46. Jozsa L, Kvist M, Balint BJ, . The role of recreational sport activity in Achilles tendon rupture. A clinical, pathoanatomical, and sociological study of 292 cases. Am J Sports Med. 1989;17(3):338-343.

47. Kader D, Saxena A, Movin T, Maffulli N. Achilles tendinopathy: some aspects of basic science and clinical management. Br J Sports Med. 2002;36(4):239-249.

48. Kannus P, Natri A. Etiology and pathophysiology of tendon ruptures in sports. Scand J Med Sci Sports. 1997;7(2):107-112.

49. Karousou E, Ronga M, Vigetti D, Barcolli D, Passi A, Maffulli N. Molecular interactions in extracellular matrix of tendon. Front Biosci (Elite Ed). 2:1-12.

50. Karousou E, Ronga M, Vigetti D, Barcolli D, Passi A, Maffulli N. Molecular interactions in extracellular matrix of tendon. Front Biosci (Elite Ed). 2010;2:1-12.

51. Khan KM, Cook JL, Bonar F, Harcourt P, Astrom M. Histopathology of common tendinopathies. Update and implications for clinical management. Sports Med. 1999;27(6):393-408.

52. Koch W, Hoppmann P, Mueller JC, Schomig A, Kastrati A. Association of transforming growth factor-beta1 gene polymorphisms with myocardial infarction in patients with angiographically proven coronary heart disease. Arterioscler Thromb Vasc Biol. 2006;26(5):1114-1119.

53. Krieger-Brauer HI, Kather H. Antagonistic effects of different members of the fibroblast and platelet-derived growth factor families on adipose conversion and NADPH-dependent H2O2 generation in 3T3 L1-cells. Biochem J. 1995;307 (Pt 2):549-556.

54. Kujala UM, Jarvinen M, Natri A, . ABO blood groups and musculoskeletal injuries. Injury. 1992;23(2):131-133.

55. Kumar K, Sharma VK, Sharma R, Maffulli N. Correction of cubitus varus by French or dome osteotomy: a comparative study. J Trauma. 2000;49(4):717-721.

56. Kvist M. Achilles tendon injuries in athletes. Sports Med. 1994;18(3):173-201.

57. Laguette MJ, Abrahams Y, Prince S, Collins M. Sequence variants within the 3'-UTR of the COL5A1 gene alters mRNA stability: implications for musculoskeletal soft tissue injuries. Matrix Biology: Journal of the International Society for Matrix Biology. 2011;30(5-6):338-345.

58. Langberg H, Skovgaard D, Petersen LJ, Bulow J, Kjaer M. Type I collagen synthesis and degradation in peritendinous tissue after exercise determined by microdialysis in humans. J Physiol. 1999;521 Pt 1:299-306.

59. Langdahl BL, Uitterlinden AG, Ralston SH, . Large-scale analysis of association between polymorphisms in the transforming growth factor beta 1 gene (TGFB1) and osteoporosis: the GENOMOS study. Bone. 2008;42(5):969-981.

60. Leadbetter WB. Cell-matrix response in tendon injury. Clin Sports Med. 1992;11(3):533-578.

61. Lewis JS, Sandford FM. Rotator cuff tendinopathy: is there a role for polyunsaturated Fatty acids and antioxidants? J Hand Ther. 2010;22(1):49.

62. Li H, Romieu I, Wu H, . Genetic polymorphisms in transforming growth factor beta-1 (TGFB1) and childhood asthma and atopy. Hum Genet. 2007;121(5):529-538.

63. Lippi G, Longo UG, Maffulli N. Genetics and sports. Br Med Bull. 2010;93:27-47.

64. Longo UG, Franceschi F, Ruzzini L, . Histopathology of the supraspinatus tendon in rotator cuff tears. Am J Sports Med. 2008;36(3):533-538.

65. Longo UG, Franceschi F, Ruzzini L, . Characteristics at haematoxylin and eosin staining of ruptures of the long head of the biceps tendon. Br J Sports Med. 2009;43(8):603-607.

66. Longo UG, Franceschi F, Ruzzini L, . Light microscopic histology of supraspinatus tendon ruptures. Knee Surg Sports Traumatol Arthrosc. 2007;15(11):1390-1394.

67. Longo UG, Oliva F, Denaro V, Maffulli N. Oxygen species and overuse tendinopathy in athletes. Disabil Rehabil. 2008;30(20-22):1563-1571.

68. Longo UG, Rittweger J, Garau G, . No influence of age, gender, weight, height, and impact profile in Achilles tendinopathy in masters track and field athletes. Am J Sports Med. 2009;37(7):1400-1405.

69. Longo UG, Ronga M, Maffulli N. Achilles tendinopathy. Sports Med Arthrosc. 2009;17(2):112-126.

70. Longo UG, Ronga M, Maffulli N. Acute ruptures of the Achilles tendon. Sports Med Arthrosc. 2009;17(2):127-138.

71. Mackey AL, Heinemeier KM, Koskinen SO, Kjaer M. Dynamic adaptation of tendon and muscle connective tissue to mechanical loading. Connect Tissue Res. 2008;49(3):165-168.

72. Mackie EJ. Molecules in focus: tenascin-C. Int J Biochem Cell Biol. 1997;29(10):1133-1137.

73. Maffulli N, Barrass V, Ewen SW. Light microscopic histology of Achilles tendon ruptures. A comparison with unruptured tendons. Am J Sports Med. 2000;28(6):857-863.

74. Maffulli N, Benazzo F. Basic sciences of tendons. Sports Medicine and Arthroscopy Review. 2000;8:1-5.

75. Maffulli N, Binfield PM, King JB. Tendon problems in athletic individuals. J Bone Joint Surg Am. 1998;80(1):142-144.

76. Maffulli N, Khan KM, Puddu G. Overuse tendon conditions: time to change a confusing terminology. Arthroscopy. 1998;14(8):840-843.

77. Maffulli N, Longo UG, Franceschi F, Rabitti C, Denaro V. Movin and Bonar scores assess the same characteristics of tendon histology. Clin Orthop Relat Res. 2008;466(7):1605-1611.

78. Maffulli N, Margiotti K, Longo UG, Loppini M, Fazio VM, Denaro V. The genetics of sports injuries and athletic performance. Muscles Ligaments Tendons J. 2013;3(3):173-189.

79. Maffulli N, Moller HD, Evans CH. Tendon healing: can it be optimised? Br J Sports Med. 2002;36(5):315-316.

80. Maffulli N, Reaper J, Ewen SW, Waterston SW, Barrass V. Chondral metaplasia in calcific insertional tendinopathy of the Achilles tendon. Clin J Sport Med. 2006;16(4):329-334.

81. Maffulli N, Sharma P, Luscombe KL. Achilles tendinopathy: aetiology and management. J R Soc Med. 2004;97(10):472-476.

82. Maganaris CN, Narici MV, Maffulli N. Biomechanics of the Achilles tendon. Disabil Rehabil. 2008:1-6.

83. Magra M, Caine D, Maffulli N. A review of epidemiology of paediatric elbow injuries in sports. Sports Med. 2007;37(8):717-735.

84. Magra M, Hughes S, El Haj AJ, Maffulli N. VOCCs and TREK-1 ion channel expression in human tenocytes. Am J Physiol Cell Physiol. 2007;292(3):C1053-1060.

85. Magra M, Maffulli N. Matrix metalloproteases: a role in overuse tendinopathies. Br J Sports Med. 2005;39(11):789-791.

86. Magra M, Maffulli N. Molecular events in tendinopathy: a role for metalloproteases. Foot Ankle Clin. 2005;10(2):267-277.

87. Magra M, Maffulli N. Nonsteroidal antiinflammatory drugs in tendinopathy: friend or foe. Clin J Sport Med. 2006;16(1):1-3.

88. Magra M, Maffulli N. Genetics: does it play a role in tendinopathy? Clin J Sport Med. 2007;17(4):231-233.

89. Magra M, Maffulli N. Genetic aspects of tendinopathy. J Sci Med Sport. 2008;11(3):243-247.

90. Mann V, Hobson EE, Li B, . A COL1A1 Sp1 binding site polymorphism predisposes to osteoporotic fracture by affecting bone density and quality. J Clin Invest. 2001;107(7):899-907.

91. Meier B, Radeke HH, Selle S, . Human fibroblasts release reactive oxygen species in response to interleukin-1 or tumour necrosis factor-alpha. Biochem J. 1989;263(2):539-545.

92. Mikic B. Multiple effects of GDF-5 deficiency on skeletal tissues: implications for therapeutic bioengineering. Ann Biomed Eng. 2004;32(3):466-476.

93. Millar NL, Hueber AJ, Reilly JH, . Inflammation is present in early human tendinopathy. Am J Sports Med. 2010;38(10):2085-2091.

94. Miyamoto Y, Mabuchi A, Shi D, . A functional polymorphism in the 5' UTR of GDF5 is associated with susceptibility to osteoarthritis. Nat Genet. 2007;39(4):529-533.

95. Mokone GG, Gajjar M, September AV, . The guanine-thymine dinucleotide repeat polymorphism within the tenascin-C gene is associated with Achilles tendon injuries. Am J Sports Med. 2005;33(7):1016-1021.

96. Mokone GG, Schwellnus MP, Noakes TD, Collins M. The COL5A1 gene and Achilles tendon pathology. Scand J Med Sci Sports. 2006;16(1):19-26.

97. Murrell GA. Oxygen free radicals and tendon healing. J Shoulder Elbow Surg. 2007 [Epub ahead of print].

98. Niyibizi C, Kavalkovich K, Yamaji T, Woo SL. Type V collagen is increased during rabbit medial collateral ligament healing. Knee Surg Sports Traumatol Arthrosc. 2000;8(5):281-285.

99. Olsen BR. New insights into the function of collagens from genetic analysis. Curr Opin Cell Biol. 1995;7(5):720-727.

100. Posthumus M, Collins M, Cook J, . Components of the transforming growth factor-{beta} family and the pathogenesis of human Achilles tendon pathology - a genetic association study. Rheumatology (Oxford). 2010.

101. Posthumus M, September AV, O'Cuinneagain D, van der Merwe W, Schwellnus MP, Collins M. The association between the COL12A1 gene and anterior cruciate ligament ruptures. Br J Sports Med. 2010.

102. Posthumus M, September AV, Schwellnus MP, Collins M. Investigation of the Sp1-binding site polymorphism within the COL1A1 gene in participants with Achilles tendon injuries and controls. J Sci Med Sport. 2009;12(1):184-189.

103. Raleigh SM, van der Merwe L, Ribbans WJ, Smith RK, Schwellnus MP, Collins M. Variants within the MMP3 gene are associated with Achilles tendinopathy: possible interaction with the COL5A1 gene. Br J Sports Med. 2009;43(7):514-520.

104. Reddy GK, Stehno-Bittel L, Enwemeka CS. Matrix remodeling in healing rabbit Achilles tendon. Wound Repair Regen. 1999;7(6):518-527.

105. Rickert M, Wang H, Wieloch P, . Adenovirus-mediated gene transfer of growth and differentiation factor-5 into tenocytes and the healing rat Achilles tendon. Connect Tissue Res. 2005;46(4-5):175-183.

106. Rocchi M, Archidiacono N, Romeo G, Saginati M, Zardi L. Assignment of the gene for human tenascin to the region q32-q34 of chromosome 9. Hum Genet. 1991;86(6):621-623.

107. Rosen GM, Pou S, Ramos CL, Cohen MS, Bratigan BE. Free radicals and phagocytic cells. FASEB J. 1995;9:200-209.

108. Ruzzini L, Abbruzzese F, Rainer A, . Characterization of age-related changes of tendon stem cells from adult human tendons. Knee Surg Sports Traumatol Arthrosc. 2013.

109. Sahnoun Z, Jamoussi K, Mounir Zeghal K. Radicaux libres et anti-oxydants: physiologie, pathologie humaine et aspects therapeutics. Therapie 1997;52:251-270.

110. Schnittger S, Herbst H, Schuppan D, Dannenberg C, Bauer M, Fonatsch C. Localization of the undulin gene (UND) to human chromosome band 8q23. Cytogenet Cell Genet. 1995;68(3-4):233-234.

111. Schwabe GC, Turkmen S, Leschik G, . Brachydactyly type C caused by a homozygous missense mutation in the prodomain of CDMP1. Am J Med Genet A. 2004;124A(4):356-363.

112. Selvanetti A, Puddu G. Overuse tendon injuries: Basic science and classification. Operative Techniques in Sports Medicine. 1997;5:110-117.

113. September AV, Cook J, Handley CJ, van der Merwe L, Schwellnus MP, Collins M. Variants within the COL5A1 gene are associated with Achilles tendinopathy in two populations. Br J Sports Med. 2009;43(5):357-365.

114. September AV, Posthumus M, van der Merwe L, Schwellnus M, Noakes TD, Collins M. The COL12A1 and COL14A1 genes and Achilles tendon injuries. Int J Sports Med. 2008;29(3):257-263.

115. September AV, Schwellnus MP, Collins M. Tendon and ligament injuries: the genetic component. Br J Sports Med. 2007;41(4):241-246; discussion 246.

116. Shah R, Hurley CK, Posch PE. A molecular mechanism for the differential regulation of TGF-beta1 expression due to the common SNP -509C-T (c. -1347C > T). Hum Genet. 2006;120(4):461-469.

117. Sharma P, Maffulli N. Basic biology of tendon injury and healing. Surgeon. 2005;3(5):309-316.

118. Sharma P, Maffulli N. The future: rehabilitation, gene therapy, optimization of healing. Foot Ankle Clin. 2005;10(2):383-397.

119. Sharma P, Maffulli N. Biology of tendon injury: healing, modeling and remodeling. J Musculoskelet Neuronal Interact. 2006;6(2):181-190.

120. Sharma P, Maffulli N. Understanding and managing Achilles tendinopathy. Br J Hosp Med (Lond). 2006;67(2):64-67.

121. Sharma S, Raby BA, Hunninghake GM, . Variants in TGFB1, dust mite exposure, and disease severity in children with asthma. Am J Respir Crit Care Med. 2009;179(5):356-362.

122. Shaw LM, Olsen BR. FACIT collagens: diverse molecular bridges in extracellular matrices. Trends Biochem Sci. 1991;16(5):191-194.

123. Somerville RP, Oblander SA, Apte SS. Matrix metalloproteinases: old dogs with new tricks. Genome Biol. 2003;4(6):216.

124. Souren JEM, Van Aken H, Van Wijk R. Enhancement of superoxide production against heat shock by HSP27 in fibroblasts. Biochem Biophys Res Commun. 1996;227:816-821.

125. Southam L, Rodriguez-Lopez J, Wilkins JM, . An SNP in the 5'-UTR of GDF5 is associated with osteoarthritis susceptibility in Europeans and with in vivo differences in allelic expression in articular cartilage. Hum Mol Genet. 2007;16(18):2226-2232.

126. Spurr NK, Gough AC, Gosden J, . Restriction fragment length polymorphism analysis and assignment of the metalloproteinases stromelysin and collagenase to the long arm of chromosome 11. Genomics. 1988;2(2):119-127.

127. Sullo A, Maffulli N, Capasso G, Testa V. The effects of prolonged peritendinous administration of PGE1 to the rat Achilles tendon: a possible animal model of chronic Achilles tendinopathy. J Orthop Science. 2001;6(4):349-357.

128. Szczaluba K, Hilbert K, Obersztyn E, Zabel B, Mazurczak T, Kozlowski K. Du Pan syndrome phenotype caused by heterozygous pathogenic mutations in CDMP1 gene. Am J Med Genet A. 2005;138(4):379-383.

129. Tallon C, Maffulli N, Ewen SW. Ruptured Achilles tendons are significantly more degenerated than tendinopathic tendons. Med Sci Sports Exerc. 2001;33(12):1983-1990.

130. Tiidus PM. Radical species in inflammation and overtraining. Can J Physiol Pharmacol. 1998;76(5):533-538.

131. Vailas AC, Pedrini VA, Pedrini-Mille A, Holloszy JO. Patellar tendon matrix changes associated with aging and voluntary exercise. J Appl Physiol. 1985;58(5):1572-1576.

132. Vishnoi M, Pandey SN, Modi DR, Kumar A, Mittal B. Genetic susceptibility of epidermal growth factor +61A>G and transforming growth factor beta1 -509C>T gene polymorphisms with gallbladder cancer. Hum Immunol. 2008;69(6):360-367.

133. Weitzman A, Gordon LI. Inflammation and Cancer: role of phagocyte-generated oxidants in carcinogenesis. J Am Soc Hematol. 1990;76:655-663.

134. Weitzman SA, Weitberg AB, Clark EP, Stossel TP. Phagocytes as carcinogens: Malignant transformation produced by human neutrophils. Science 1985;227:1231-1233.

135. Wolfman NM, Hattersley G, Cox K, . Ectopic induction of tendon and ligament in rats by growth and differentiation factors 5, 6, and 7, members of the TGF-beta gene family. J Clin Invest. 1997;100(2):321-330.

136. Yamada M, Suzuki K, Kudo S, . Effects of exhaustive exercise on human neutrophils in athletes. Luminescence. 2000;15:15-20.

137. Ye S, Eriksson P, Hamsten A, Kurkinen M, Humphries SE, Henney AM. Progression of coronary atherosclerosis is associated with a common genetic variant of the human stromelysin-1 promoter which results in reduced gene expression. J Biol Chem. 1996;271(22):13055-13060.

138. Ye S, Patodi N, Walker-Bone K, Reading I, Cooper C, Dennison E. Variation in the matrix metalloproteinase-3, -7, -12 and -13 genes is associated with functional status in rheumatoid arthritis. Int J Immunogenet. 2007;34(2):81-85.

139. Young BB, Zhang G, Koch M, Birk DE. The roles of types XII and XIV collagen in fibrillogenesis and matrix assembly in the developing cornea. J Cell Biochem. 2002;87(2):208-220.

140. Yuan X, Liao Z, Liu Z, . Single nucleotide polymorphism at rs1982073:T869C of the TGFbeta 1 gene is associated with the risk of radiation pneumonitis in patients with non-small-cell lung cancer treated with definitive radiotherapy. J Clin Oncol. 2009;27(20):3370-3378.

"The force is what gives a Jedi his power. It's an energy field created by all living things. It surrounds us and penetrates us. It binds the universe together."

Obi-Wan Kenobi, Star Wars Episode IV: A New Hope

Chapter 5

Biomechanical Aspects of the Achilles Tendon

Michael R. Carmont, Karin Grävare Silbernagel, Jón Karlsson, Nicola Maffulli

Take Home Message

• *Tendinopathy is a complex pathological process, which affects the biomechanical properties of the Achilles tendon.*

• *Eccentric loading and management of the predisposing factors for tendinopathy provide an effective way of managing the problem in the early stages.*

• *The optimal management of an Achilles tendon rupture involves approximating the ruptured tendon ends and then permitting early loading and controlled active movement.*

Introduction

The Achilles tendon has an important role both during stance and for propulsion during walking and running. This chapter will discuss the biomechanical aspects of the Achilles tendon following rupture and during the repair process, and the important factors related to treatment for tendinopathy of both the mid-portion and the insertion. Finally, we will comment on the principles related to the reconstruction of the Achilles tendon.

Knowledge of some basic biomechanical terms is useful in understanding the processes involved in the rupture and pathology of Achilles tendon injuries (Table 1).

Term	Definition	Units
Stress	Force applied per unit area	N/m^2
Strain	Change in length compared to original length	None
Modulus of Elasticity	Ratio of stress compared to strain, gradient of the biomechanical curve	N/m^2
Ultimate Tensile Strength	The force at which the tendon ruptures	N
Resilience	The energy required to deform the tendon elastically, the area beneath the straight portion of the curve	
Toughness	The energy required to deform the tendon until failure occurs; the area beneath the straight curve elastic deformation and the plastic deformation	
Hysteresis	The area between the loading and unloading portion of the curves, dissipated as heat	
Fatigue Failure	When the tendon fails due to the repetitive application of force considerably lower than the ultimate tensile force	
Creep	Permanent deformation due to the continued application of lad	
Viscoelasticity	The altered biomechanical properties of the tendon due to the rate i.e. time dependent, application of force	

Table 1. Biomechanical terms.

The biomechanical anatomy of the healthy Achilles tendon

The Achilles tendon, gastrocnemius and soleus muscles comprise a musculo-tendinous unit spanning three joints: the knee, the ankle and the sub-talar joint. The Achilles tendon develops from the epimysial fibres of the gastrocnemius and soleus muscles at the musculo-tendinous junction forming a tendon, and progresses distally becoming narrower to a typical thickness of approximately 6 mm. The tendon consists of fascicles, fibrils, sub-fibrils and micro-fibrils (Figure 1). The tendon fascicles rotate externally through 90° at the mid-portion, before the tendon broadens to insert over a relatively large area (Figure1). The insertion site of the calcaneus is 19.8 mm long and 23.8 mm wide proximally[8]. It broadens distally to 31.2 mm wide and inserts dorsally and distally to the postero-superior tubercle on the calcaneus [8].

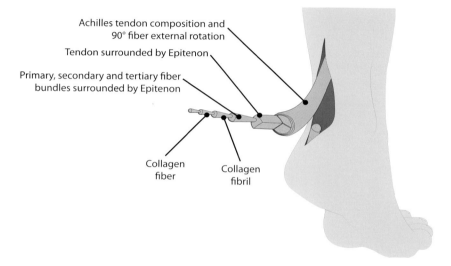

Figure 1. Structure of the Achilles tendon demonstrating the 90° rotational nature of the fascicles.

The biomechanics of the healthy Achilles tendon

Rather than acting as a simple check rein between the muscle and the insertion of the tendon, the viscoelastic biomechanical properties of the tendon direct its function. One of the principal aspects is the composition of the tendon and the orientation of the tendon fibres. These allow energy to be absorbed during the stance phase of gait and released during push off. The 90° spiralization of the fascicles provides a mechanical advantage by concentrating mechanical stresses and then realizing them [14].

The factors that influence the storage and subsequent release of energy include the state of the tissue itself, the length of the tendon and the duration of application and release of load. The mechanical properties of all the biological tissues can be appreciated by examining their stress-strain relationship. The energy stored by a biological structure corresponds to the area beneath the stress-strain curve (Figure 2). When the collagen fibre orientation is compared to the stress strain curve, the fibres are initially relatively slack and relaxed (Figure 2). Following the application of load, the fibres become more aligned, increasing in length: this status corresponds to a 2% strain, and is represented as the toe region of the curve [56]. With additional load, the fibrils absorb this load and have increased tension, without increasing strain. When the load is released and the tendon returns to its original relaxed state, it follows a hysteresis pattern, i.e., it does not follow the same path along the stress strain curve but at a lower level. The reduction in the area beneath this curve represents the loss of energy dissipated principally as heat during the loading and unloading processes. This viscoelastic behaviour features microphysical deformation in the loading and recruitment of collagen fibres, and the rearrangement of the microstructure of collagens type I and III proteoglycans and water. In normal walking, this accounts for 6% of the total energy. During one-legged hopping, 74% of the mechanical energy is stored, and the subsequent energy release or elastic recoil from the tendon contributes to 16% of the energy during push off [14]. This steady state behaviour is obtained after a warm up periodof at least six minutes or 270 loading cycles after a period of inactivity [24]. The failure of the Achilles tendon occurs at about 8-10% strain, typically at the mid-portion rather than the insertion.

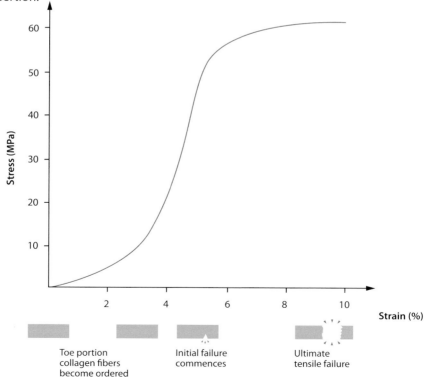

Figure 2. The biomechanical properties of an Achilles tendon until failure/rupture.

The cross-sectional area of the tendon is dependent upon both the loads to which it is subjected [40] and the presence of pathological processes.

The greater the cross-sectional area of a tendon, the larger its capacity to withstand heavy loads before failure; longer tendons have a greater capacity to elongate before failure in comparison to shorter tendons [82]. At low rates of loading, tendons are more viscous or ductile. Tendons therefore absorb more energy at lower rates of loading. At high rates of loading, tendons become more brittle and absorb less energy, but they are more effective in moving high loads [33]. The tendon therefore reacts differently to slow stretch when compared with jumping activity. The tensile strength of healthy tendons increases during childhood and adolescence, and peaks between 25 and 35 years of age, after which the tensile strength slowly decreases [27].

In vivo measurements of loading the Achilles tendon, during various types of activity, were performed using a buckle-type transducer [38]. The forces in the Achilles tendon varied considerably between individuals, and the forces were well above the range of the single load ultimate tensile strength of the tendon. During gait, the Achilles tendon force was built up before heel contact, with a sudden momentary release of the force at early impact [38]. Thereafter, the force in the Achilles tendon was built up relatively quickly during the stance phase, with the peak force measured at push-off. They measured a force of 2.6 kN during walking, while during running the force was 9 kN, corresponding to approximately 12 times body weight. Cycling only produced a force of less than 1 kN [38].

The response of the tendon to resistance loading and physical training

Human tendons are metabolically active and respond to repetitive loading. During this process, both synthesis and degradation are increased. Degradation has been shown in the initial phase of increased loading [83] but is followed by a dramatic increase in synthesis in the following days [44]. Whether resistance or endurance training alters the cross-sectional area is still a subject of discussion. Resistance training increases tendon stiffness by 65% with unchanged tendon dimensions, and produces a 22% reduction in mechanical hysteresis [69]. Habitual long-distance running, for more than five years, enlarges the tendon cross-sectional area by up to 22% compared with non-runners [57]. This increase in size was, however, not found after nine months of endurance training in previously untrained individuals [24].

The biomechanical aspects of rupture

The rupture of the Achilles tendon typically occurs following the rapid eccentric loading of the musculo-tendinous unit. Rupture typically occurs in an elongated abnormal tendon fibril. This reduces the remaining thickness of the tendon over which the force is applied, and this force is likely to be greater than the ultimate tensile strength of the remaining tendon tissue, leading to further failure (i.e., ending in a total rupture). Relative elongation and, thus, increasing strain with the same force being applied but with increasing stress (i.e., a reduction in area), corresponds to the stress/strain curve prior to failure.

Rupture will start at one particular point and progress from there. This initial failure may occur with the mechanical weakening of the tendon, perhaps with reduced collagen content. The fibrillar structure of the tendon means that, during failure, sequential fibrils will elongate with subsequent separation and delamination before ultimately failing. This sliding behaviour is an important aspect of the failure pattern of the Achilles tendon and, with 10% of the applied load and evidence of sub- and post-fascicle sliding, is clearly visible [39]. This may be one of the mechanisms that produces the "mop head" appearance of the ruptured tendon-end (Figure 3). For a partial rupture to occur, it is likely that the load would have to be released by muscular relaxation in response to the pain stimulus almost instantaneously. This hypothesis of the mechanism of failure could explain why partial ruptures are very rare. Ruptures occur at the narrowest point in the tendon, typically located at the most hypovascular area [40].

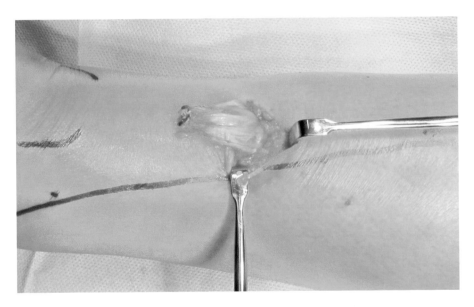

Figure 3. The "mop head" appearance of a ruptured Achilles tendon.

The biomechanical aspects of healing and repair

The general principles of rupture management consist of the approximation of the tendon-ends, permitting early movement and tendon loading.

With non-surgical management, ultrasonography may be used to visualize the tendon-ends to ensure that they are in apposition. If this does not occur, surgical repair should be considered [41, 89]. Non-surgical management has the advantage of avoiding surgical complications. The haematoma is also preserved. There is concern, however, over the separation of the tendon-ends during early movement rehabilitation programmes. Expensive serial ultrasonography may be required to ensure that the tendon-ends remain opposed during early rehabilitation. On the other hand, Schepull and co-workers found no significant difference in the amount of tendon elongation between patients treated surgically and non-surgically, where both groups were allowed early weight-bearing from the beginning [78].

The outcome of surgical repair in the form of open or percutaneous repair will be discussed at length elsewhere in the text. Open repair has the advantage that the surgeon can see directly whether the tendon-ends are opposed, with varying suture techniques and the ability to use a reinforcing peripheral running suture and augment the repair with either autograft or synthetic materials. Percutaneous repair techniques minimize incision length and wound healing problems, and reduce the direct visualisation of tendon-end opposition. Obviously, the configurations of the suture that can be used in percutaneous techniques are limited. In general, with using the same suture material of the same diameter, the strength on the suture is proportional to the number of strands passing longitudinally through the tendon. Modern studies have ascertained that, if the above principles are followed, percutaneous techniques impart to the repair a comparable initial mechanical strength as open techniques.

The literature concerning the different suture methods is reported in Table 2. It must be appreciated that these studies are on tenotomy models rather than true ruptures, and the appearance of ragged mop-ends to the tendon is, therefore, not produced in these models.

Author	Tendon	Repair Construct	Suture	Failure	Conclusions
Hockenbury 1990 [25]	Human cadaveric	Bunnell open vs. Percutaneous		Open has twice strength Percutaneous	Percutaneous has 50% of the initial strength of open repairs
Mortensen 1991 [60]	Human cadaveric	Continuous [6] strand suture Bunnell technique			Continuous 6 strand suture stronger
Watson 1995 [87]	Human cadaveric	Kessler vs. Bunnell with the addition of locking loop	1 Ethibond	85N vs. 93N	The addition of locking loop significantly added strength to repair
Cretnik 2000 [12]	Human cadaveric	Bunnell/Box vs. modified configuration with circumferential whip stitch	2 Vicryl		New modified configuration greater tensile strength and gapping resistance
Jaakkola 2000 [30]	Human cadaveric	Triple bundle repair vs. Krakow locking loop	1 Ethibond	161N	Triple bundle stronger P0.001

Author[26]	Tendon	Repair Construct	Suture	Failure	Conclusions
Kangas 2001[34]	Rabbits	Polyglyconate (Maxon) Strength of suture material rather than the construct	Polygly-conate (Maxon) vs. Poly L/D Lactide		PLDLA lower initial tensile strength than Maxon, PLDLA showed prolonged strength retention
Yildririm 2002[90]	48 sheep fresh frozen	Bunnell vs. Kessler locking	5 Ticron		
Lewis 2003[47]	Human cadavericc	Tenofix repair vs. 2 strand modified 2 Kessler		Kessler Gap 0.3N/mm2 Peak 1.03 N/mm2, TenoFix Gap 0.8N/mm2 Peak 1.19 N/mm2	Gap formation in 29% and 67% of peak tensile stress
Zandbergen 2005[91]	Human cadaveric	Open Bunnell vs. Percutaneous Calcaneal tunnel and Percutaneous Bone Anchor	1 PDS II	No difference in techniques P=0.5	Mode failure suture breakage in non-anchors and anchor pull out
Benthuen 2006[5]	Bovine cadaveric	Using 4 strand Krakow repair	2 Fibrew-ire Poly-blend vs. 2 Ethibond Polyester	582N vs. 222N	Poly blend resulted in stronger repairs and less gap formation (P 0.001) All failed at knots
Shepard 2007[79]	Human cadaveric	2 Ethibond Krakow locking suture vs. the addition of a 4,0 Nylon suture			With running suture the initial stiffness 173% greater and load to failure stronger 119%
Gebauer 2007[19]	Human cadaveric	Bunnell vs. Kessler with and without Plantaris tendon augmentation	PDS Thread and PDS Cord	Bunnell thread 139N, cord 291N/ Kessler thread 137N, Cord 180N Bunnell PDS thread with Plantaris augmentation 326N	The PDS Cord was mechanically strong method, however the augmentation added more stability
Ismail 2008[26]	Ovine	Achillon vs. 2 strand Kessler	2 Ticron	Achillon 153N Kessler 123N	Comparable strength, Achillon sound method of repair
Shepherd 2008[80]	Human cadaveric	Epitenon cross stitch vs. simple running stitch			Gaping resistance and initial stiffness were comparable however the cross stitch had improved failure strength

Author	Tendon	Repair Construct	Suture	Failure	Conclusions
Labib 2009 [43]		Gift box technique (with knots tied away from the rupture site) vs. Krakow		Load to failure Giftbox 168N Traditional Krakow 81N	Recommends Gift box technique.
Lee 2009 [47]	Human cadaveric	Early post op forces were simulated by cyclical loading for: Percutaneous, 4 strand Krakow, or epitendinous augmented 4 strand Krakow technique.			The use of an epitendinous suture increased the strength of repair, Percutaneous repair failed after 1000cycles of 100N, the 4 strand Krakow all failed at 190N whereas the augmented repairs were all intact
Lee 2009 [46]		Augmented with cross stitch weave vs. 3 figure 8 sutures and 4 strand Krakow			Force to failure, stiffness and gapping resistance were increased with the augmented suture
Cook 2010 [11]	Human cadaveric	Modified Krakow suture	2-0 Fibre-loop vs. No 2 Ethibo-nd	Mean yield loads were Fibreloop 233N and Ethibond 134N. Mean ultimate loads were Fibreloop 283N and Ethibond 135N.	Cross sectional area of one pass of 2-0 Fibreloop was calculated to be 0.21mm^2, one pass of Ethibond was 0.28mm^2. The smaller calibre fibreloop was significantly stronger than No 2 Ethibond suggesting there is no advantage is using a larger material in terms of strength.
McCoy 2010 [58]	Human cadaveric	Double Krakow locking loop vs. Bunnell single Kessler suture	2 Mersi-lene 4 strands	Double Krakow 200N, Double Bunnell 196N, Double Kessler 167N	No difference
Ortiz 2012 [65]	Bovine cadaveric	Triple strand Dresden vs. Dresden vs. Krakow vs. Oblique		Triple Dresden 246N Dresden 180N Krakow 22.6N Oblique 437N	Triple strand Dresden increased tensile strength (P0.0001) and gap resistance (P0.01)

67

Author	Tendon	Repair Construct	Suture	Failure	Conclusions
Pilson 2012 [67]	Human cadaveric	Single vs. double row repair of the distal Achilles tendon	No difference in load to failure sP =0.46 Or energy expenditure P= 0.069		No mechanical advantage of double over single row.
Longo 2012 [50]	Human cadaveric	Achillon vs. modified percutaneous repair		Similar biomechanical performance	No difference in mean strength, mean maximum load, mean failure elongation, tension, stiffness and mode of failure between the two groups.

Table 2. Literature of the strength of differing suture materials and techniques used for Achilles tendon repair.

The strongest open repairs are obtained using a locking core suture (Krakow) tied using a gift box method [43], away from the repair site, together with a peripheral running suture. This may be augmented with a fascial or aponeurosis turndown [20] or else a plantaris tendon weave [19]. However, the additional strength of these augmentations must be balanced by the risks of increased wound length for exposure, especially considering that clinical studies have shown that the clinical outcome is no different whether an augmentation is performed or not. Augmentation using the flexor hallucis longus will be covered in the chapter on reconstruction.

The role of the suture material is important. The use of absorbable suture materials has been recommended to minimize nerve injury [37], and there are different opinions regarding the use of non-absorbable or absorbable sutures. Not only is the behaviour of the suture itself over time important, but the response of the tissue to the suture must also be considered. Polydioxanone sutures (PDSs) have a higher tendon holding strength than polyester-blended sutures [88]. This becomes most apparent with the lowest pull-out strength found during the third post-operative week [89]. In terms of the suture strength for non-absorbable sutures, polyblend sutures are stronger than polyester [11]. As to absorbable sutures, although poly-L/D-lactide sutures are have an initial lower tensile strength, they have a prolonged tensile strength compared to polyglyconate sutures [34].

The augmentation of the repair site with graft jacket matrices significantly increases the repair site strength and stiffness [4]. Whether these techniques result in better outcomes is, however, still unknown.

Similar studies have shown a higher stiffness failure load and greater energy to failure following augmentation with broad adhesive coated scaffolds; however, the use of fibrin sealant by itself has no influence on healing [51].

Once the initial/post-operative resting tone has been established, the next aims of management are to promote healing and restore the strength and function of the injured tendon. The maintenance of the apposition of the tendon ends is important during healing and the early movement of the tendons [34]. Following surgery or apposition during non-surgical management, healing goes through the phases of haematoma, inflammation and organization. In the early stage, the regenerating tendon forms a sleeve around the ruptured tendon-ends. In sheep models, this early sleeve has a greatly reduced load to failure, but a near-normal hysteresis in terms of energy storage [85]. In a rat model, healing during the inflammatory phase is aided by intermittent mechanical loading [15].

Unfortunately, elongation occurs with all forms of management, and much more research is required so that this aspect of tendon healing and rehabilitation can be understood. Hyper-dorsiflexion occurs in chronic cases with gapping and symptomatic elongation. The precise effects of immediate weight bearing and early movement will be discussed elsewhere in the text. However, both of these promote tendon healing, and do not appear to have a deleterious effect on outcomes [35, 60].

The separation of the tendon-ends during loading – termed 'gapping' – leads to worse outcomes [35], and a gap greater than 5 mm may lead to failure [46]. Schepull and co-workers have measured the modulus of elasticity in healing tendons and found it to correlate with late function [78].

Protection of the healing tendon

Re-rupture is generally considered to occur during two mechanisms. The first is uncontrolled loading early in the post-operative period. This typically appears as a cut tendon-end at the rupture site. Late re-rupture typically occurs due to fatigue failure proximal to the original rupture site [59, 76].

In the early post-operative and injury period, the healing tendon may be protected by a dorsal shell [6] to prevent uncontrolled dorsiflexion or else a protective boot with heel wedges. Both permit the loading of the tendon, however with wedges the load on the tendon is reduced by bypassing the tendon being stress-shielded by the tibia [17]. The use of a 2.5 cm heel lift has been shown to reduce the force through the Achilles tendon by 191 N [69], as well as a 12% reduction in the maximum voluntary contraction that can be performed by the triceps surae [2].

The biomechanical aspects of tendinopathy

Achilles tendinopathy may be caused by micro-injury, with small tears and an inadequate healing response. As detailed elsewhere in the text, the process leads to the formation of a thicker, painful, dysfunctional tendon [53]. Tenocytes within a tendinopathic tendon have an abnormal morphology, and morphological changes occur in the matrix of the collagen in response to increased mechanical load [1].

Changes within the tendon substance have also been characterized by intra-tendinous degenerative lesions, voids and – in very chronic cases – the formation of calcification [73]. The relative transfer of loads through the tendon is significant. Loads preferentially pass through the side of the tendon not affected by tendinopathy [55]; thus, the tendinopathic area of the tendon is stress-shielded. As the Achilles tendon spans two joint distally, the alignment of the hind foot and the spatial orientation of the sub-talar joint is a factor. Alignment and biomechanical faults have been shown to play a causative role in two thirds of Achilles tendon problems in athletes [16, 22, 28, 31, 42]. Patients with Achilles tendon pathology were found to have a significantly increased deviation angle of the sub-talar joint (18°) compared to those who did not have such a pathology (10°) [72]. The sagittal plane biomechanics may play a more important role in insertional Achilles tendinopathy. A prominent posterior superior calcaneal tuberosity and the lateral process of the calcaneus have been associated with insertional tendinopathy. The role of an increased deviation angle has already been discussed in relation to mid-portion tendinopathy but, conversely, a cavus foot may be associated with insertional tendinopathy. Cavus feet have increased calcaneal pitch and the insertion may move relatively distally, placing increased tension on the Achilles tendon and increasing the angle of insertion [48]. Similarly, the postero-superior prominence will be brought closer to the tendon, increasing local pressure.

These changes will affect the biomechanical properties of the tendon. A thicker tendon, with a larger cross-sectional area, suffers reduced stress when loads are applied; however, such a tendon would be much less able to change in length compared with its original length and strain. As a result, the tendon becomes stiffer with an increasing modulus of elasticity.

The development of the structural changes of tendinopathy also alters the mechanical properties of the Achilles tendon (Figure 4). Tendinopathic Achilles tendons are less stiff than healthy tendons, despite their increased cross-sectional area [10].

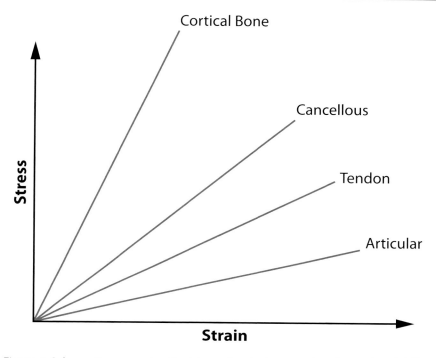

Figure 4. Schematic comparing the biomechanical properties of samples of different biological materials.

The insertion of the Achilles tendon consists of a transition through fibrocartilage to mineralized fibrocartilage and, ultimately, bone. In insertional Achilles tendinopathy, the nearby tendon suffers a reduction in collagen content, increased water content and a relatively young collagenous matrix is also present [13]. The insertional area develops chondral metaplasia and produces abnormally high quantities of collagen type II and III, and so may be less resistant to tensile forces [54].

Ultimately, in chronic cases, the changes progress to the formation of ossified tissue at the tendon insertion [62, 73]. This change from degenerate to calcified tissue will make the insertion site stiffer, increasing the modulus of elasticity. The presence of calcification and ossification further changes the mechanical properties of the tendon. Failure may occur suddenly with fracture rather than the narrowing and elongation of a non-calcified tendon.

Eccentric loading exercises lead to decreased tendon thickness and a normalized structure in most patients [63, 70]. A 12 week programme of eccentric exercises increases the rate of collagen synthesis in tendinopathic tendons [44]. These exercises are beneficial in patients with both mid-portion and insertional Achilles tendinopathy (though the latter give less good clinical results than the former) [32]. The avoidance of dorsiflexion may also reduce impingement from the prominent posterior superior calcaneal tubercle.

How these effects occur has been discussed in terms of whether it is the increase in length/strain or the addition of increased force (i.e., stress in the tendon) resulting in increased muscular strength that is efficacious[3]. Mechanical stretching of 4% strain promotes the differentiation of tenocyte stem cells into tenocytes; however, increased strain up to 8% leads to differentiation towards adipogenic, chondrogenic and osteogenic lineages [91]. High-frequency oscillations in tendon force occur during eccentric exercises, but were rare during concentric exercises [71]. Lower-frequency vibrations have been found in Achilles tendinopathy during eccentric rehabilitation exercises[21].

Conclusions

The key biomechanical function of the Achilles tendon is the storage and elastic recoil of energy. This process is disturbed with the changes occurring in tendinopathy and following rupture. More research is required in the loading and unloading of the Achilles tendon, particularly during rehabilitation following injury, before this process is understood.

References

1. Abraham T, Fong G, Scott A. Second harmonic generation analysis of early Achilles tendinosis in response to in vivo mechanical loading. BMC Musculoskeletal Disorders. 2011; 12: 26.

2. Akizuki KH, Gartman EJ, Nisonson B, Ben-Avi S, McHugh MP. The relative stress on the Achilles tendon during ambulation in an ankle immobiliser: implications for rehabilitation of Achilles tendon repair. Br J Sports Med. 2001; 35: 329-334.

3. Allison GT, Purdham C. Eccentric loading for Achilles tendinopathy- strengthening or stretching? Br J Sports Med. 2009; 43(4): 276-9.

4. Barber FA, McGarry JE, Herbert MA, Anderson RB. A biomechanical study of Achilles tendon repair augmentation using GaftJacket matrix. Foot Ankle Int. 2008; 29(3): 329-33.

5. Benthien RA, Aronov MS, Doran-Diaz V, Sullivan RJ, Naujoks R, Adams DJ. Cyclic loading of Achilles tendon repairs: a comparison of polyester and polyblend sutures. Foot Ankle Int. 2006; 27(7): 512-8.

6. Carden DG, Noble J, Chalmers J, Lunn P, Ellis J. Rupture of the calcaneal tendon; the early and late management. J Bone Joint Surg Br. 1987; 69(3): 416-20.

7. Chan AP, Chan YY, Fong DT, Wong PY, Lam HY, Lo CK, Yung PS, Fung KY, Chan KM. Clinical and biomechanical outcome of minimal invasive and open repairs of the Achilles tendon. Sports Med Arthrosc Rehabil Ther Technol. 2011; 3(1): 32.

8. Chao W, Deland JT, Bates JE, Kenneally SM. Achilles tendon insertion: an in vitro anatomic study. Foot Ankle Int. 1997; 18(2): 81-89.

9. Cheng HY, Lin CL, Wang HW, Chou SW. Finite element analysis of plantar fascia under stretch. The relative contribution of the windlass mechanism and Achilles tendon force. J Biomech. 2008; 419: 1937-44.

10. Child S, Bryant AL, Clark RA, Crossley KM. Mechanical properties of the Achilles tendon aponeurosis are altered in athletes with Achilles tendinopathy. Am J Sports Med 2010; 38(9): 1885-93.

11. Cook KD, Clark G, Lui E, Vajaria G, Wallace GF. Strength of braided polyblend polyethylene suture versus braided polyester sutures in Achilles tendon repair: a cadaveric study. J Am Podiatr Med Assoc. 2010; 100(3): 185-8.

12. Cretnik A, Zlajpah L, Smrkolj V, Kosanovic M. The strength of percutaneous methods of repair of the Achilles tendon: a biomechanical study. Med Sci Sports Exerc. 2000; 32(1): 16-20.

13. e Mos M, van El B, De Groot J, Jahr H, van Shie HT, van Arkel ER, Tol H, Heijboer R, van Osch GJ, Verhaar JA. Achilles tendinosis: changes in biochemical composition and collagen turnover rate. Am J Sports Med. 2007; 35(9): 1549-56.

14. Doral MN, Alam M, Bozkurt M ,Turhan E, Atay OA, Dunmez G, Maffulli N. Functional anatomy of the Achilles tendon. Knee Surg Sports Traumatol Arthrosc. 2010; 18(5): 638-42.

15. Eliasson P, Andersson Aspenberg R. Achilles tendon healing in rats is improved by intermittent mechanical loading during the inflammatory phase. J Orthop Res. 2012; 30(2): 274-9.

16. Fahlstrom M, Lorentzon R, Alfredson H. Painful conditions in the Achilles tendon region: a common problem in middle aged competitive badminton players. Knee Surg Sports Traumatol Arthrosc. 2002; 10(1): 57-60.

17. Farris DJ, Buckeridge E, Trewarble G, McGuigan MP. The effects of athletic heel lifts on the Achilles tendon force during running. J Appl Biomech. 2012; 28(5): 511-519.

18. Finni T, Kami PV, Lukkariniemi J. Achilles tendon loading during walking: application of a novel optic fibre technique. Eur J Appl Physiol. 1998; 77: 289-291.

19. Gebauer M, Bell FT, Beckamnn J, Sarvary AM, Ueblacker P, Ruecker AH, Hoiste J, Meenen NM. Mechanical evaluation of different techniques for Achilles tendon repair. Arch Orthop Trauma Surg. 2007; 127(9): 795-9.

20. Gerdes MH, Brown TD, Bell AL, Baker JA, Levson M, Layer S. A flap augmentation technique for Achilles tendon repair. Postoperative strength and functional outcome. Clin Orthop Relat Res. 1992; 280: 241-6.

21. Grigg NL, Wearing SC, Smeathers KE. Eccentric calf muscle exercise produces a greater acute reduction in thickness than concentric exercises. Br J Sports Med. 2009; 43(4): 280-3.

22. Haglund-Akerlind Y, Eriksson E. Range of movement, muscle torque and training habits in runners with and without Achilles tendon problems. Knee Surg Sports Traumatol Arthrosc. 1993; 3(4): 195-9.

23. Hansen P, Asgaard P, Kjaer M, Larsson B, Magnusson SP. Effect of habitual running on human Achilles tendon load deformation and cross sectional area. J Appl Physiol. 2003; 95: 2375-80.

24. Hawkins D, Lim C, Gaydos D, Dunning R. Dynamic creep and preconditioning of the Achilles tendon in vivo. J Biomech. 2009; 42(16): 2813-7.

25. Hockenbury RT, Johns JC. A biomechanical in vitro comparison of open versus percutaneous repair of tendon Achilles. Foot Ankle. 1990; 11(2): 67-72.

73

26. Ismail M, Karim A, Shulman R, Amis A, Calder J. The Achillon Achilles tendon repair: is it strong enough? Foot Ankle Int. 2008; 29(8): 808-13.

27. Ippolito E, Natali PG, Postacchini F, Accinni L, De Martino C. Morphological immunochemical and biochemical study of rabbit Achilles tendon at various ages. J Bone Joint Surg Am. 1980; 62(4): 583-98.

28. Järvinen M. Lower leg overuse injuries in athletes. Knee Surg Sports Traumatol Arthrosc. 1993; 1(2): 126-30.

29. Järvinen TA, Järvinen TL, Kanus P, Józsa L, Järvinen M. Collagen fibres of the spontaneously ruptured human tendons display decreased thickness and crimp angle. J Orthop Res. 2004; 22(6): 1303-9.

30. Jaakkola JI, Hutton WC, Beskin JL, Lee GP. Achilles tendon rupture repair: biomechanical comparison of the triple bundle technique versus the Krakow locking loop technique. Foot Ankle Int. 2000; 21: 14-17.

31. Johansson C. Injuries in elite orienteers. Am J Sports Med. 1986; 14: 410-5.

32. Jonsson P, Alfredson H, Snding K, Fahlström m, Cook J. New regime of eccentric muscle training in patients with chronic insertional Achilles tendinopathy: Results of a pilot study. Br J Sports Med. 2008; 42(9): 746-9.

33. Józsa L, Kannus P. Histopathological findings in spontaneous tendon ruptures. Scand J Med Sci Sports. 1997; 7(2): 113-8.

34. Kangas J, Paasimaa S, Makela P, Leppilahti J, Tormala P, Waris T, Ashammakhi N. Comparison of strength properties of poly-L/D-Lactide (PLDLA) 96/4 and polyglyconate (Maxon) suturs: in vitro, in the subcutis and in the Achilles tendon of rabbits. J Biomater Res. 2001; 58(1): 121-6.

35. Kangas J, Paajala A, Ohtenen P, Leppilahti J. Achilles tendon elongation after rupture repair: a randomized comparison of two post-operative regimens. Am J Sports Med. 2007; 35(1): 59-64.

36. Khan CJ, Wang X, Rahouadj R. Non-linear model for the viscoelastic behaviour of the Achilles tendon. J Biomech Eng. 2010; 132(11): 111002.

37. Klein W, Lang DM, Saleh. The use of the Ma_Griffiths technique for the percutaneous repair of the fresh ruptured tendo Achillis. Chir Organi Mor. 1991; 76(3): 223-8.

38. Komi PV, Fukashiro S, Järvinen M. Biomechanical loading of the Achilles tendon during normal locomotion. Clin Sports Med. 1992; 11(3): 521-31.

39. Komolafe OA, Doehring TC. Fascicle scale loading and failure behaviour of the Achilles tendon. J Biomech Eng. 2010; 132(2): 021004.

40. Kongsgaard P, Asgaard P, Kjaer M, Magnusson SP. Structural Achilles tendon properties in athletes subjected to different modes and in Achilles tendon rupture patients. J Appl Physiol. 2005; 99: 1965-71.

41. Kotnis R, David S, Hadnley R, Willett K, Ostiere S. Dynamic ultrasound as a selection tool for reducing Achilles tendon re-ruptures. Am J Sports Med. 2006; 34(9): 1395-400.

42. Kvist J. Achilles tendon injuries in athletes. Sports Med. 1994; 18: 173-201.

43. Labib SA, Rolf R, Dacus R, Hutton WC. The "Giftbox" repair of the Achilles tendon: a modification of the Krakow technique. Foot Ankle Int. 2009; 30(5): 410-4.

44. Langberg H, Ellingsgaard H, Madesn T, Jansson J, Magnusson SP, Aagaard P, Kjaer M. Eccentric rehabilitation exercise increases peritendinous type 1 collagen synthesis in humans with Achilles tendinosus. Scand J Med Sci Sports. 2007; 17(1): 61-6.

45. Lee J, Guarino V, Gloria A, Ambrosio L, Tae G, Kim YH, Jung Y, Kim SH, Kim SH. Regeneration of Achilles tendon: the role of dynamic stimulation for enhanced cell proliferation and mechanical properties. J Biomater Sci Polym Ed. 2010; 21(8-9): 1173-90.

46. Lee SJ, Goldsmith S, Nicholas SJ, McHugh M, Kremenic I, Ben-Avi S. Optimising Achilles tendon repair: the effect of epitendinous suture augmentation on the strength of Achilles tendon repairs. Foot Ankle International. 2008; 29(4): 427-432.

47. Lee SJ, Sileo MJ, Kremenic IJ, Orishimo K, Ben-Avi S, Nicholas SJ, McHugh M. Cyclic loading of 3 Achilles tendon repairs simulating early post-operative forces. Am J Sports Med. 2009; 37(4): 786-90.

48. Lersch C, Grotsch A, Segesser B, Koebke, Brüggemann CP, Potthast W. Influence of the calcaneal angle and muscle forces on the strain distribution in the human Achilles tendon. Clin Biomech (Bristol Avon). 2012; 27(9): 955-61.

49. Lewis N, Quitkin HM. Strength analysis and comparison of the Teno Fix tendon repair system with the two strand modified Kessler repair in the Achilles tendon. Foot Ankle Int. 2003; 24(11): 857-60.

50. Longo UG, Forriol F, Campi S, Maffulli N, Denaro V. A biomechanical comparison of the primary stability of two minimally invasive techniques for repair of ruptured Achilles tendon. Knee Surg Sports Traumatol Arthrosc 2012; 20(7): 1392-7.

51. Lusardi DA, Cain JE Jr. The effect of fibrin sealant on the strength of tendon repair of full thickness tendon laceration in the rabbit Achilles tendon. J Foot Ankle Surg. 1994; 33(5): 443-7.

52. Lysholm J, Wiklander J. Injuries in runners. Am J Sports Med. 1987; 15: 168-71.

53. Maffulli N, Khan KM, Puddu G. Overuse tendon condition: time to change a confusing terminology. Arthroscopy. 1998; 14(8): 840-3.

54. Maffulli N, Reaper J, Ewen SW, Waterston SW, Barras V. Chondral metaplasia in calcific insertional tendinopathy of the Achilles tendon. Clin J Sports Med. 2006; 16(4): 329-34.

55. Magnaris CN, Naria MV, Maffulli N. Biomechanics of the Achilles tendon. Disabil Rehabil. 2008; 30(20-22): 1542-7.

56. Magnusson SP, Qvotrup K, Larsen JO et al. Collagen fibril size and crump morphology in ruptured and intact Achilles tendons. Matrix Biol. 2002; 21(4): 369-77.

57. Magnusson SP, Kjaer M. Region specific differences in Achilles tendon cross sectional area in runners and non-runners. Eur J Appl Physiol. 2003; 90: 549-53.

58. McCoy BW, Haddad SL. The strength of Achilles tendon repair: a comparison of three suture techniques in human cadaver tendons. Foot Ankle Int. 2010; 31(8): 701-5.

59. Molloy A, Wood EV. Complications of the treatment of Achilles tendon ruptures. Foot Ankle Clin. 2009; 14(4): 45-59.

60. Mortensen NH, Saether J. Achilles tendon repair: a new method of Achilles tendon repair tested on cadaverous materials. J Trauma. 1991; 31(3): 381-4.

61. Mullaney MJ, McHugh MP, Tyler TF, Nicholas SJ, Lee SJ. Weakness in end-range plantar flexion after Achilles tendon repair. Am J Sports Med. 2006; 34(7): 1120-5.

62. O'Brien EJ, Frank CB, Shrive NG, Hallgrimison B, Hart DA. Heterotrophic mineralisation (ossification or calcification) in tendinopathy or following surgical tendon trauma. Int J Exp Pathol. 2012; 93(5): 319-31.

63. Ohberg L, Lorentzen R, Alfredson H. Eccentric training in patients with chronic Achilles tendinosis: normalised tendon structure and decreased thickness at follow up. Br J Sports Med. 2004; 38(1): 8-11.

64. Oliva F, Via AG, Maffulli N. Physiopathology of intra-tendinous calcific deposition. BMC Med. 2012; 10: 95.

65. Ortiz C, Wagner E, Mococain P, Labarca G, Keller A, Del Buono A, Maffulli N. Biomechanical comparison of four methods of repair of the Achilles tendon: a laboratory study with bovine tendons. J Bone Joint Surg Br. 2012; 94(5): 663-7.

66. Paavola M, Kannus P, Paakkala T, Pasonen M, Järvinen M. Long-term prognosis of patients with Achilles tendinopathy. An observational 8 year follow-up study. Am J Sports Med. 2000; 28(5): 634-42.

67. Pilson H, Brown P, Stitzel J, Scott A. Single row versus double row repair of the distal Achilles tendon: a biomechanical comparison. J Foot Ankle Surg. 2012; 51(6): 762-6.

68. Pollock CM, Shadwick RE. Relationship between the body mass and biomechanical properties of limb tendon in adult mammals. Am J Physiol. 1994; 266: R1016-21.

69. Reeves ND, Marici MV, Maganaris CN. Strength training alters the viscoelastic properties of tendons in elderly humans. Muscle Nerve. 2003; 28(1): 74-81.

70. Rees JD, Lichtwark GA, Wolman RL, Wilson AM. The mechanism for efficacy of eccentric loading of Achilles tendon injury: an in vivo study in humans. Rheumatology (Oxford). 2008; 47(10): 1493-7.

71. Rees JD, Wilson AM, Wolman RL. Current concepts in the management of tendon disorders. Rheumatology (Oxford). 2006; 45(5): 508-21.

72. Reule CA, Alt WW, Lohrer H, Hochwold H. Spatial orientation of the sub-talar joint axis is different in subjects with or without Achilles tendon disorders. Br J Sports Med. 2011; 45(13): 1029-34.

73. Richards PJ, Braid JC, Carmont MR, Maffulli N. Achilles tendon ossification: pathology, imaging and aetiology. Disabil Rehabil. 2008; 30(20-22): 1651-65.

74. Roberts JM, Goldstrohm GL, Brown TD, Mears DC. Comparison of unrepaired, primarily repaired and polyglactin mesh reinforced Achilles tendon lacerations in rabbits. Clin Orthop Relat Res. 1983; 181: 244-9.

75. Rosso C, Valderabano . Biomechanics of the Achilles tendon. Chapter 4. In Calder J, Karlsson J, Maffulli N, Thermann H, van Dijk CN. Achilles tendinopathy: Current Concepts. DJO publications London. 2010. pp. 25-34.

76. Rushton PR, Singh AK, Deskmukh RG. A case of "fresh rupture" after open repair of a ruptured Achilles tendon. J Foot Ankle Surg. 2012; 51(1): 95-8.

77. Schepsis AA, Jones H, Haas AL. Achilles tendon disorders in athletes. Am J Sports Med. 2002; 30(2): 287-305.

78. Schepull T, Kvist J, Aspenberg P. Early E modulus of healing Achilles tendons correlates with late function. Scand J Med Sci Sports. 2012; 22(1): 18-23.

79. Shepard ME, Lindsey DP, Chou LB. Biomechanical testing of epitenon suture in Achilles tendon repairs. Foot Ankle Int. 2007; 28(10): 1074-7.

80. Shepard ME, Lindsey DP, Chou LB. Biomechanical comparison of the simple running and cross-stitch sutures in Achilles tendon repairs. Foot Ankle Int. 2008; 29(5): 513-7.

81. Soma CA, Mendelbaum BR. Achilles tendon disorders. Clin Sports Med. 1994; 13: 811-23.

82. Stanish WD, Rubinovich RM, Curwin S. Eccentric exercise in chronic tendonitis. Clin Orthop Relat Res. 1986; 208: 65-8.

83. Tardioli A, Malliaras P, Maffulli N. Immediate and short-term effects of exercise on tendon structure: biochemical, biomechanical and imaging responses. Br Med Bull 2012; 103(1): 169-202.

84. Thermann H, Frerichs O, Holch M, Biewener A. Healing of Achilles tendon an experimental study: Part 2 histological, immunohistological and ultrasound analysis. Foot Ankle Int. 2002; 23(7): 606-13.

85. Virchenko O, Fahlgreen A, Rundgren M, Aspenberg P. Early Achilles tendon healing in sheep. Arch Orthop Trauma Surg. 2008; 128(9): 1001-6.

86. Wang HK, Lin KH, Su Sc, Shih TT, Huang YC. Effects of tendon viscoelasticity in Achilles tendinosis on explosive performance and clinical severity in athletes. Scand J Med Sci Sports. 2012; 22(6): e147-55.

87. Watson TW, Jurist KA, Yang KH, Shen KL. The strength of Achilles tendon repair: an in vitro study of the biomechanical behaviour in human cadaver tendons. Foot Ankle Int. 1995; 16(4): 191-5.

88. Virchenko O, Fahlgreen A, Rundgren M, Aspenberg P. Early Achilles tendon healing in sheep. Arch Orthop Trauma Surg. 2008; 128(9): 1001-6.

89. Yildirim Y, Esemenli T. Initial pull out strength of tendon sutures: an in vitro study in sheep Achilles tendon. Foot Ankle Int. 2002; 23(12): 1126-30.

90. Yildirim Y, Kara H, Cabukoglu C, Esemenli T. Suture holding capacity of the Achilles tendon during the healing period: an in vivo experimental study in rabbits. Foot Ankle Int. 2006; 27(2): 121-4.

91. Zandbergen RA, de Boer SF, Swiestra BA, Day J, Kleinrensink GJ, Beumer A. Surgical treatment of Achilles tendon rupture: examination of strength of 3 types of suture techniques in a cadaver model. Acta Orthop. 2005; 76(3): 408-11.

92. Zhang J Wang JH. Mechanobiological response to tendon stem cells: implications of tendon homeostasis and pathogenesis in tendinopathy. J Orthop Res. 2010; 28(5): 639-43.

"Scientia potentia est."

Thomas Hobbes 1658
(Sir Francis Bacon)

CHAPTER 6

Healing and Repair Mechanism

Paul W. Ackermann

Take Home Message

• *Tendon healing entails five essential and overlapping processes:*
  1) *Induction*
  2) *Production*
  3) *Orchestration*
  4) *Conduction*
  5) *Modification*

• *The repair process may fail in any one of the above-mentioned phases, and targeted therapies are being developed to overcome repair failure.*

• *Most new treatment options (e.g., platelet rich plasma (PRP)), however, still need rigorous scientific evidence before general clinical usage can be recommended.*

Introduction

Tendon healing is initiated at the wound site by blood-derived cells (platelets, leukocytes, monocytes and lymphocytes), which interact in an intricate manner with tissue-derived cells (macrophages, fibroblasts, myofibroblasts, endothelial cells, mast cells and stromal stem cells). Reparative signalling entails vascular, cellular and neuronal mediators, which orchestrate in overlapping sequences the different phases of healing. The immediate goal in the healing process is to achieve tissue integrity, homeostasis and load-bearing capability. The instant

77

inflammatory response may, however, not always be in harmony with the ultimate repair goal – the restoration of optimal tissue function. Repair may, therefore, sometimes result in fibrotic scar formation leading to inferior tissue properties. In addition, healing events are influenced by a multitude of factors, such as the site of the injury, the age, sex, genetics, nutrition and health status of the patient, including neuro-vascular status and the supply of mediators [19].

The repair process can principally be divided in five important overlapping sequences; 1) Induction, 2) Production, 3) Orchestration, 4) Conduction and 5) Modification (Figure 1). The understanding of the interacting healing phases is critical for the physician in order to optimize the treatment outcome.

Figure 1. Tendon repair.
a) Induction – Blood-derived cells.
b) Production – Tissue-derived cells.
c) Orchestration – Neuro-vascular ingrowth.
d) Conduction – Tissue matrix.
e) Modification – Mechanical stimulation.

Induction of healing

After injury, the wound site is infiltrated with blood-derived cells (Table 1) acting as "traffic police", stopping bleeding, cleaning-up tissue debris and directing further traffic by the release of inflammatory mediators (e.g., cytokines, nitric oxide and growth factors). This is the initiation of the inflammatory healing phase.

BLOOD-DERIVED CELLS		
CELL	**ACTION**	**MEDIATOR**
Platelets	Wound Haemostasis	PDGF, TGF-B, FGF, EGF, B-thromboglobulin, histamine, serotonin, bradykinin, prostaglandins, prostacyclin, and thromboxane. PF4, C5a complement, PAF, leukotriene B4
Neutrophils	Neutrophils Phagocytosis and Wound Debridement	Proteolytic enzymes
Monocytes	Monocytes Transform into Macrophages	IL-2, TNF-a, PDGF, and IFN-y stimulate transformation
Lymphocytes	Anti-Inflammatory Helper T Cells	

Table 1. Infiltration of wound site with blood derived cells in response.

Platelets

Platelets release a wide variety of growth factors at the site of injury. A great number of these growth factors (such as PDGF, VEGF, IGF-1, TGF-beta and FGF), promote repair in various soft tissue models. One experimental study demonstrated that one injection of a moderate amount of activated platelets into the haematoma six hours after rat tendon injury increased the force at failure after one week, with the most prominent effects seen at three weeks after injury [10]. Moreover, collagen organization was significantly improved [80]. Thus, blood-derived cells (e.g., platelets) and the subsequently-released growth factors are essential for the initiation of the healing process [19].

Platelet rich plasma (PRP)

In case of injury or repetitive injuries without bleeding, it is reasonable to consider whether there is lack of essential substances starting and modulating the healing process. Deficient healing without bleeding is also a rationale for the more recently popular treatment with PRP [9]. This treatment, however, is still not well validated in clinical studies. PRP is is the cellular component of plasma that settles after centrifugation of whole blood. It contains numerous growth factors, such as TGF-β1, IGF-1 and 2, VEGF basic fibroblast growth factor and HGF [61]. Experimental studies have found positive effects in tendinopathy and tendon healing, possibly by PRP influencing neovascularization, collagen production and fibroblast proliferation in the early phase of tendon healing [43, 48, 61]. There is still no consensus as to the best means of administrating PRP with regards to the volume, preparation, injection technique, timing, number of injections, or the best rehabilitation protocol following injection. Moreover, in patients with acute Achilles tendon injuries, PRP injections may even produce detrimental effects [66]. Overall, there is a need for rigorous basic and clinical studies on the effect of PRP supply in relation to both acute and chronic Achilles tendon injuries.

NSAIDs

How does the inhibition of the inflammatory healing phase afflict tendon healing? If a cox inhibitor (NSAID) is given to the patient during early healing, the fibrous callus can lose a third of its strength due to inferior material properties [50]. Experimental studies have shown its effect on collagen synthesis, MMP expression and the reduced expression of cytokines [3, 27, 74]. The results are conflicting, possibly depending on timing of administration. Virchenko and co-workers experimentally demonstrated the detrimental effects of NSAIDs on callus strength in the first 14 days following injury, but an increased stress of failure if administered later than 14 days from the time of injury [81]. Thus, as anticipated, it appears that inhibiting the early inflammatory healing phase may impair the healing process. Similarly, a clinical study demonstrated the decreased production of collagen after exercise and NSAID intake [25]. However, there are no clinical studies demonstrating the benefits to the tendon after NSAID intake. On the whole, NSAIDs have not, at present, shown a clinical effect in enhancing tendon healing and should therefore be used moderately, especially given their known side-effects [63].

Laser Therapy

The use of low-level laser therapy (LLLT, laser sources at powers too low to cause measurable temperature increases) has been suggested as augmenting early tendon healing by the down-regulation of inflammation [34]. Moreover, recent experimental studies suggest that LLLT affects tendon healing by reducing inflammatory mediators in number and improving matrix reorganization during healing [56, 71]. Five RCTs have studied the effect of LLLT on human Achilles tendinopathy with varying results, and a systematic review on four RCTs concluded that the evidence for the beneficial effects of LLLT in Achilles tendinopathy is so far inconclusive [76], with two studies demonstrating beneficial effects and two showing no effect. Recently, one fairly small clinical study (20 patients in each group) performed on humans did not find any significant beneficial effect of adding LLLT to eccentric exercises for Achilles tendinopathy [75]. It may prove that the diverging results of LLLT derive from the fact that inflammatory mediators are not present in all cases of end stage tendinopathy.

Production of calluses

The inflammatory mediators released by the blood clot attract tissue-derived cells (Table 2) which, during the following 72 hours, are triggered to transform, *inter alia*, fibroblasts into myofibroblasts, and subsequently activate the production of tendon callus [53]. Accordingly, granulation tissue (i.e., extracellular matrix and collagen type III (scar collagen)) is formed from the tissue-derived cells, which normally reside in the extrinsic peritendinous tissues and the intrinsic tissue of the epitenon and endotenon. During the first week, collagen synthesis commences and reaches its maximum by week four – the reparative, collagen-forming phase. The glycoprotein - fibronectin - acts as a chemotactic agent for fibroblasts, which are the predominant cell type for the production of type III collagen.

The tissue- and blood-derived cells that infiltrate the wound area also release a cascade of mediators (growth factors, cytokines, BMPs and neuropeptides) which, in several experimental studies where supplements of these factors have been used, have demonstrated promising results for the optimization of the repair process [2]. The demonstrated increase in load results from an increase in the cross-sectional area of tendon, suggesting a generalized surge in matrix synthesis rather than improved matrix organization. However, and by analogy with PRP, there is no consensus regarding the modus or timing of administration, nor regarding the tendon loading regime. Growth factors (GFs) typically have a very short half-life in the tissues; hence the development of a number of different methods of prolonged GF release, such as GF-saturated sponges, scaffolds and lately GF-coated sutures.

TISSUE-DERIVED CELLS		
CELL	**ACTION**	**MEDIATOR**
Macrophages	Orchestrate healing by regulating angiogenesis, fibroplasia, and extracellular matrix synthesis. Wound debridement.	Fibroblast chemotaxis and proliferation: PDGF Myofibroblast activation: TGF-B1, fibronectin Other growth factors: EGF, IGF Cytokines: TNF-a, IL-1,6, IFN-y Debridement: Collagenase, elastase Antimicrobial: NO, oxygen radicals
Fibroblasts	Collagen synthesis and myofibroblast transformation	PDGF released from macrophages stimulates proliferation of fibroblasts into the wound from the surrounding tissue
Myofibroblast	Type III collagen synthesis and contraction	The myofibroblast is derived from the fibroblast by macrophage release of TGF-B1 and adhesion to the extracellular matrix molecule, fibronectin
Endothelial Cells	Forming of capillary tubes by VEGF stimuli	Endothelial cells synthesize NO, which increases VEGF production
Mast Cells	Vascular permeability, tissue remodelling, neurotrophic	Vascular permeability: Histamine Tissue remodelling: TGF-beta, IL-1 and IL-4, tryptase Neurotrophic: NGF

Table 2. Tissue derived cells, triggered to transform and activate production of extracellular matrix and collagen type III.

Insulin-like growth factor (IGF)

IGF promotes cell proliferation, collagen synthesis and decreases swelling in healing tendons [47]. Experimental studies have shown higher Achilles tendon function scores and accelerated recovery in rats following IGF administration [45].

Transforming growth factor-β (TGF-β)

The growth factor TGF-β is abundant in healing and scar formation. Its fetal isoforms (TGF-β2 and β3) promote healing without scar tissue formation. This might suggest that the inhibition of TGF-β1 and the exogenous administration of β2 and β3 would promote healing in the absence of excessive scar tissue formation. Experimental studies have shown that TGF-β1 administration and the suppression of β2 and β3 results in an increased cross-sectional area but a lower failure load (i.e., mechanically inferior tissue quality) [55]. Higher levels of TGF-β have been found in tendinopathic humans, complicating the understanding of its role in human tendon healing [29].

Bone morphogenetic proteins (BMPs)

BMPs - a group of growth factors - were discovered by their ability to induce the formation of bone and cartilage. Two BMPs (BMP-2 and -7) have been approved for clinical application to promote bone regeneration. In Achilles tendon healing, a local injection of BMP -12,-13 or -14 into the haematoma six hours after Achilles tendon transection leads to an approximately 30% increase in total strength after one week in rats [31]. In rabbits, similar effects have been observed at two weeks [30]. These two models used unsutured tendon defects allowing full weight-bearing.

Neuropeptides

In addition to growth factors, neuromediators (so-called neuropeptides) that are released by ingrowing nerve fibres during tendon repair have an essential effect on the healing process [1, 5, 6]. Nerve sprouting and growth within the tendon proper is followed by a time-dependent expression of neuropeptides during the tendon healing process [5]. During inflammatory and early proliferative healing, sensory neuropeptides (e.g., substance P) are mainly released, while during the proliferative phase autonomic neuropeptides emerge [5]. Subsequently, after the healing process is finished, sprouting nerve fibres within the tendon proper retract to the surrounding structures (i.e., the paratenon and surrounding loose connective tissue). Injections of substance P in physiological concentrations into the healing Achilles tendon have be shown to enhance fibroblast aggregation and collagen production and organization, and to increase tensile strength by more than 100% compared with controls (Figure 2) [20, 22, 72].

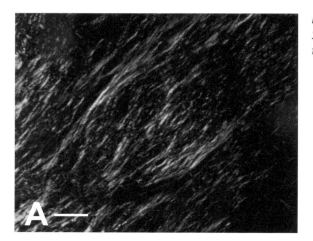

Figure 2A.
Substance P + captopril/
thiorphan-

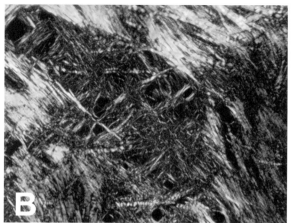

Figure 2B.
Captopril/thiorphan-

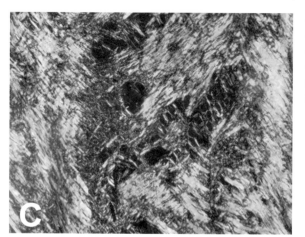

Figure 2C.
Saline-treated rats.
Short green fibres
denote collagen III-like
structures. Scale
bar=200 um.

Figure 2. Sirius red-polarized light micrographs of longitudinal sections through a healing Achilles tendon at one week post-injury of:

Stem cells and gene therapy

Since the optimal delivery of growth factors as yet has been of limited clinical success, molecular approaches have been developed. Mesenchymal stem cells (MSCs) [58], bone marrow stem cells (BMCs) [59] and genetically modified cells, which synthesize and deliver the desired growth factor in a temporally and spatially orchestrated manner to the wound site would be a powerful means to overcome the limitations of various delivery systems [7]. Based on the available gene therapy experiments that have demonstrated the enhancement of tendon repair, the growth factor genes for TGF-B1 [39, 52], PDGF [78, 73], bFGF [28, 79], BMP-2 [62], BMP-12 [51], BMP-13 [41] and BMP-14 [11, 64] may also be good candidates for the promotion of repair.

Orchestration of callus formation

During cell activation and the initiation of matrix production, the healing tendon proper – which is normally practically devoid of nerves and vessels – is successively infiltrated by new nerves and vessels, providing essential neuro-vascular mediators that can orchestrate the repair process (Figures 3-4) [1, 4, 53].

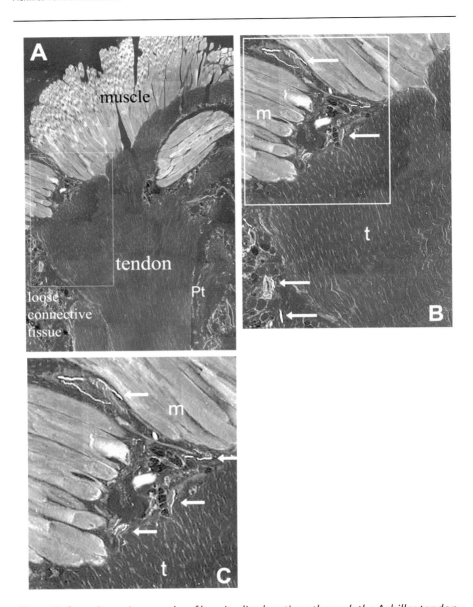

Figure 3. Overview micrographs of longitudinal sections through the Achilles tendon. Incubation with antisera to the general nerve marker PGP 9.5. Micrographs depict the proximal half of the Achilles tendon at increasing magnification in figures (A-C). Arrows denote varicosities and nerve terminals. The typical vascular localization of autonomic neuropeptides is depicted in the lower left (B), whereas the free nerve endings are a typical localization of sensory neuropeptides (C). The immunoreactivity is seen in the paratenon and surrounding loose connective tissue, whereas the proper tendinous tissue, notably, is almost devoid of nerve fibres (pt = paratenon).

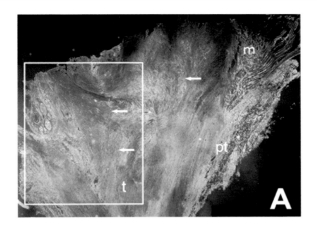

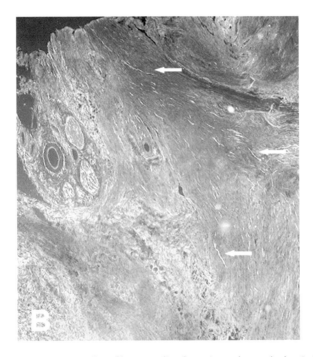

Figure 4. Overview micrographs of longitudinal sections through the Achilles tendon at two weeks post-injury (rupture). Incubation with antisera to a nerve growth marker, GAP-43. Micrographs depict the proximal half of the Achilles tendon at increasing magnification in figures (A-B). Arrows denote varicosities and nerve terminals. The GAP-positive fibres, indicating wound re-innervation, are abundantly observed in the healing tendon tissue.

Neoinnervation and Neovascularization

Our knowledge has evolved regarding the neuronal regulation of tendon repair [6]. New nerve ingrowth within the tendon proper – which is normally aneuronal - is followed by a time-dependent expression of neuropeptides during the tendon healing process (Figure 5) [4]. During the inflammatory and early proliferative phase (i.e., 2-6 weeks after injury), there is a conspicuously increased occurrence of sensory neuropeptides, substance P (SP) and calcitonin gene-related peptide (CGRP) in the healing tendon tissue. SP and CGRP are located partly in free sprouting nerve endings among fibroblasts in the healing tendinous tissue, and partly perivascular to newly-formed blood vessels (Figure 6). These observations possibly reflect a stimulatory role for sensory neuropeptides in cell proliferation, as demonstrated in cultured fibroblasts [57] and endothelial cells [35]. Thus, SP is known to enhance neoangiogenesis [35]. A stimulatory effect on tendon healing has been strengthened by studies demonstrating that the supplementation of SP clearly promoted tendon repair, partly by increasing tensile strength by more than 100% as compared with controls [20, 21, 72]. Accordingly, selective denervation resulting in a lower amount of SP results in impaired tendon healing [15]. Recently, it has been additionally elucidated that SP improves repair by homing stromal stem cells to the site of injury [37]. Therefore, one might conclude that nerve ingrowth and orchestrated SP release guide stem cells to the site of injury.

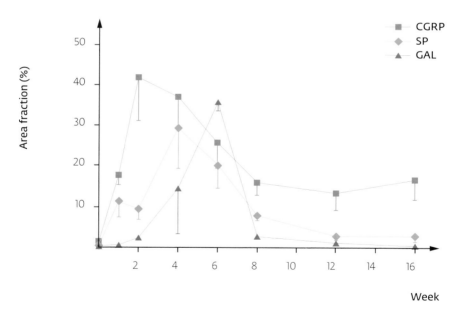

Figure 5. Area occupied by nerve fibres (%) immunoreactive to SP, CGRP and GAL in relation to the total healing area, over 16 weeks post-tendon injury (mean±SEM).

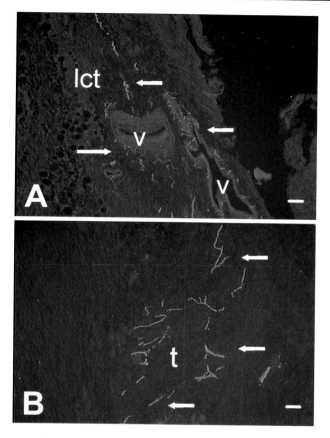

Figure 6. Immunofluorescence micrograph of a healing Achilles tendon 1- (A) and 2- (B) weeks post-rupture after incubation with antisera to CGRP. Nerve fibres immunopositive to CGRP at week one are seen as vascular and free nerve endings in the loose connective tissue (A). At week two, CGRP-immunoreactivity is localized predominantly in the healing tendinous tissue as sprouting free nerve fibres (B). v = blood vessel; lct = loose connective tissue; t = proper tendon tissue; Bar = 50 µm.

However, for healing to progress, the ingrown nerves and vessels have to retract – a process which is promoted by adequate mechanical stimuli. In the case of tendinopathy, an increased number of vessels and sensory nerves with elevated SP-levels have been observed within the tendon proper, indicating an unaccomplished healing process. Thus, signals that regulate nerve and blood vessel retraction are critical in the understanding of preventing tendinopathy. Factors that may regulate nerve retraction and are released upon mechanical stimulus during tendon healing include IL-6 family members [3, 8, 46], neurotrophic factors [12], glutamate [33] and their receptors [18, 38, 69, 70].

Extracorporeal shock wave therapy

Extracorporeal shock wave therapy has been demonstrated to enhance angiogenesis and peripheral nerve regeneration [36, 54]. Novel research efforts to improve tendon and tendon-to-bone healing have included biomedical energy applications such as extracorporeal shock wave therapy, which has shown encouraging clinical effects [65]. Extracorporeal shock wave therapy has also demonstrated positive effects on tendon-to-bone healing by stimulating tenocyte proliferation and collagen synthesis, which are related to an up-regulated gene expression of TGF-beta1, IGF-I and NO release [23, 24]. Shock wave treatment has been shown to be superior to gene therapy for wound healing [40].

Other biomedical applications, such as ultrasound, have also shown promising effects on tendon-to-bone healing by improving osteo-integration and vascularity [77]. Although biophysical methods have demonstrated the potential to promote tendon-to-bone healing, the optimal protocols and underlying mechanisms are far from fully understood.

Conduction of ingrowth

A prerequisite for healing to commence is an existing and functioning tissue matrix into which cells, vessels and nerves can grow, and where the production of new granulation tissue can occur. If a tissue defect exists, the repair process will be prolonged or else will not be able to take place at all. Hence, in non-surgical as well as in the surgical treatment of patients with tendon injuries, it is an important principle to bring the disrupted tendon parts close together for the regulation of fibril fusion and new tissue ingrowth. Small-sized defects can mostly be managed by autologous methods (i.e., repair by the remaining tendon tissue, flap techniques or tendon grafts). Larger defects sometimes need free tendon grafts (e.g., the semitendinosus tendon) and/or scaffolding techniques - either biogenic or synthetic (e.g., bioresorbable polymers) scaffolds. At present, autologous grafts remain the gold standard, while the development of new biogenic and synthetic scaffolds is still under investigation [47].

Modification of the healing callus

Loading

Mechanical loading is the most well-known extrinsic factor adapted to regulate tendon protein synthesis and degradation [49]. One exercise bout in human tendons activates an initial increase in both the synthesis and degradation of collagen. The initial loss of collagen after loading is thus, over time, ensued by a net gain in collagen. Increasing mechanical loading activates myofibroblasts and fibroblasts, to increase the production of collagen type I and increase the callus size, and to enhance the capacity to withstand high mechanical loads. With the loading of the tendon, the orientation of the fibroblasts and collagen changes towards the longitudinal axis of the tendon by four weeks after injury. By then, the mechanical strength of the repairing tendon increases, as there is consolidation and the remodelling of the maturing granulation tissue under tension, and the collagen synthesis under load changes from type III to type I. Various factors influence the rate and quality of tendon healing. The most important is the mechanical tension across the repair, which speeds the realignment of collagen fibres, increases tensile strength and minimizes deformation at the repair site [32]. Early motion accelerates nerve plasticity (i.e., nerve regeneration), the expression of neuromediators and their receptors, and nerve retraction (Figure 7) [16, 17].

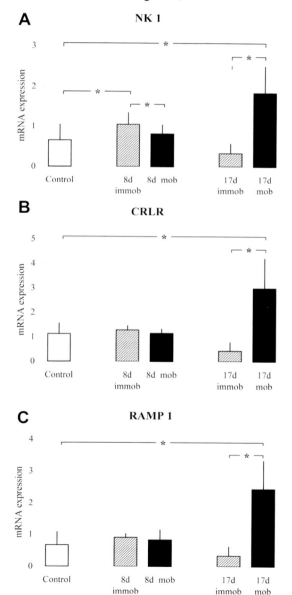

Figure 7. Normalized expression of mRNA for the SP- (NK1) (A) and CGRP- (CRLR (B) and RAMP-1 (C)) receptors in the healing area in the Achilles tendon of rats subjected to two different levels of physical activity (freely mobilized versus plaster immobilized) at eight and 17 days post-rupture (mean+SD). *= p<0.05; n.s. = p>0.05. Between eight and 17 days, there was an immense increase of the receptor expression in the mobile healing group, while the expression in the immobilized healing group fell back to levels comparable to the intact tendon control group.

Immobilization

Mechanical stimuli promote tendon repair, while immobilization is detrimental for healing. In a rat model with the plaster cast immobilization of the hind-limb after Achilles tendon rupture, the ultimate tensile strength was reduced by 80% at two weeks post-rupture compared with a freely-mobilized group [67]. Moreover, in the same model of hind-limb immobilized rats, the mRNA expression of essential sensory neuropeptide receptors (NK-1, RAMP), growth factors (BDNF, bFGF) and extracellular matrix molecules (collagen type I and III, versican, decorin, biglycan) were all down-regulated at two weeks post-rupture [13, 16]. In the same studies, it was demonstrated that a shorter period of immobilization (viz., one week) did not affect the mRNA expression of the above-mentioned molecules (Figure 7). These reports support the notion that prolonged immobilization post-injury hampers the healing process by compromising the up-regulation of repair gene expression in the healing tendon. Moreover, the data also suggest that endogenous as well as exogenously-given growth factors and PRP-therapies may not be effective until mechanical stimulation is initiated, since their receptors are not up-regulated [14].

External tendon activation

One novel method of applying mechanical stimulation to an immobilized tendon could be applied by using external intermittent pneumatic compression (IPC). IPC, which is clinically adapted to prevent thrombosis and increase blood circulation [42], has experimentally-proven positive effects on wound and fracture healing [44, 68], although the mechanisms are still largely unknown. Recently, however, IPC was demonstrated to enhance neuro-vascular ingrowth in a tendon repair model such as to increase the expression of sensory neuropeptides by up to 100% [26]. In the same model, IPC was able – during immobilization – to improve the maximum force by 65%, energy by 168%, the organized collagen diameter by 50%, and collagen III-LI occurrence by 150%, compared with immobilization only [68]. Whether IPC can reverse the negative effects of immobilization in patients still needs to be explored further.

Conclusion

Data after Achilles tendon rupture in patients and results in tendinopathy treatment suggest that there is room for improving healing [60]. However, we still do not know which parameters are most important for an optimal functional outcome. It may prove that the underlying pathology, e.g., tendinopathy, at the time of rupture is one predictor for the outcome after rupture. There is a need for better markers of tendon healing that can be used to predict outcomes and to direct the therapy. Currently, there are no evidence-based therapies except for exercise to promote tendon healing. Well-defined, large clinical studies are necessary to abandon less effective or non-effective therapies and to introduce evidence-based therapy to optimize the outcome after tendon injury.

References

1. Ackermann PW, Ahmed M, Kreicbergs A. Early nerve regeneration after Achilles tendon rupture - a prerequisite for healing? A study in the rat. J Orthop Res. 2002;20(4):849-56.
2. Ackermann PW, Calder J, Aspenberg P. Healing and Repair Mechanisms. DJO Publications; 2008.
3. Ackermann PW, Domeij-Arverud E, Leclerc P, Amoudrouz P, Nader GA. Anti-inflammatory cytokine profile in early human tendon repair. Knee surgery, sports traumatology, arthroscopy: official journal of the ESSKA. 2012.
4. Ackermann PW, Li J, Lundeberg T, Kreicbergs A. Neuronal plasticity in relation to nociception and healing of rat Achilles tendon. J Orthop Res. 2003;21(3):432-41.
5. Ackermann PW, Li J, Lundeberg T, Kreicbergs A. Neuronal plasticity in relation to nociception and healing of rat Achilles tendon. J Orthop Res. 2003;21(3):432-41.
6. Ackermann PW, Salo PT, Hart DA. Neuronal pathways in tendon healing. Front Biosci. 2009;14:5165-87.
7. Ackermann PW, Salo PT, Hart DA. Gene Therapy. In: Van Dijk N, Karlsson J, Maffulli N, editors. Achilles Tendinopathy Current Concept. London: DJO Publications 2010. pp. 165-75.
8. Andersen MB, Pingel J, Kjaer M, Langberg H. Interleukin-6: a growth factor stimulating collagen synthesis in human tendon. J Appl Physiol. 2011;110(6):1549-54.
9. Andia I, Sanchez M, Maffulli N. Tendon healing and platelet-rich plasma therapies. Expert Opin Biol Ther. 10(10):1415-26.
10. Aspenberg P, Virchenko O. Platelet concentrate injection improves Achilles tendon repair in rats. Acta Orthop Scand. 2004;75(1):93-9.
11. Bolt P, Clerk AN, Luu HH, Kang Q, Kummer JL, Deng ZL, et al. BMP-14 gene therapy increases tendon tensile strength in a rat model of Achilles tendon injury. The Journal of Bone and Joint Surgery. 2007;89(6):1315-20.
12. Bring, Reno, Renstrom, Salo, Hart, Ackermann. Prolonged immobilization compromises up-regulation of repair genes after tendon rupture in a rat model. Scand J Med Sci Sports. 2009; 20(3), 411-417.
13. Bring D, Reno, Renstrom, Salo, Hart, Ackermann PW. Prolonged immobilization compromises up-regulation of repair genes after tendon rupture in a rat model. Scand J Med Sci Sports. 2010;20(3):411-7.
14. Bring D, Reno C, Renstrom P, Salo P, Hart D, Ackermann P. Prolonged immobilization compromises up-regulation of repair genes after tendon rupture in a rat model. Scand J Med Sci Sports. 2010;20(3):411-7.
15. Bring DK, Paulson K, Renstrom P, Salo P, Hart DA, Ackermann PW. Residual substance P levels after capsaicin treatment correlate with tendon repair. Wound Repair Regen. 2012;20(1):50-60.
16. Bring DK, Reno C, Renstrom P, Salo P, Hart DA, Ackermann PW. Joint immobilization reduces the expression of sensory neuropeptide receptors and impairs healing after tendon rupture in a rat model. J Orthop Res. 2009;27(2):274-80.
17. Bring DKI, Kreicbergs A, Renstrom PAFH, Ackermann PW. Physical activity modulates nerve plasticity and stimulates repair after Achilles tendon rupture. J Orthop Res. 2007;25(2):164-72.
18. Bring DKI, Reno C, Renstrom P, Salo P, Hart DA, Ackermann PW. Joint immobilization reduces the expression of sensory neuropeptide receptors and impairs healing after tendon rupture in a rat model. J Orthop Res. 2009;27(2):274-80.
19. Broughton G, 2nd, Janis JE, Attinger CE. Wound healing: an overview. Plast Reconstr Surg. 2006;117(7 Suppl):1e-S-32e-S.
20. Burssens P, Steyaert A, Forsyth R, van Ovost EJ, De Paepe Y, Verdonk R. Exogenously administered substance P and neutral endopeptidase inhibitors stimulate fibroblast proliferation, angiogenesis and collagen organization during Achilles tendon healing. Foot Ankle Int. 2005;26(10):832-9.
21. Carlsson O, Schizas N, Li J, Ackermann PW. Substance P Injections Enhance Tissue Proliferation and Regulate Sensory Nerve Ingrowth in Rat Tendon Repair. Scand J Med Sci Sports. 2010;Mar 10. [Epub ahead of print].
22. Carlsson O, Schizas N, Li J, Ackermann PW. Substance P Injections Enhance Tissue Proliferation and Regulate Sensory Nerve Ingrowth in Rat Tendon Repair. Scand J Med Sci Sports. 2011;21(4):562-9.
23. Chao YH, Tsuang YH, Sun JS, Chen LT, Chiang YF, Wang CC, et al. Effects of shock waves on tenocyte proliferation and extracellular matrix metabolism. Ultrasound Med Biol. 2008;34(5):841-52.
24. Chen YJ, Wang CJ, Yang KD, Kuo YR, Huang HC, Huang YT, et al. Extracorporeal shock waves promote healing of collagenase-induced Achilles tendinitis and increase TGF-beta1 and IGF-I expression. J Orthop Res. 2004;22(4):854-61.
25. Christensen B, Dandanell S, Kjaer M, Langberg H. Effect of anti-inflammatory medication on the running-induced rise in patella tendon collagen synthesis in humans. J Appl Physiol. 2011;110(1):137-41.
26. Dahl J, Li J, Bring DK, Renstrom P, Ackermann PW. Intermittent pneumatic compression enhances neurovascular ingrowth and tissue proliferation during connective tissue healing: a study in the rat. J Orthop Res. 2007;25(9):1185-92.

27. Dohnert MB, Venancio M, Possato JC, Zeferino RC, Dohnert LH, Zugno AI, et al. Gold nanoparticles and diclofenac diethylammonium administered by iontophoresis reduce inflammatory cytokines expression in Achilles tendinitis. Int J Nanomedicine. 2012;7:1651-7.

28. Feng Y, Zheng D, Yang S, Li J. Construction of eukaryotic expression plasmid of bFGF gene in rats and its expression in tenocytes. J Huazhong Univ Sci Technolog Med Sci. 2007;27(1):27-30.

29. Fenwick SA, Curry V, Harrall RL, Hazleman BL, Hackney R, Riley GP. Expression of transforming growth factor-beta isoforms and their receptors in chronic tendinosis. J Anat. 2001;199(Pt 3):231-40.

30. Forslund C, Aspenberg P. Improved healing of transected rabbit Achilles tendon after a single injection of cartilage-derived morphogenetic protein-2. The American Journal of Sports Medicine. 2003;31(4):555-9.

31. Forslund C, Rueger D, Aspenberg P. A comparative dose-response study of cartilage-derived morphogenetic protein (CDMP)-1, -2 and -3 for tendon healing in rats. J Orthop Res. 2003;21(4):617-21.

32. Gelberman RH, Manske PR, Akeson WH, Woo SL, Lundborg G, Amiel D. Flexor tendon repair. J Orthop Res. 1986;4(1):119-28.

33. Greve K, Domeij-Arverud E, Labruto F, Edman G, Bring D, Nilsson G, et al. Metabolic activity in early tendon repair can be enhanced by intermittent pneumatic compression. Scand J Med Sci Sports. 2012;22(4):e55-63.

34. Guerra FD, Vieira CP, Dos Santos de Almeida M, Oliveira LP, Claro AC, Simoes GF, et al. Pulsed LLLT improves tendon healing in rats: a biochemical, organizational, and functional evaluation. Lasers in medical science. 2013.

35. Haegerstrand A, Dalsgaard CJ, Jonzon B, Larsson O, Nilsson J. Calcitonin gene-related peptide stimulates proliferation of human endothelial cells. Proc Natl Acad Sci U S A. 1990;87(9):3299-303.

36. Hausner T, Pajer K, Halat G, Hopf R, Schmidhammer R, Redl H, et al. Improved rate of peripheral nerve regeneration induced by extracorporeal shock wave treatment in the rat. Exp Neurol. 2012;236(2):363-70.

37. Hong HS, Lee J, Lee E, Kwon YS, Ahn W, Jiang MH, et al. A new role of substance P as an injury-inducible messenger for mobilization of CD29(+) stromal-like cells. Nat Med. 2009;15(4):425-35.

38. Hou ST, Jiang SX, Smith RA. Permissive and repulsive cues and signalling pathways of axonal outgrowth and regeneration. Int Rev Cell Mol Biol. 2008;267:125-81.

39. Hou Y, Mao Z, Wei X, Lin L, Chen L, Wang H, et al. Effects of transforming growth factor-beta1 and vascular endothelial growth factor 165 gene transfer on Achilles tendon healing. Matrix Biol. 2009;28(6):324-35.

40. Huemer GM, Meirer R, Gurunluoglu R, Kamelger FS, Dunst KM, Wanner S, et al. Comparison of the effectiveness of gene therapy with transforming growth factor-beta or extracorporeal shock wave therapy to reduce ischemic necrosis in an epigastric skin flap model in rats. Wound Repair Regen. 2005;13(3):262-8.

41. Jelinsky SA, Li L, Ellis D, Archambault J, Li J, St Andre M, et al. Treatment with rhBMP12 or rhBMP13 increase the rate and the quality of rat Achilles tendon repair. J Orthop Res. 2011;29(10):1604-12.

42. Kakkos SK, Caprini JA, Geroulakos G, Nicolaides AN, Stansby GP, Reddy DJ. Combined intermittent pneumatic leg compression and pharmacological prophylaxis for prevention of venous thromboembolism in high-risk patients. Cochrane Database Syst Rev. 2008;(4):CD005258.

43. Kaux JF, Drion PV, Colige A, Pascon F, Libertiaux V, Hoffmann A, et al. Effects of platelet-rich plasma (PRP) on the healing of Achilles tendons of rats. Wound Repair Regen. 2012;20(5):748-56.

44. Khanna A, Gougoulias N, Maffulli N. Intermittent pneumatic compression in fracture and soft-tissue injuries healing. Br Med Bull. 2008;88(1):147-56.

45. Kurtz CA, Loebig TG, Anderson DD, DeMeo PJ, Campbell PG. Insulin-like growth factor I accelerates functional recovery from Achilles tendon injury in a rat model. Am J Sports Med. 1999;27(3):363-9.

46. Legerlotz K, Jones ER, Screen HR, Riley GP. Increased expression of IL-6 family members in tendon pathology. Rheumatology (Oxford). 2012;51(7):1161-5.

47. Longo UG, Lamberti A, Maffulli N, Denaro V. Tissue engineered biological augmentation for tendon healing: a systematic review. British Medical Bulletin. 2011;98:31-59.

48. Lyras DN, Kazakos K, Verettas D, Polychronidis A, Tryfonidis M, Botaitis S, et al. The influence of platelet-rich plasma on angiogenesis during the early phase of tendon healing. Foot Ankle Int. 2009;30(11):1101-6.

49. Magnusson SP, Langberg H, Kjaer M. The pathogenesis of tendinopathy: balancing the response to loading. Nat Rev Rheumatol. 2010;6(5):262-8.

50. Magra M, Maffulli N. Nonsteroidal antiinflammatory drugs in tendinopathy: friend or foe. Clin J Sport Med. 2006;16(1):1-3.

51. Majewski M, Betz O, Ochsner PE, Liu F, Porter RM, Evans CH. Ex vivo adenoviral transfer of bone morphogenetic protein 12 (BMP-12) cDNA improves Achilles tendon healing in a rat model. Gene therapy. 2008;15(16):1139-46.

52. Majewski M, Porter RM, Betz OB, Betz VM, Clahsen H, Fluckiger R, et al. Improvement of tendon repair using muscle grafts transduced with TGF-beta1 cDNA. Eur Cell Mater. 2012;23:94-101; discussion -2.

53. Martin P. Wound healing - aiming for perfect skin regeneration. Science (New York, NY). 1997;276(5309):75-81.

54. Mittermayr R, Antonic V, Hartinger J, Kaufmann H, Redl H, Teot L, et al. Extracorporeal shock wave therapy (ESWT) for wound healing: technology, mechanisms, and clinical efficacy. Wound Repair Regen. 2012;20(4):456-65.

55. Molloy T, Wang Y, Murrell G. The roles of growth factors in tendon and ligament healing. Sports Med. 2003;33(5):381-94.

56. Neves MA, Pinfildi CE, Wood VT, Gobbato RC, da Silva FM, Parizotto NA, et al. Different power settings of LLLT on the repair of the calcaneal tendon. Photomed Laser Surg. 2011;29(10):663-8.

57. Nilsson J, von Euler AM, Dalsgaard CJ. Stimulation of connective tissue cell growth by substance P and substance K. Nature. 1985;315(6014):61-3.

58. Nourissat G, Diop A, Maurel N, Salvat C, Dumont S, Pigenet A, et al. Mesenchymal stem cell therapy regenerates the native bone-tendon junction after surgical repair in a degenerative rat model. PLoS One. 2010;5(8):e12248.

59. Okamoto N, Kushida T, Oe K, Umeda M, Ikehara S, Iida H. Treating Achilles tendon rupture in rats with bone-marrow-cell transplantation therapy. J Bone Joint Surg Am. 2010;92(17):2776-84.

60. Olsson N, Nilsson-Helander K, Karlsson J, Eriksson BI, Thomee R, Faxen E, et al. Major functional deficits persist 2 years after acute Achilles tendon rupture. Knee Surg Sports Traumatol Arthrosc. 2011;19(8):1385-93.

61. Paoloni J, De Vos RJ, Hamilton B, Murrell GA, Orchard J. Platelet-rich plasma treatment for ligament and tendon injuries. Clin J Sport Med. 2011;21(1):37-45.

62. Pelled G, Snedeker JG, Ben-Arav A, Rigozzi S, Zilberman Y, Kimelman-Bleich N, et al. Smad8/BMP2-engineered mesenchymal stem cells induce accelerated recovery of the biomechanical properties of the Achilles tendon. J Orthop Res. 2012;30(12):1932-9.

63. Randelli P, Randelli F, Cabitza P, Vaienti L. The effects of COX-2 anti-inflammatory drugs on soft tissue healing: a review of the literature. J Biol Regul Homeost Agents. 2010;24(2):107-14.

64. Rickert M. BMP-14 gene therapy increases tendon tensile strength in a rat model of Achilles tendon injury. The Journal of Bone and Joint Surgery. 2008;90(2):445; author reply -6.

65. Rompe JD, Furia J, Maffulli N. Eccentric loading compared with shock wave treatment for chronic insertional Achilles tendinopathy. A randomized, controlled trial. The Journal of Bone and Joint Surgery. 2008;90(1):52-61.

66. Schepull T, Kvist J, Norrman H, Trinks M, Berlin G, Aspenberg P. Autologous platelets have no effect on the healing of human Achilles tendon ruptures: a randomized single-blind study. Am J Sports Med. 2011;39(1):38-47.

67. Schizas N, Li J, Andersson T, Fahlgren A, Aspenberg P, Ahmed M, et al. Compression therapy promo010;28(7):852-8.

68. Schizas N, Li J, Andersson T, Fahlgren A, Aspenberg P, Ahmed M, et al. Compression therapy promotes tes proliferative repair during rat Achilles tendon immobilization. J Orthop Res. 2 proliferative repair during rat Achilles tendon immobilization. J Orthop Res. 2010;28(7):852-8.

69. Schizas N, Lian O, Frihagen F, Engebretsen L, Bahr R, Ackermann PW. Coexistence of up-regulated NMDA receptor 1 and glutamate on nerves, vessels and transformed tenocytes in tendinopathy. Scand J Med Sci Sports. 2010;20(2):208-15.

70. Schizas N, Weiss R, Lian O, Frihagen F, Bahr R, Ackermann PW. Glutamate receptors in tendinopathic patients. J Orthop Res. 2012;30(9):1447-52.

71. Silva DF, Gomes AS, de Campos Vidal B, Ribeiro MS. Birefringence and Second Harmonic Generation on Tendon Collagen Following Red Linearly Polarized Laser Irradiation. Ann Biomed Eng. 2012.

72. Steyaert AE, Burssens PJ, Vercruysse CW, Vanderstraeten GG, Verbeeck RM. The effects of substance P on the biomechanical properties of ruptured rat Achilles' tendon. Arch Phys Med Rehabil. 2006;87(2):254-8.

73. Suwalski A, Dabboue H, Delalande A, Bensamoun SF, Canon F, Midoux P, et al. Accelerated Achilles tendon healing by PDGF gene delivery with mesoporous silica nanoparticles. Biomaterials. 2010;31(19):5237-45.

74. Tsai WC, Hsu CC, Chang HN, Lin YC, Lin MS, Pang JH. Ibuprofen upregulates expressions of matrix metalloproteinase-1, -8, -9, and -13 without affecting expressions of types I and III collagen in tendon cells. J Orthop Res. 2010;28(4):487-91.

75. Tumilty S, McDonough S, Hurley DA, Baxter GD. Clinical effectiveness of low-level laser therapy as an adjunct to eccentric exercise for the treatment of Achilles' tendinopathy: a randomized controlled trial. Archives of Physical Medicine and Rehabilitation. 2012;93(5):733-9.

76. Tumilty S, Munn J, McDonough S, Hurley DA, Basford JR, Baxter GD. Low level laser treatment of tendinopathy: a systematic review with meta-analysis. Photomedicine and Laser Surgery. 2010;28(1):3-16.

77. Walsh WR, Stephens P, Vizesi F, Bruce W, Huckle J, Yu Y. Effects of low-intensity pulsed ultrasound on tendon-bone healing in an intra-articular sheep knee model. Arthroscopy. 2007;23(2):197-204.

78. Wang XT, Liu PY, Tang JB. Tendon healing in vitro: genetic modification of tenocytes with exogenous PDGF gene and promotion of collagen gene expression. The Journal of Hand Surgery. 2004;29(5):884-90.

79. Wang XT, Liu PY, Xin KQ, Tang JB. Tendon healing in vitro: bFGF gene transfer to tenocytes by adeno-associated viral vectors promotes expression of collagen genes. The Journal of Hand Surgery. 2005;30(6):1255-61.

80. Virchenko O, Aspenberg P. How can one platelet injection after tendon injury lead to a stronger tendon after 4 weeks? Interplay between early regeneration and mechanical stimulation. Acta Orthopaedica. 2006;77(5):806-12.

81. Virchenko O, Skoglund B, Aspenberg P. Parecoxib impairs early tendon repair but improves later remodeling. The American Journal of Sports medicine. 2004;32(7):1743-7.

"Everything that can be counted does not necessarily count; everything that counts cannot necessarily be counted."

Albert Einstein

Chapter 7

Assessment and Outcome Measures

Karin Grävare Silbernagel, Annelie Brorsson, Jón Karlsson

Take Home Message

- *To evaluate outcomes following an Achilles tendon injury, it is important to use reliable, valid and responsive outcome measures.*

- *It is important not to use just one outcome measure, since the aspects of patients' satisfaction and function are multifactorial.*

- *Proper evaluations with validated tests are not only for scientific purposes, but also of importance to the practitioner and the patient in following the progress of treatment and rehabilitation.*

Introduction

Evidence-based medicine is widely accepted, and for evaluating and comparing research studies, valid and reliable outcome measures are needed. Such assessment parameters can also be used as guidelines for prognosis and assist physicians, physical therapists and patients in the decision-making process. In recent years, the demand for validated, reliable and responsive outcome measures that are injury-specific has been growing.

In this chapter, our overall aim is to review valid and reliable outcome measures for evaluating pain, symptoms, physical parameters, strength, endurance and function in patients with Achilles tendon problems.

Patient-reported outcome measures

Clinical measures that can evaluate and quantify patients' symptoms and impairments in body function, activity limitations and participation restrictions, are useful both in the clinical setting and for research. Such measures can be used to determine the severity of injury and evaluate the progression of treatment. Patient-reported outcome measures that are either injury-specific or more general can both be useful. The most important aspect is, however, that the measurements be reliable, valid and responsive for the patient population in question. In this chapter, we will review the outcome measures that are designed for evaluating outcomes in patients with Achilles tendon injuries along with other more general foot and ankle measures that have been used in the literature for this patient group.

Injury-specific questionnaires

Achilles tendinopathy – insertional and mid-portion
The Victorian Institute of Sports Assessment – Achilles questionnaire (VISA-A) [51]

In 2001, this questionnaire was developed as an index of the clinical severity of Achilles tendinopathy [51]. This questionnaire has become well established for evaluating patient-reported outcomes in patients with Achilles tendinopathy. A recent systematic review, analysing the use of the VISA-A score for measuring outcomes in patients with Achilles tendinopathy, found 26 studies that had used VISA-A as an outcome measure [17]. Even though this questionnaire was designed for patients with both mid-portion and insertional injuries, it is not as frequently used in studies on insertional Achilles tendon injuries. It has been used as an outcome measure in a study of the surgical treatment of calcific insertional Achilles tendinopathy [32]. The VISA-A questionnaire is based on and adapted from a similar questionnaire for patellar tendinopathy (the VISA) [63]. In the original VISA-A study [51], validity and reliability were evaluated on a mixed group of patients with diagnoses of Achilles tendinosis, paratendinitis or partial ruptures with or without a retrocalcaneal or Achilles bursitis. It was found to be valid and reliable for evaluating the severity of symptoms in this mixed patient group. The questionnaire has also been cross-culturally adapted and translated into various languages, including Swedish, Italian, German and Turkish [9, 29, 31, 59]. Further evaluations have found the questionnaire to be primarily capable of evaluating two factors, namely *pain/symptoms* and *physical activity*. VISA-A is responsive to changes over time, with an effect size of 2.1 [58, 59]. The results from the various studies support the use of the VISA-A questionnaire as an outcome measure both in research studies and in the clinical setting.

The VISA-A is a self-administered questionnaire. The score ranges between 0-100, and a lower score indicates worse symptoms and greater limitations on physical activity. In the initial study, healthy individuals had a mean score of 97, pre-surgical patients had a mean score of 44, and the non-surgical patients had a mean score of 64 [51]. In the clinic, the VISA-A questionnaire can be used to assess the clinical severity of the patient's symptoms and provide a basic guideline for treatment, as well as for monitoring the effect of treatment over time.

Achilles tendon rupture
The Achilles tendon total rupture score (ATRS) [43]

Until recently, there has not been any injury-specific questionnaire available for evaluating outcome after treatment for acute an Achilles tendon rupture. In 2007, Nilsson-Helander and co-workers [43] developed a patient-reported instrument for evaluating outcomes in patients with a total Achilles tendon rupture – the ATRS. The ATRS evaluates aspects of symptoms and physical activity. The questionnaire consists of 10 items, where the score for each item ranges between 0-10 on a Likert scale, with a maximal score of 100. The total score for patients in their study ranged from 17 to 100, with a mean of 77 (SD 21.4). A significantly ($p < 0.0001$) higher total score was found for the healthy subjects, ranging from 94 to 100 with a mean of 99.8 (SD 1.1). The questionnaire was further evaluated and was shown to have good reliability (test-retest reliability ICC=0.98), validity and responsiveness (an effect size of 0.87-2.21) for evaluating outcomes after treatment in patients with an acute Achilles tendon rupture. The English version of the ATRS has also been shown to have excellent reliability (ICC=0.99) and the results of the Swedish and English versions are comparable both at six and 12 months after injury [8]. Furthermore the effect size for the English version was 0.93, with a minimal detectable change of 6.75 points [8]. A recent systematic review of patient-reported outcome measures for patients with an Achilles tendon rupture concluded that the ATRS was the only outcome measure that had demonstrated validity for use in this patient group [20]. In summary, this questionnaire can be recommended for use both in research and everyday clinical work.

Region-specific questionnaires

Foot- and ankle-specific
The foot and ankle outcome score (FAOS)

The FAOS is a questionnaire that assesses patients' symptoms, functionality and foot- and ankle-related quality of life [52]. The FAOS content is based on the knee injury and osteoarthritis outcome score (KOOS) and has been shown to have good content validity and reliability in patients with ankle injuries [52]. It assesses five different dimensions, such as pain, other symptoms (stiffness, swelling and range of motion), activities of daily living, sports and recreational activities, and foot- and ankle-related quality of life. It has, however, not been validated for patients with Achilles tendon injuries. When used as an outcome measure for patients with Achilles tendinopathy, it has been shown to be responsive to changes over time with treatment [52, 23, 53].

Several questions in the FAOS appear to have low surface validity for evaluating patients with Achilles tendon injury, and it is also more time consuming, making its clinical utility lower in comparison with injury-specific questionnaires. However, certain parts of the FAOS – such as the quality of life section – may be useful in evaluating other aspects of patient satisfaction with treatment. This questionnaire might, therefore, be a good addition to the injury-specific questionnaires in both the clinic and in research.

American orthopaedic foot and ankle -hind foot scale (AOFAS)

The AOFAS scales for various regions of the foot were designed in 1994 by Kitaoka and co-workers [22] with the purpose of providing uniform assessments of outcomes after various types of treatment. These scales incorporate both subjective scores of pain and functionality provided by the patient (either by verbal history descriptions or by written questionnaire) and objective measures of range of motion, stability and alignment measured during the physical examination. The AOFAS ankle-scale is recommended for use in patients with various diagnoses and post-surgery, such as ankle replacement, ankle arthrodesis, ankle instability operations, sub-talar arthrodesis, sub-talar instability operations, talo-navicular arthrodesis, calcaneo-cuboid arthrodesis, calcaneal osteotomy, calcaneus fracture, talus fracture and ankle fracture [22]. The subjective portion has been shown to have satisfactory reliability and responsiveness [16]. It has been validated against SF-36, the foot function index and the Maryland foot score [60]. The scores are normalized to 100, whereby a lower score indicates greater disability. For patients with insertional Achilles tendon injury, these questionnaires have been used as an outcome measure in surgical studies [7, 18, 28, 47, 50]. In these studies (which evaluate a variety of different surgical techniques), the pre-surgical scores ranged between 53 and 62, and the post-surgical scores ranged between 86 and 98. Even though the AOFAS ankle-hind foot scale has been used as an outcome measure in studies of Achilles tendon injuries, it cannot be recommended as the only outcome measure since it has not been evaluated for reliability, validity or responsiveness in this patient population.

The foot and ankle ability measure (FAAM)

This is a questionnaire, filled out by the patient, designed to evaluate the patient's ability to perform activities of daily living (ADLs) and sports [35, 36]. It has been validated for patients with general foot and ankle disorders, and is reported as having good validity, reliability and responsiveness [36]. This score also ranges from 0-100, where the lower score indicates greater disability. For this questionnaire, the minimal clinically important difference is reported to be 8 points for the ADL scale and 9 points for the sport scale [36]. This questionnaire has, however, not been evaluated for use in patients with Achilles tendon injury.

Functional assessment

Patients with Achilles tendon injury have been reported to demonstrate deficits in the joint range of motion, strength, endurance, flexibility and jumping ability [21, 42, 46, 54]. When evaluating the final outcome of treatment, it is therefore important to also include such measurements. To evaluate functional outcomes, it is common to compare the injured side with the healthy side and establish the limb symmetry index expressed as a percentage (involved/uninvolved x100=LSI). For determining the return to sport, a frequently-used criterion is that the LSI for strength and functionality should be at least 85-90%. When using these types of criteria, it is important to have functional measurements that are both reliable and valid.

Range of motion

In the literature, abnormalities in the ankle or sub-talar joint range of motion have been identified as intrinsic risk factors for Achilles tendon injury, and therefore such measurements are often recommended [27,40]. A comparison between the injured and healthy side is usually performed to determine if any deficits exist. The measurement techniques vary from goniometric evaluations to measurements with passive motion in a hydraulic isokinetic dynamometer [15,19,33]. Both types of measurements have their inherit limitations.

Goniometric measurements of ankle dorsiflexion and plantar flexion can be performed with the patient supine or standing, and both passively or actively with the foot carefully placed in a sub-talar neutral position. The arms of the goniometer should be aligned, with the proximal arm along the mid-line of the fibula, the fulcrum at the lateral malleolus, and the distal arm parallel to the fifth metatarsal [44]. When measuring dorsiflexion with the patient standing in a weight-bearing position, the knee can be extended or flexed. Measurements taken with the patient supine are not interchangeable with the measurements taken in a standing weight-bearing position [44]. It has also been shown that measuring ankle joint dorsiflexion with a digital inclinometer placed on the anterior tibial border in a standing position with the knee extended is a reliable method [39]. For evaluating the sub-talar joint range of motion, the patient is in the prone position. The sub-talar joint neutral position is used as the starting position, from where inversion and eversion are measured [11,12]. The sub-talar joint neutral position was defined by Elveru and co-workers [11] as the relative zero position of the sub-talar joint, when the forefoot is passively pronated and the ankle is in dorsiflexion until reaching a soft end-feel, and when the head of the talus is equally extended medially and laterally (neutral position). The goniometer is aligned with the mid-line of the lower leg and the mid-line of the calcaneus [12]. The goniometric range of motion evaluations have been shown to have good intra-tester reliability of the ankle and sub-talar joint, with ICCs ranging from 0.74-0.9 [11]. In terms of inter-tester reliability, the ICCs range from 0.17-0.25 for the sub-talar joint and 0.5-0.72 for the ankle joint [11].

Calf circumference

Circumference measurements are often used in the clinical setting to determine gross muscular hypotrophy. It is important to remember that circumference measurements are affected by swelling and body composition (fat versus muscle). Therefore, increases in circumference may not indicate increased muscle mass or vice versa. Techniques include documenting maximum circumference or measuring at predetermined positions relating to bony landmarks. The maximum calf circumference measurement has been shown to have good reliability (ICC 0.97) [38]. However, this measure has been shown to have a weak correlation to calf muscle endurance and strength [37].

Strength

Strength measurements with dynamometry have been performed in patients with Achilles tendon injury, in both aetiological and prospective treatment studies [37] [1, 2, 15, 34, 41, 49, 62]. Isokinetic dynamometry has been used to test ankle plantarflexion and dorsiflexion strength, both concentrically and eccentrically at various angular velocities, such as 30o/s, 50o/s, 60o/s, 120o/s, 180o/s and 225o/s [1, 2, 15, 34, 41]. Paavola and co-workers [49], on the other hand, measured the isometric strength of the lower limb in an isometric leg press dynamometer. Testa and co-workers [62] measured the maximum isometric muscle activation as well as isometric muscular endurance in patients with Achilles tendinopathy.

The various body positions described in the literature and used in the clinical setting to measure plantarflexion and dorsiflexion strength are supine with the knee and hip extended, sitting with the hip in 100-110 degrees of flexion and the knee in either 40 degrees or 90 degrees of flexion, and a closed-chain position in which the measurement pad is placed on the knee [1, 2, 15, 34, 38, 41]. The reliability of the isokinetic and isometric dynamometry is generally high, and the various testing positions for plantarflexion and dorsiflexion have good test-retest reliability [2, 38]. A test for measuring the muscular strength and power of the ankle plantarflexion in a regular weight-training machine has also been shown to be reliable and valid for patients with Achilles tendinopathy [54]. In this test, muscle power development (i.e., the ability to produce a high force quickly) was evaluated both concentrically and eccentrically-concentrically. The reason for evaluating muscle power was that power is considered to be more important for both sports performance and injury protection compared to the ability to produce a high force [26].

It is, however, important to remember that although strength tests are valid for measuring improvements in strength, they are only moderately correlated to functional performance and they need to be complemented with other types of functional assessment [3].

Endurance test

Muscular endurance testing is another type of muscle function measurement. In a heel-rise test (also called 'heel-raise', 'heel-drop' or 'toe-raise'), the repetitive plantarflexion of the ankle is performed upon standing until fatigued. It is the most commonly-used test for measuring the muscular endurance of the calf musculature. The normal number of heel-rise repetitions on one healthy leg is regarded as being approximately 25, but it can range from six to 70 in healthy individuals [30]. The testing position for the subject is standing on one leg while maintaining a straight knee, supported with the fingertips for balance and avoiding body sway forward. It is important to instruct the patient to go as high as possible for every heel-rise. A metronome can be used to ensure consistent rhythm and a frequency of 30 heel-rises per minute has been used in some research studies [54, 55]. This test has been used in several research studies and has shown good reliability (ICC 0.78-0.84) [38, 61]. The heel-rise test has been used in evaluations of patients with all types of Achilles tendon injury [6, 42, 46, 57]. In patients with Achilles tendon rupture, Häggmark and co-workers [14] used a light beam at a height of 5 cm above the floor, and only the number of heel rises above the light beam was counted. One method to evaluate heel-rise endurance measures not only the number of repetitions that the patients can perform but also the height of each heel-rise [55]. In patients with Achilles tendinopathy, no side-to-side differences in heel-rise height were found, but in patients with Achilles tendon rupture the injured side had a significant deficit compared to the healthy side [55]. The side-to-side differences in heel-rise height, when comparing the injured and healthy sides in patients with an Achilles tendon rupture, have also been shown to correlate with the occurrence of tendon elongation on the injured side [56]. A correlation between isokinetic strength measurement and heel rise test has been reported by Möller and co-workers [38].

Jump tests

Various jump tests are often used to evaluate functionality in patients with lower extremity injuries, as well as to evaluate functional performance in athletes [10, 45, 48]. High loads occur on the Achilles tendon during activities in which the so-called 'stretch-shortening cycle' (SSC) is utilized [13, 25]. The SSC is a combination of an eccentric muscle action (with the lengthening of the muscle and tendon), immediately followed by a concentric muscle action (a shortening of the muscle-tendon complex) [5,4]. The concentric force production will be higher when preceded by an eccentric muscle action compared with a pure concentric muscle action [5, 24]. The efficiency of utilizing the SSC in various types of jumps reportedly ranges from 17-34% [4,13]. The Achilles tendon's elasticity is important for storing and releasing energy during the SSC, and thereby improves the economy and performance of the motion [13, 24]. Changes in lower leg functions, such as muscle-tendon strength, endurance, flexibility and motor control, could all affect the various mechanisms in the SSC [15, 61].

Jump tests, such as counter-movement jumps (CMJs), squat jumps (SJs) and hopping, have been used to evaluate the loading of the Achilles tendon [25]. CMJs and SJs are vertical jumps, where the jump height is used for the evaluation. In a CMJ, the starting position is upright whereas for an SJ the starting position is with the knees bent. Hopping is a continuous rhythmical jump, similar to a jumping rope, and here the contact times and flight times are usually evaluated [13,25]. A drop counter-movement jump (drop CMJ) is performed jumping down from a box/step and, directly upon landing, then performing a maximal vertical jump. This type of jump is often used in training to improve jumping ability in athletes, and it also places high demands on the ability to utilize the SSC. All these jump tests have been used to evaluate the functional outcome in patients with both Achilles tendinopathy and Achilles tendon rupture [42, 46, 54, 57]. Another frequently-used jump test is the one-legged hop for distance, which has also been used in a prospective study to identify the intrinsic risk factors for Achilles tendon overuse injury [34].

Summary

Achilles tendon injury causes pain, difficulty with physical activity and impairments in various aspects of lower leg function. It is, therefore, important to continuously evaluate the patients' progress with both validated subjective scoring systems and various validated functional tests. Moreover, the patients' ability to return to previous physical activity and sports are important outcome measures. Proper evaluations with validated tests are not only for scientific purposes, but also of importance to the practitioner and the patient in following the progress of treatment and rehabilitation.

References

1. Alfredson H, Pietilä T, Jonsson P, Lorentzon R. Heavy-load eccentric calf muscle training for the treatment of chronic Achilles tendinosis. Am J Sports Med. 1998; 26: 360-6.
2. Alfredson H, Pietilä T, Öhberg L, Lorentzon R. Achilles tendinosis and calf muscle strength. The effect of short-term immobilization after surgical treatment. Am J Sports Med. 1998; 26: 166-71.
3. Augustsson J, Thomeé R. Ability of closed and open kinetic chain tests of muscular strength to assess functional performance. Scand J Med Sci Sports. 2000; 10: 164-8.
4. Belli A, Bosco C. Influence of stretch-shortening cycle on mechanical behaviour of triceps surae during hopping. Acta Physiol Scand. 1992; 144: 401-8.
5. Bosco C, Tarkka I, Komi PV. Effect of elastic energy and myoelectrical potentiation of triceps surae during stretch-shortening cycle exercise. Int J Sports Med. 1982; 3: 137-40.
6. Bostick GP, Jomha NM, Suchak AA, Beaupre LA. Factors associated with calf muscle endurance recovery 1 year after Achilles tendon rupture repair. J Orthop Sports Phys Ther. 2010; 40: 345-51.
7. Brunner J, Anderson J, O'Malley M, Bohne W, Deland J, Kennedy J. Physician and patient based outcomes following surgical resection of Haglund's deformity. Acta Orthop Belg. 2005; 71: 718-23.
8. Carmont MR, Silbernagel KG, Nilsson-Helander K, Mei-Dan O, Karlsson J, Maffulli N. Cross cultural adaptation of the Achilles tendon total rupture score with reliability, validity and responsiveness evaluation. Knee Surg Sports Traumatol Arthrosc. 2012. 21(6):1356-60
9. Dogramaci Y, Kalaci A, Kucukkubas N, Inandi T, Esen E, Yanat AN. Validation of the VISA-A questionnaire for Turkish language: the VISA-A-Tr study. Br J Sports Med. 2011; 45: 453-5.
10. Eastlack ME, Axe MJ, Snyder-Mackler L. Laxity, instability, and functional outcome after ACL injury: copers versus noncopers. Med Sci Sports Exerc. 1999; 31: 210-5.
11. Elveru RA, Rothstein JM, Lamb RL. Goniometric reliability in a clinical setting. Subtalar and ankle joint measurements. Phys Ther. 1988; 68: 672-7.
12. Elveru RA, Rothstein JM, Lamb RL, Riddle DL. Methods for taking subtalar joint measurements. A clinical report. Phys Ther. 1988; 68: 678-82.
13. Fukashiro S, Komi PV, Järvinen M, Miyashita M. In vivo Achilles tendon loading during jumping in humans. Eur J Appl Physiol Occup Physiol. 1995; 71: 453-8.
14. Haggmark T, Liedberg H, Eriksson E, Wredmark T. Calf muscle atrophy and muscle function after non-operative vs. operative treatment of Achilles tendon ruptures. Orthopedics. 1986; 9: 160-4.
15. Haglund-Åkerlind Y, Eriksson E. Range of motion, muscle torque and training habits in runners with and without Achilles tendon problems. Knee Surg Sports Traumatol Arthrosc. 1993; 1: 195-9.
16. Ibrahim T, Beiri A, Azzabi M, Best AJ, Taylor GJ, Menon DK. Reliability and validity of the subjective component of the American Orthopaedic Foot and Ankle Society clinical rating scales. J Foot Ankle Surg. 2007; 46: 65-74.
17. Iversen JV, Bartels EM, Langberg H. The Victorian Institute of Sports Assessment - Achilles questionnaire (VISA-A) - a reliable tool for measuring Achilles tendinopathy. International Journal of Sports Physical Therapy. 2012; 7: 76-84.
18. Johnson KW, Zalavras C, Thordarson DB. Surgical management of insertional calcific Achilles tendinosis with a central tendon splitting approach. Foot Ankle Int. 2006; 27: 245-50.
19. Kaufman KR, Brodine SK, Shaffer RA, Johnson CW, Cullison TR. The effect of foot structure and range of motion on musculoskeletal overuse injuries. Am J Sports Med. 1999; 27: 585-93.
20. Kearney RS, Achten J, Lamb SE, Plant C, Costa ML. A systematic review of patient-reported outcome measures used to assess Achilles tendon rupture management: what's being used and should we be using it? Br J Sports Med. 2012; 46: 1102-9.
21. Khan RJ, Carey Smith RL. Surgical interventions for treating acute Achilles tendon ruptures. Cochrane database of systematic reviews (Online). 2010: CD003674.
22. Kitaoka HB, Alexander IJ, Adelaar RS, Nunley JA, Myerson MS, Sanders M. Clinical rating systems for the ankle-hind foot, mid-foot, hallux and lesser toes. Foot Ankle Int. 1994; 15: 349-53.
23. Knobloch K, Schreibmueller L, Longo UG, Vogt PM. Eccentric exercises for the management of tendinopathy of the main body of the Achilles tendon with or without the AirHeel Brace. A randomized controlled trial. A: effects on pain and microcirculation. Disabil Rehabil. 2008; 30: 1685-91.
24. Komi PV. Stretch-shortening cycle: a powerful model to study normal and fatigued muscle. J Biomech. 2000; 33: 1197-206.
25. Komi PV, Fukashiro S, Järvinen M. Biomechanical loading of Achilles tendon during normal locomotion. Clin Sports Med. 1992; 11: 521-31.
26. Kraemer WJ, Adams K, Cafarelli E, Dudley GA, Dooly C, Feigenbaum MS, Fleck SJ, Franklin B, Fry AC, Hoffman JR, Newton RU, Potteiger J, Stone MH, Ratamess NA, Triplett-McBride T. American College of Sports Medicine position stand. Progression models in resistance training for healthy adults. Med Sci Sports Exerc. 2002; 34: 364-80.

27. Kvist M. Achilles tendon injuries in athletes. Ann Chir Gynaecol. 1991; 80: 188-201.

28. Leitze Z, Sella EJ, Aversa JM. Endoscopic decompression of the retrocalcaneal space. J Bone Joint Surg Am. 2003; 85-A: 1488-96.

29. Lohrer H, Nauck T. Cross-cultural adaptation and validation of the VISA-A questionnaire for German-speaking Achilles tendinopathy patients. BMC Musculoskelet Disord. 2009; 10: 134.

30. Lunsford BR, Perry J. The standing heel-rise test for ankle plantar flexion: criterion for normal. Phys Ther. 1995; 75: 694-8.

31. Maffulli N, Longo UG, Testa V, Oliva F, Capasso G, Denaro V. Italian translation of the VISA-A score for tendinopathy of the main body of the Achilles tendon. Disabil Rehabil. 2008; 30: 1635-9.

32. Maffulli N, Testa V, Capasso G, Sullo A. Calcific insertional Achilles tendinopathy: reattachment with bone anchors. Am J Sports Med. 2004; 32: 174-82.

33. Mahieu NN, Witvrouw E, Stevens V, Van Tiggelen D, Roget P. Intrinsic risk factors for the development of Achilles tendon overuse injury: a prospective study. Am J Sports Med. 2006; 34: 226-35.

34. Mahieu NN, Witvrouw E, Stevens V, Van Tiggelen D, Roget P. Intrinsic Risk Factors for the Development of Achilles Tendon Overuse Injury: A Prospective Study. Am J Sports Med. 2005.

35. Martin RL, Irrgang JJ. A survey of self-reported outcome instruments for the foot and ankle. J Orthop Sports Phys Ther. 2007; 37: 72-84.

36. Martin RL, Irrgang JJ, Burdett RG, Conti SF, Van Swearingen JM. Evidence of validity for the foot and ankle ability measure (FAAM). Foot Ankle Int. 2005; 26: 968-83.

37. Moller M, Lind K, Movin T, Karlsson J. Calf muscle function after Achilles tendon rupture. A prospective, randomised study comparing surgical and non-surgical treatment. Scand J Med Sci Sports. 2002; 12: 9-16.

38. Möller M, Lind K, Styf J, Karlsson J. The reliability of isokinetic testing of the ankle joint and a heel-raise test for endurance. Knee Surg Sports Traumatol Arthrosc. 2005; 13: 60-71.

39. Munteanu SE, Strawhorn AB, Landorf KB, Bird AR, Murley GS. A weightbearing technique for the measurement of ankle joint dorsiflexion with the knee extended is reliable. J Sci Med Sport. 2009; 12: 54-9.

40. Myerson MS, McGarvey W. Disorders of the Achilles tendon insertion and Achilles tendinitis. Instr Course Lect. 1999; 48: 211-8.

41. Niesen-Vertommen S, Taunton J, Clement D, Mosher R. The effect of eccentric versus concentric exercise in the management of Achilles tendonitis. Clin J Sport Med. 1992; 2: 109-13.

42. Nilsson-Helander K, Silbernagel KG, Thomee R, Faxen E, Olsson N, Eriksson BI, Karlsson J. Acute Achilles tendon rupture: a randomized, controlled study comparing surgical and nonsurgical treatments using validated outcome measures. Am J Sports Med. 2010; 38: 2186-93.

43. Nilsson-Helander K, Thomee R, Gravare-Silbernagel K, Thomee P, Faxen E, Eriksson BI, Karlsson J. The Achilles tendon total rupture score (ATRS): development and validation. Am J Sports Med. 2007; 35: 421-6.

44. Norkin CC, White DJ. Measurement of joint motion: a guide to goniometry. Philadelphia: Davis; 1985.

45. Noyes FR, Barber SD, Mangine RE. Abnormal lower limb symmetry determined by function hop tests after anterior cruciate ligament rupture. Am J Sports Med. 1991; 19: 513-8.

46. Olsson N, Nilsson-Helander K, Karlsson J, Eriksson BI, Thomee R, Faxen E, Silbernagel KG. Major functional deficits persist 2 years after acute Achilles tendon rupture. Knee Surg Sports Traumatol Arthrosc. 2011; 19: 1385-93.

47. Ortmann FW, McBryde AM. Endoscopic bony and soft-tissue decompression of the retrocalcaneal space for the treatment of Haglund deformity and retrocalcaneal bursitis. Foot Ankle Int. 2007; 28: 149-53.

48. Östenberg A, Roos E, Ekdahl C, Roos H. Isokinetic knee extensor strength and functional performance in healthy female soccer players. Scand J Med Sci Sports. 1998; 8: 257-64.

49. Paavola M, Kannus P, Paakkala T, Pasanen M, Järvinen M. Long-term prognosis of patients with Achilles tendinopathy. An observational 8-year follow-up study. Am J Sports Med. 2000; 28: 634-42.

50. Philippot R, Wegrzyn J, Grosclaude S, Besse JL. Repair of insertional Achilles tendinosis with a bone-quadriceps tendon graft. Foot Ankle Int. 2010; 31: 802-6.

51. Robinson JM, Cook JL, Purdam C, Visentini PJ, Ross J, Maffulli N, Taunton JE, Khan KM. The VISA-A questionnaire: a valid and reliable index of the clinical severity of Achilles tendinopathy. Br J Sports Med. 2001; 35: 335-41.

52. Roos EM, Brandsson S, Karlsson J. Validation of the foot and ankle outcome score for ankle ligament reconstruction. Foot Ankle Int. 2001; 22: 788-94.

53. Roos EM, Engström M, Lagerquist A, Söderberg B. Clinical improvement after 6 weeks of eccentric exercise in patients with mid-portion Achilles tendinopathy - a randomized trial with 1-year follow-up. Scand J Med Sci Sports. 2004; 14: 286-95.

54. Silbernagel KG, Gustavsson A, Thomee R, Karlsson J. Evaluation of lower leg function in patients with Achilles tendinopathy. Knee Surg Sports Traumatol Arthrosc. 2006; 14: 1207-17.

55. Silbernagel KG, Nilsson-Helander K, Thomee R, Eriksson BI, Karlsson J. A new measurement of heel-rise endurance with the ability to detect functional deficits in patients with Achilles tendon rupture. Knee Surg Sports Traumatol Arthrosc. 2010; 18: 258-64.

56. Silbernagel KG, Steele R, Manal K. Deficits in heel-rise height and Achilles tendon elongation occur in patients recovering from an Achilles tendon rupture. Am J Sports Med. 2012; 40: 1564-71.

57. Silbernagel KG, Thomee R, Eriksson BI, Karlsson J. Continued sports activity, using a pain-monitoring model, during rehabilitation in patients with Achilles tendinopathy: a randomized controlled study. Am J Sports Med. 2007; 35: 897-906.

58. Silbernagel KG, Thomee R, Eriksson BI, Karlsson J. Full symptomatic recovery does not ensure full recovery of muscle-tendon function in patients with Achilles tendinopathy. Br J Sports Med. 2007; 41: 276-80;.

59. Silbernagel KG, Thomeé R, Karlsson J. Cross-cultural adaptation of the VISA-A questionnaire, an index of clinical severity for patients with Achilles tendinopathy, with reliability, validity and structure evaluations. BMC Musculoskelet Disord. 2005; 6: 12.

60. Suk M. Musculoskeletal outcomes measures and instruments. New York: Thieme; 2005.

61. Svantesson U, Carlsson U, Takahashi H, Thomeé R, Grimby G. Comparison of muscle and tendon stiffness, jumping ability, muscle strength and fatigue in the plantar flexors. Scand J Med Sci Sports. 1998; 8: 252-6.

62. Testa V, Capasso G, Benazzo F, Maffulli N. Management of Achilles tendinopathy by ultrasound-guided percutaneous tenotomy. Med Sci Sports Exerc. 2002; 34: 573-80.

63. Visentini PJ, Khan KM, Cook JL, Kiss ZS, Harcourt PR, Wark JD. The VISA score: an index of severity of symptoms in patients with jumper's knee (patellar tendinosis). Victorian Institute of Sport Tendon Study Group. J Sci Med Sport. 1998; 1: 22-8.

"The eye of the master will do more work than both his hands."

Benjamin Franklin

CHAPTER 8

IMAGING OF THE ACHILLES TENDON

Ruben Zwiers, Maayke N. van Sterkenburg, C. Niek van Dijk

Take Home Message

• *Imaging plays a pivotal role in Achilles tendon pathology because, on clinical examination, the exact origin of pain can often be hard to elucidate.*

• *An Achilles tendon rupture is diagnosed clinically. In doubtful or partial rupture cases, ultrasonography can be performed to confirm the diagnosis.*

• *Ultrasound and MRI both play important roles in the assessment of mid-portion Achilles tendinopathy.*

Introduction

A rupture of the Achilles tendon is easily diagnosed clinically. With the increasing interest in the disorders of the Achilles tendon and the increase in specialized imaging modalities, physicians are now aware of a number of further disorders affecting the main body of the Achilles tendon, which include mid-portion or insertional tendinopathy and paratendinopathy. Complex chronic trauma and/or partial ruptures may hamper clinical examination and the sensitivity of the clinical diagnosis [10]. Tendinopathy and paratendinopathy may also result in a thickening of the heel, and may not be accurately differentiated by clinical examination alone.

The imaging modalities that are primarily used in patients with Achilles tendinopathy are ultrasonography (US) and/or magnetic resonance imaging (MRI) [5, 11, 21]. Conventional radiographs are useful in evaluating possible bony abnormalities, such as a postero-superior calcaneal prominence [11, 29]. Imaging is useful for documenting tendon pathology and outlining other causes of patients' symptoms [5, 11, 21, 32, 33]. An overview of the advantages and disadvantages is provided in Table 1.

	Radiograph	Ultrasound	MRI
Insertional Achilles Tendinopathy			
Pros	– Detection of bony spurs, calcifications	– Detection of bony spurs, calcifications	– Allows analysis of all possible pain generators
Cons	– Not useful in detecting soft-tissue abnormalities		
Retrocalcaneal Bursitis			
Pros	– Both high sensitivity and specificity – Detection of postero-superior calcaneal prominence	– High specificity	– Superior diagnostic tool for retrocalcaneal bursitis
Cons		– Low sensitivity	
Mid-Portion Tendinopathy			
Pros		– Neo-vascularization can be detected using colour Doppler	– Excellent sensitivity (94%) – Good specificity (84%)
Cons	– Not useful	– Difficult to diagnose paratendinopathy	
Achilles Tendon Ruptures			
Pros		– Dynamic examination in dorsiflexion and plantarflexion: differentiation between partial and complete ruptures. – Differentiate synovial thickening from fluid around the tendon – Useful in localising tendon ends for pre-operative planning	– Clear image of internal splits and tears
Cons	– Not useful		

Table 1. Overview of the advantages and disadvantages of the different imaging modalities.

In this chapter, the radiography, ultrasound and MRI of the Achilles tendon will be described. The characteristic imaging findings in the various pathologies around the Achilles tendon will be illustrated and described.

Imaging modalities

Radiography

Plain radiography has long been abandoned for assessing Achilles tendinopathy, although it is still frequently performed in patients with heel pain. Plain radiographs can be valuable in demonstrating calcification or spurs and other possible causes for heel pain, including the obliteration of the retrocalcaneal recess in the case of retrocalcaneal bursitis [37].

Ultrasound

Ultrasound is quick, safe and inexpensive, but it is regarded as user-dependent and requires an experienced radiologist [27]. Ultrasound is valuable in detecting the occurrence and location of tendon lesions, but it is unable to differentiate between partial tendon ruptures and focal degenerative tendinopathy [2, 22]. Sometimes, mild to moderate changes can be found in both symptomatic and asymptomatic tendons, and the changes seen are not always related to patients' symptoms [7, 22, 24].

MRI

MRI is less user-dependent, and is regarded as accurate at visualizing the pathological conditions of the tendon and peritendinous structures [11, 21, 27]. Since ultrasound images are dynamic and can only be interpreted by the manufacturer, MRI – and especially its three-dimensional element – is valuable for pre-operative planning.

Normal appearance of Achilles tendon

Radiography

A normal Achilles tendon appears as a stripe of soft tissue density, with smooth and parallel margins from the soleus origin to the calcaneal insertion. The contour of the tendon is easily visualized because the pre-Achilles fat pad provides a high contrast interface with the anterior tendon surface. The pre-Achilles fat pad, formerly known as Kager's fat pad, is less dense than the tendon, appears as a black triangle between the tendon and the muscles and tendons of the ankle. The pre-Achilles fat pad is an important landmark, since it can be obliterated by inflamed tissue, scar tissue and post-traumatic bleeding [15, 25] (Figure 1).

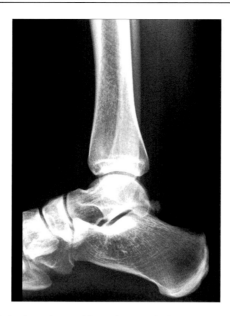

Figure 1. Lateral weight-bearing ankle radiograph showing the normal appearance of the Achilles tendon and calcaneus.

Ultrasound

The Achilles tendon normally demonstrates a homogeneous fibrillar structure on the sagittal scans, with approximately 6-8 characteristic undulating lines of internal echoes that reflect the acoustic borders between the collagen fibrils and loose connective tissue between the fascicles [12]. Axial imaging demonstrates the oval shape of the tendon, which has a superficial convexity and a deep concavity. Occasionally, in some individuals, the tendon is divided by a hyperechogenic septum. The tendon is well demonstrated as bordering its subcutaneous fatty tissue by the paratendon, a visible hyperechogenic line situated at the anterior and posterior borders (Figure 2).

Anterior to the Achilles tendon, the pre-Achilles fat pad can be found. Along with the Achilles tendon, the fat pad fills the distal part of the triceps surae compartment of the calf. This structure typically shows a mottled echo texture; however, there is marked individual variability.

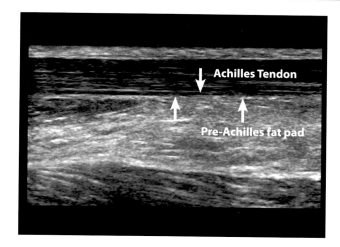

Figure 2. Longitudinal ultrasound image of the normal appearance of the mid-portion of the Achilles tendon. The arrowheads point to the hyperechogenic paratendon.

In one series, normal tendon thickness ranged from 4.0-6.7 mm (mean 5.2 mm) in 24 subjects[12]. In subjects with asymptomatic tendons, a sonographic thickness of more than 6 mm was related to intensive sport, suggesting physiological adaptation to mechanical stress.

The sonographic findings of the insertion of the Achilles tendon are demonstrated as a strong echogenic border against the bone (Figure 3). The tendon flattens and covers the calcaneus. Interestingly, in children, a broad layer of hyaline cartilage covers the posterior aspect of the calcaneus, and by using high resolution probes the structure of the hyaline cartilage can be demonstrated as speckled hyperechogenic foci within a relatively hypoechogenic matrix. Between the Achilles tendon and the supero-posterior aspect of the calcaneus, a small crescent-shaped bursa (retrocalcaneal bursa) can be demonstrated as a thin hypoechogenic structure (Figure 3). The shape and position of this bursa will vary depending on the degree of flexion and extension of the ankle.

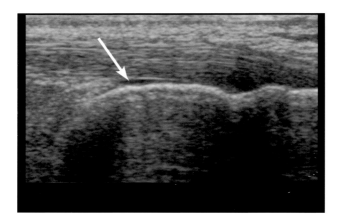

Figure 3. Longitudinal ultrasound image showing the normal appearance of the retrocalcaneal bursa. The bursa appears as a thin hypoechoic structure.

MRI

Typical MRI findings of the Achilles tendon indicate a low signal homogeneous structure on both T1- and T2-weighted images (Figure 4). Occasionally, punctuated and short linear high foci are seen, especially on the anterior aspect of the tendons in the axial series [17].

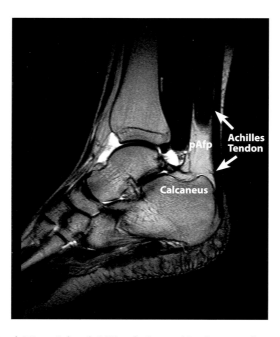

Figure 4. Sagittal T1-weighted MRI of the ankle. Image showing the normal appearance or the Achilles tendon.

The plantaris tendon may be visible as a linear structure passing through the medial distal portion of the pre-Achilles fat pad. It arises from the lower part of the lateral supracondylar line and has a small fusiform belly, which forms a long slender tendon that obliquely crosses the calf between the gastrocnemius and the soleus and inserts onto the calcaneus medial to the Achilles tendon. This may be absent in 10% of patients. Occasionally, the tendon may blend into the medial fibres of the Achilles in the lower third of the calf (Figure 5).

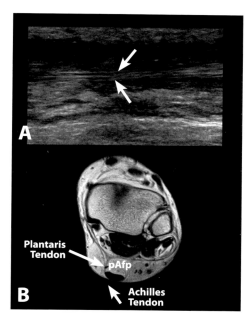

Figure 5. Plantaris tendon: (A) Longitudinal ultrasound images showing the Plantaris tendon; (B) Axial T1-weighted MRI showing the plantaris tendon located at the medial side of the pre-Achilles fat pad.

The use of intravenous gadolinium demonstrates the normal enhancing synovium in the bursa. The tendon and the paratendon do not enhance in normal individuals, and enhancement may be demonstrated around the paratendon on pathological states. Further developments using ultra-short TE (UTE) in higher field strength MRI scanners can produce a signal from the tendon in orthogonal planes [36].

Mid-portion Achilles tendinopathy

Ultrasound

Excluding the paratendon, there are four typical sonographic findings in patients with clinical Achilles signs and symptoms. Sonographic findings include normal tendons, enlarged tendons (spindle-shape/fusiform thickening), hypoechoic and hyperechogenic lesions within the tendons, and power Doppler imaging showing neo-vascularization (Figure 6).

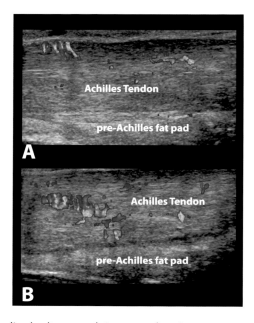

Figure 6. Longitudinal ultrasound images showing neo-vascularization of the mid-portion of the Achilles tendon located at: (A) the paratendon; (B) central part of the tendon.

In patients with a clinical diagnosis of Achilles tendinopathy, Archambault and co-workers demonstrated a significant longer recovery time in enlarged tendons and tendons with hypoechoic lesions compared with tendons with normal appearance [1]. Furthermore, patients without sonographic changes had significantly better clinical outcomes after non-surgical treatment [20]. Moreover, patients with tendon thickening and circumscribed lesions had higher rates of spontaneous tendon rupture. Achilles tendinopathy typically affects the middle third of the Achilles tendon. Gibbon and co-workers demonstrated that small micro-ruptures, indicative of a tendinopathic process were present in approximately 28% of normal individuals [8]. Conversely, only 18% of athletes with chronic Achilles tendinopathy did not show ultrasonographic evidence of intra-tendinous damage. Patients with a partial tendon rupture all had micro-ruptures in the middle third of the Achilles tendon. The increased frequency of micro-ruptures was significantly associated with Achilles tendon rupture.

A more recent study performed by Leung and co-workers [14] concluded that Achilles tendinopathy results in enlargement and, more particularly, in the mid- and distal-portions of the tendon, with damage to the normal intratendinous fibrillar pattern and an associated increase in tendon vascularity. Additional signs included increased Kager's fat pad echogenicity and paratendon thickening. Tendon calcification and changes in the retrocalcaneal bursa and calcaneal contour were not specific for Achilles tendinopathy. Over the last ten years, there has been increasing interest in the neo-vascularization of the Achilles tendon, and a number of studies have assessed the usefulness of colour Doppler ultrasound [26, 39]. Neo-vascularization is specific for patient's pain, but it does not indicate an unfavourable outcome, although tendon inhomogeneity does. Furthermore, power Doppler imaging demonstrates significantly greater microvascularity than colour Doppler imaging. All neo-vascularity appears to arise from the ventral side of the Achilles tendon, with a non-linear relationship between tendinopathy, tendon size and microvascularity. However, there is a direct relationship between power Doppler imaging and the duration of symptoms. Moreover, it was unlikely that neo-vascularization occurs in tendons smaller than 6 mm. Symptoms of Achilles tendinopathy may be indistinguishable from those of paratendinopathy. The typical findings are a normal Achilles tendon with a circumferential hypoechogenic halo around the tendon, often combined with an (echogenic) thickening of the paratendon (Figure 7). Power Doppler imaging may reveal hyper-vascularity. Ultrasound is superseded by contrast-enhanced MRI for the detection of Achilles paratendinopathy. Frequently, Achilles tendinopathy and paratendinopathy co-exist.

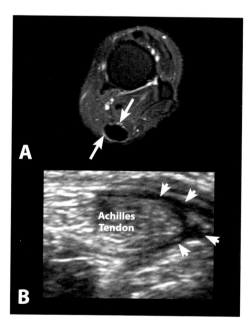

Figure 7. Paratendinopathy of the Achilles tendon: (A) Axial T2-weighted MRI showing a high signal at the paratendon; (B) Axial ultrasound image showing a hypoechogenic halo around the Achilles tendon.

MRI

Over the last decade, MRI has proven to be a sensitive and specific technique for assessing the Achilles tendon and tendon abnormalities.

For Achilles tendon abnormalities, the overall sensitivity of MRI is 94%, with a specificity of 81% and a positive predicted value of 90% [14] (Figure 8). With more refined imaging sequences, sensitivity and specificity are likely to improve. Furthermore, as many as 68% of patients in that study with an associated intratendinous lesion also exhibited evidence of paratendinopathy, a finding supporting in the earlier work of Schepsis and co-workers [28].

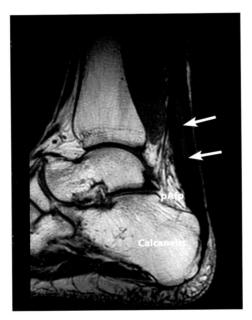

Figure 8. Sagittal T1-weighted MRI showing the thickening of the Achilles tendon mid-portion, central enhancement is seen, consistent with intra-tendinous neo-vascularization.

Achilles tendon ruptures

Radiography

Plain radiological examinations have their main value in diagnosing an avulsion rupture, calcaneal exostoses or any other bony pathology at the calcaneal tuberosity.

Ultrasound

With ultrasound, the tendon should be examined in both longitudinal and axial planes [38]. An acute tendon rupture mostly appears as a focal lucency in the tendon, with a small amount of fluid in and surrounding the tendon. The frayed ends of the tendons can be detected, and they separate in dorsiflexion. In 75% of acute cases, a nearly complete juxtaposition of the stumps can be seen (Figure 9). In dorsiflexion, a visible gap can be shown in patients with a complete rupture. In partial ruptures, the proximal gliding of the tendon and tendon muscle unit can be depicted. In plantarflexion, the full juxtaposition of the tendon stumps that has been used as a basis for non-surgical treatment can be assessed [34, 35]. In chronic ruptures, complete juxtaposition is not possible, and a haematoma is seen between the tendon stumps, even in plantar flexion.

Ultrasound is effective in differentiating synovial thickening from the fluid around the tendon. As a rule of thumb, in a healthy tendon, fluid in the tendon sheath or thickening is not visible. Another application of ultrasound is in the possibility of dynamic examination in dorsiflexion and plantarflexion [34, 35]. Partial tendon ruptures will not separate on ankle movement, and the tendon ends will not show paradoxical movement [38].

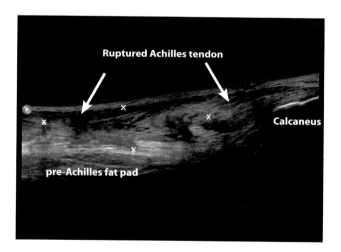

Figure 9. Longitudinal ultrasound image showing the complete rupture of the Achilles tendon.

Ultrasound can be of additional value in localizing the tendon ends when surgery is planned. This might assist the surgical procedure when small incisions are used in the case of a large haematoma. The precise location of the tendon ends at a given position of the flexion of the ankle should be noted in relation to the postero-superior corner of the calcaneus [38].

119

MRI

For chronic Achilles tendon ruptures, MRI is a useful investigation. The setting depends on the differential diagnosis. The T1-weighted images will provide anatomic details, whereas T2-weighted images are useful in evaluating the alterations in water content [4].

The average thickness of the Achilles tendon is approximately 6 mm, and 1 mm slices in the sagittal plane are mandatory in order to accurately depict the pathology.

The normal retrocalcaneal area is visible on MR imaging, and should be at most 6 mm (superior to inferior), 3 mm (medial to lateral) and 2 mm (anterior to posterior). In comparison with ultrasound, conventional MRI is less valuable in differentiating synovial thickening due to free fluid. A superior image will be obtained by injecting Gadolinium DTPA, which increases the signal within most areas of synovitis. Internal splits and ruptures can be clearly seen as lines in T1-weighted images and/or oedema within the tendon in T2-weighted images [38].

In complete Achilles tendon rupture with retraction, MRI will demonstrate a tendon gap with the fraying of the tendon ends [13]. In acute ruptures, the tendon gap demonstrates an intermediate signal on T1-weighted images, hyper-intensity, oedema and haemorrhage, and on T2-weighted images (Figure 10). In chronic ruptures, the tendon may be replaced by scar or fat tissue [18].

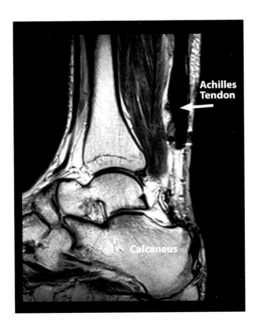

Figure 10. Sagittal T2- weighted turbo spin echo MRI of a five day old complete rupture of the Achilles tendon.

120

A diagnostic pitfall can be a heterogeneous area from the presence of connective tissue with intratendinous vessels between the collagen bundles. On T1-weighted and gradient echo images, it results in punctuated and short, linear, hyper-intense foci[6]. This heterogeneity is given by the confluence of the gastrocnemius and soleus tendon into the Achilles tendon, which is normal. It can be distinguished from partial rupture, because the tendon demonstrates no morphological changes and maintains its flat-to-concave anterior surface on axial MR images.

Pathologies around the Achilles tendon insertion

Imaging plays a pivotal role in the management of insertional Achilles tendon pathology, as the exact origin of the pain can often be hard to elucidate using clinical means alone. There is frequently more than one pain generator at the Achilles insertion, all of which may need to be addressed to achieve a good clinical outcome from the various treatment strategies that are available.

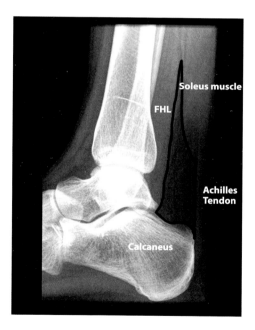

Figure 11. Lateral weight-bearing radiograph of the ankle with the normal appearance of the pre-Achilles fat pad.

121

Radiography

Conventional radiography is indicated in all causes of pain around the Achilles tendon insertion. The radiographs should include a lateral weight-bearing view of the foot and ankle (Figure 11), and an axial view of the heel (Figure 12).

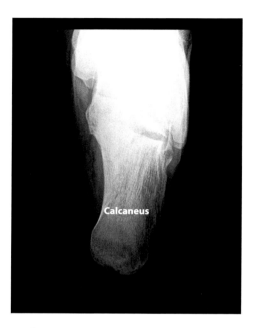

Figure 12. Axial view radiograph of the calcaneus.

On conventional radiography, the Achilles tendon has well-defined margins, particularly anteriorly, due to the interface between the anterior surface of the tendon and the pre-Achilles fat pad (Figure 11). Van Sterkenburg en co-workers have found an obliteration of the normally fat-filled retrocalcaneal recess on lateral weight-bearing radiographs in patients with retrocalcaneal bursitis [37] (Figure 13).

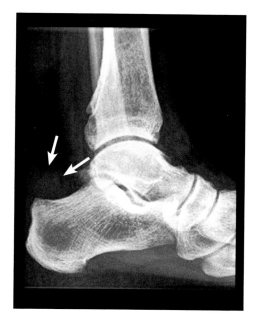

Figure 13. Lateral weight-bearing radiograph of the ankle with the obliteration of the retrocalcaneal recess of the pre-Achilles fat pad.

Pavlov and co-workers described the 'parallel pitch lines' method used to define the presence of a postero-superior calcaneal prominence on a lateral radiograph of the heel [23] (Figure 14).

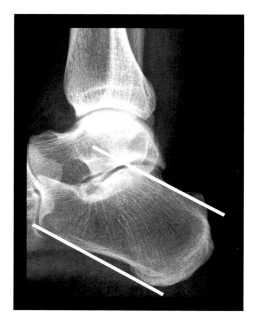

Figure 14. Lateral weight-bearing radiograph of the ankle. The 'parallel pitch lines' show a postero-superior calcaneal prominence.

Plain radiography can also demonstrate calcification or ossification within the Achilles tendon, or a bony spur at the distal tendon insertion onto the posterior calcaneus, which can be a feature of chronic tendinitis or previous tendon rupture (Figure 15).

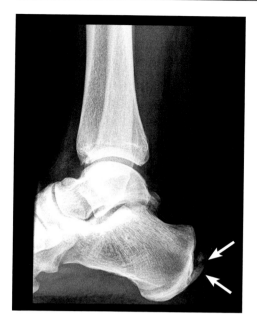

Figure 15. Lateral weight-bearing radiograph of the ankle showing calcifications and a bony spur at the insertion site of the Achilles tendon.

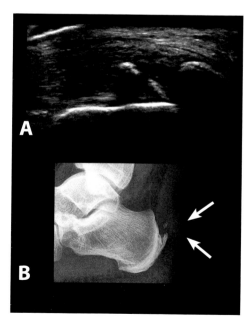

Figure 16. (A) Longitudinal ultrasound image showing calcifications in and the thickening of the Achilles tendon insertion; (B) Lateral weight-bearing radiograph of the same ankle showing local thickening at the level of the insertion.

Ultrasound

Ultrasound is useful in demonstrating calcifications at the insertion site of the Achilles tendon (Figure 16). Ultrasound is poorly sensitive but highly specific in establishing the diagnosis of retrocalcaneal bursitis when compared with MRI [16]. When visible, the bursa is typically distended with fluid, but may be diffusely thickened by synovial hypertrophy [19] (Figure 17). Colour Doppler or power Doppler imaging typically reveals increased blood flow at the margin of the bursa [3]. When present, the superficial calcaneal bursa resides between the posterior aspect of the Achilles tendon insertion and the skin. Ultrasound and MRI show the subcutaneous fat between the tendon and the skin, and the absence of this fat may represent superficial calcaneal bursitis. MRI and ultrasound may demonstrate inflammatory change within the bursa and – occasionally – bursal distension can be revealed.

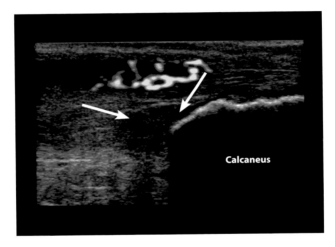

Figure 17. Longitudinal colour Doppler ultrasound image showing thickened retro-calcaneal bursa (arrows) with increased blood flow at the margin of the bursa (red).

MRI

Despite its low resolution images, the sensitivity of MRI in detecting soft-tissue and bone inflammatory changes allows for the contemporaneous analysis of the various pain generators around the Achilles insertion (i.e., the tendon, bone, bursa and fat pad). The choice of sequences varies between institutions, but the conventional imaging of the Achilles tendon should include a combination of T1-weighted and fluid sensitive sequences in the axial and sagittal planes [30]. Fluid-sensitive sequences include short-tau inversion recovery (STIR) and fat-suppressed T2-weighted or intermediate (proton) density-weighted sequences.

Sagittal MRI is the optimal imaging tool in making the diagnosis and imaging findings, including excessive fluid in the retrocalcaneal and superficial calcaneal bursa, and enlarged calcaneal tuberosity along with signal changes within the tendon [9, 28, 30, 31] (Figure 18). Patients with isolated insertional tendinopathy (without enlarged postero-superior calcaneal tuberosity) are typically older than patients with an enlarged calcaneal tuberosity [19]. This group of patients frequently has an underlying inflammatory arthropathy. Ultrasound will demonstrate an expanded hypoechoic distal tendon, which frequently shows florid vascularization on Doppler imaging (Figure 18).

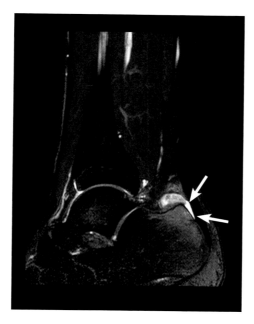

Figure 18. Sagittal T2-weighted TSE SPAIR MRI showing postero-superior calcaneal prominence, with an enlarged retrocalcaneal bursa indicating retrocalcaneal bursitis.

Conclusion

Disorders around the Achilles tendon insertion do not usually involve a single tissue. Most commonly, the Achilles tendon, retrocalcaneal bursa and superficial calcaneal bursa are typically inflamed simultaneously. These conditions are optimally assessed with MRI. However, plain radiographs are recommended to assess the postero-superior tuberosity of the calcaneus and detect intra-tendinous calcifications and enthesophyte formation. Ultrasound allows a dynamic assessment of the tendon and can be used to guide needle therapies.

Regarding mid-portion Achilles tendinopathy, ultrasound has two specific functions. The first is to exclude other potential causes and mimics of Achilles tendinopathy. Secondly, it can confirm paratendinopathy, fusiform tendon swelling, focal areas of pain and the reduction of new vessels, and may be important in long-term follow-up. MRI remains important in establishing the diagnosis of mid-portion Achilles tendinopathy.

In suspected Achilles tendon ruptures, imaging examinations should not be used routinely for diagnosis, and are probably overused, with the consequence that multiple normal anatomic variants may be erroneously interpreted as pathological. The familiarity of the examiner with normal anatomic variants is important for the accurate diagnostic interpretation of ultrasound and MR images. The advantages of ultrasound, such as dynamic assessment potential, wide availability, and favourable speed and cost factors, are important considerations in selecting an ultrasound examination as the first additional step to establishing an acute Achilles tendon rupture in doubtful cases. MRI shows greater detail as to the extent of tendon degeneration, but is hardly ever indicated in the diagnostic evaluation of acute Achilles tendon ruptures.

References

1. Archambault JM, Wiley JP, Bray RC, Verhoef M, Wiseman DA, Elliott PD. Can sonography predict the outcome in patients with achillodynia? J. Clin. Ultrasound. 1998; 26(7): 335-339.

2. Åström M, Gentz CF, Nilsson P, Rausing A, Sjöberg S, Westlin N. Imaging in chronic Achilles tendinopathy: a comparison of ultrasonography, magnetic resonance imaging and surgical findings in 27 histologically verified cases. Skeletal Radiol. 1996; 25(7): 615-620.

3. Balint PV, Sturrock RD. Inflamed retrocalcaneal bursa and Achilles tendonitis in psoriatic arthritis demonstrated by ultrasonography. Ann Rheum Dis, 2000; 59(12): 931-934.

4. Bencardino J, Rosenberg ZS, Delfaut E. MR imaging in sports injuries of the foot and ankle. Magn Reson Imaging Clin N Am. 1999; 7(1): 131.

5. Bleakney RR, White LM, Maffulli N. Imaging of the Achilles tendon. The Achilles Tendon, 2007; 25-38.

6. Dussault RG, Kaplan PA, Roederer G. MR imaging of Achilles tendon in patients with familial hyperlipidemia: comparison with plain films, physical examination, and patients with traumatic tendon lesions. AJR Am J Roentgenol. 1995; 164(2): 403-407.

7. Fredberg U, Bolvig L. Significance of ultrasonographically detected asymptomatic tendinosis in the patellar and Achilles tendons of elite soccer players: a longitudinal study. Am J Sports Med. 2002; 30(4): 488-491.

8. Gibbon WW, Cooper JR, Radcliffe GS. Sonographic incidence of tendon microtears in athletes with chronic Achilles tendinosis. Br J Sports Med. 1999; 33(2): 129-130.

9. Harris CA, Peduto AJ. Achilles tendon imaging. Australas Radiol. 2006; 50(6): 513-525.

10. Inglis AE, Scott WN, Sculco TP, Patterson AH. Ruptures of the tendo Achillis. J Bone Joint Surg Am. 1976; 58: 990-993.

11. Kader D, Saxena A, Movin T, Maffulli N. Achilles tendinopathy: some aspects of basic science and clinical management. Br J Sports Med. 2002; 36(4): 239-249.

12. Kainberger FM, Engel A, Barton P, Huebsch P, Neuhold A, Salomonowitz E. Injury of the Achilles tendon: diagnosis with sonography. AJR Am J Roentgenol. 1990; 155(5): 1031.

13. Keene JS, Lash EG, Fisher DR, De Smet AA. Magnetic resonance imaging of Achilles tendon ruptures. Am J Sports Med. 1989; 17(3): 333-337.

14. Leung JL, Griffith JF. Sonography of chronic Achilles tendinopathy: a case-control study. J Clin Ultrasound. 2008; 36(1): 27-32.

15. Ly JQ, Bui-Mansfield LT. Anatomy of and abnormalities associated with Kager's fat Pad. AJR Am J Roentgenol. 2004; 182(1): 147-154.

16. Mahlfeld K, Kayser R, Mahlfeld A, Grasshoff H, Franke J. Value of ultrasound in diagnosis of bursopathies in the area of the Achilles tendon. Ultraschall Med. 2001; 22(2): 87.

17. Mantel D, Flautre B, Bastian D, Delforge PM, Delvalle A, Leclet H. Structural MRI study of the Achilles tendon. Correlation with microanatomy and histology. Journal de Radiologie. 1996; 77(4): 261.

18. Marcus DS, Reicher MA, Kellerhouse LE. Achilles tendon injuries: the role of MR imaging. J Comput Assist Tomogr. 1989; 13(3): 480-486.

19. Narváez JA, Narváez J, Ortega Rl, Aguilera C, Sánchez A, Andía E. Painful Heel: MR Imaging Findings. Radiographics. 2000; 20(2): 333-352.

20. O'Connor PJ, Grainger AJ, Morgan SR, Smith KL, Waterton JC, Nash AFP. Ultrasound assessment of tendons in asymptomatic volunteers: a study of reproducibility. Eur Radiol. 2004; 14(11): 1968-1973.

21. Paavola M, Kannus P, Järvinen TA, Khan K, Józsa L, Järvinen M. Achilles tendinopathy. J Bone Joint Surg Am. 2002; 84(11): 2062-2076.

22. Paavola M, Paakkala T, Kannus P, Järvinen M. Ultrasonography in the differential diagnosis of Achilles tendon injuries and related disorders: A comparison between pre-operative ultrasonography and surgical findings. Acta Radiol. 1998; 39(6): 612-619.

23. Pavlov H, Heneghan MA, Hersh A, Goldman AB, Vigorita V. The Haglund syndrome: initial and differential diagnosis. Radiology. 1982; 144(1): 83-88.

24. Peers KH, Brys PP, Lysens RJ. Correlation between power Doppler ultrasonography and clinical severity in Achilles tendinopathy. Int Orthop. 2003; 27(3): 180-183.

25. Pierre-Jerome C, Moncayo V, Terk MR. MRI of the Achilles tendon: a comprehensive review of the anatomy, biomechanics, and imaging of overuse tendinopathies. Acta Radiol. 2010; 51(4): 438-454.

26. Richards PJ, Win T, Jones PW. The distribution of microvascular response in Achilles tendonopathy assessed by colour and power Doppler. Skeletal Radiol. 2005; 34(6): 336-342.

27. Sandmeier R, Renström PAFH. Diagnosis and treatment of chronic tendon disorders in sports. Scand J Med Sci Sports. 1997; 7(2): 96-106.

28. Schepsis AA, Wagner C, Leach RE. Surgical management of Achilles tendon overuse injuries. A long-term follow-up study. Am J Sports Med. 1994; 22(5): 611-619.

29. Schunck J, Jerosch J. Operative treatment of Haglund's syndrome. Basics, indications, procedures, surgical techniques, results and problems. Foot Ankle Surg. 2005; 11: 123-130.

30. Schweitzer ME, Karasick D. MR imaging of disorders of the Achilles tendon. AJR Am J Roentgenol. 2000; 175(3): 613-625.

31. Sella EJ, Caminear DS, McLarney EA. Haglund's syndrome. J Foot Ankle Surg. 1998; 37(2): 110-114.

32. Shalabi A, Kristoffersen GÇÉ, Wiberg M, Aspelin P, Movin T. MR evaluation of chronic Achilles tendinosis. Acta Radiologica. 2001; 42(3): 269-276.

33. Shalabi A. Magnetic resonance imaging in chronic Achilles tendinopathy. Acta Radiologica. 2004; 45(suppl 432): 1-45.

34. Thermann H, Hoffmann R, Zwipp H, Tscherne H. The use of ultrasonography in the foot and ankle. Foot Ankle Int. 1992; 13(7): 386-390.

35. Thermann H, Zwipp H, Tscherne H. Functional treatment concept of acute rupture of the Achilles tendon. 2 years results of a prospective randomized study]. Unfallchirurg. 1995; 98(1): 21.

36. Tyler DJ, Robson MD, Henkelman RM, Young IR, Bydder GM. Magnetic resonance imaging with ultrashort TE (UTE) PULSE sequences: technical considerations. J Magn Reson Imaging. 2007; 25(2): 279-289.

37. van Sterkenburg MN, Muller B, Maas M, Sierevelt IN, van Dijk CN. Appearance of the weight-bearing lateral radiograph in retrocalcaneal bursitis. Acta Orthop. 2010; 81(3): 387-390.

38. Wilson DJ. Injuries of the ligaments and tendons in the ankle and foot. Imaging of Orthopedic Sports Injuries. Springer. 2007; 321-335.

39. Zanetti M, Metzdorf A, Kundert HP. Achilles tendons: clinical relevance of neovascularization diagnosed with power Doppler US. Radiology. 2003; 227(2): 556-560.

"Use it or lose it."

Jimmy Connors

Chapter 9

Non-Invasive Non-Surgical Treatment and Rehabilitation for Achilles Tendinopathy

Karin Grävare Silbernagel, Peter Malliaras, Annelie Brorsson, Jón Karlsson

Take Home Message

- *The majority of patients with both mid-portion and insertional Achilles tendinopathy recover fully with non-invasive non-surgical treatment.*

- *There is evidence that exercise for at least 12 weeks can be recommended as the initial treatment for both mid-portion and insertional Achilles tendinopathy.*

- *Insertional Achilles tendinopathy is a more complex syndrome than mid-portion Achilles tendinopathy and, therefore, the non-invasive non-surgical treatment for these patients ought to be individualized.*

Introduction

In the literature, non-surgical treatment is recommended as the initial treatment for patients with mid-portion and insertional Achilles tendinopathy [16, 32, 39, 42, 73, 84, 86]. The non-invasive non-surgical treatment recommendations include – but are not limited to – rest, activity modification, shoe modification, ice, anti-inflammatory medications, orthotics, ultrasound, low level laser therapy, shockwave therapy and exercises [32, 43, 80, 86]. Although considered distinct pathological entities, it is also common to combine descriptions of treatment for both mid-portion Achilles tendinopathy and insertional Achilles tendinopathy. Since insertional Achilles tendinopathy is a complex syndrome with at least three sub-diagnoses (insertional Achilles tendinopathy, retrocalcaneal bursitis and superficial calcaneal bursitis), the non-surgical treatment might also vary, depending on the specific patient's diagnosis.

The purpose of non-surgical treatment is to address possible risk factors and other contributing factors, and to treat functional impairments to facilitate a return to function and promote healing. In this chapter, the evidence of effectiveness and the theory and mechanisms behind the most commonly-suggested treatments are reviewed. Extra-corporal shockwave therapy (ESWT) will be discussed in a separate chapter.

Immobilization and rest

A period of rest from painful activities is often recommended with all types of injuries. The purpose is to refrain from causing further damage and minimize the patient's pain and discomfort, while promoting the healing of the damaged tissue. Often, the patients themselves modify their activity level - for instance by avoiding activities that cause increased pain – prior to seeking medical assistance. The level of symptoms and pain are often used as a guide when determining the appropriate level of activity participation [78]. Patients vary in pain perception and tolerance, but avoiding moderate and severe pain and worsening symptoms over time is a priority when considering the activity level. Since physical activity is important for staying healthy, recommending alternative activities that impart lower load on the Achilles tendon and the Achilles tendon insertion might be better than rest in general.

Complete unloading of a tendon has been shown to have detrimental effects on tendon structure and healing [37]. For mid-portion Achilles tendinopathy, it has been found that immediate exercise and allowing continued running and jumping - but limiting the amount by the use of a pain-monitoring model – is not negative for recovery [78]. This has not been evaluated in insertional Achilles tendinopathy, and since this type of injury might be more inflammatory in nature if the retrocalcaneal bursa is involved, for these patients a period of rest might be beneficial. When prescribing exercise and loading, it is important to understand the origin and cause of the pain in order to make appropriate recommendations.

Heel lifts and shoe modification

Mid-portion Achilles tendinopathy

In patients with mid-portion Achilles tendinopathy, there is rarely any compression from the shoe on the area of the tendinopathy unless the patient is wearing high top shoes. However, if there is compression on the area of tendinopathy there might be increased pain, and shoes that avoid the compression might be beneficial. Heel lifts or shoes with a higher heel-to-toe gradient are also commonly used in the clinical setting. This is mainly to provide pain relief by decreasing the amount of stretch placed on the tendon by keeping the ankle in a greater degree of plantarflexion. There is minimal evidence to support the use of a heel-lift as treatment; however, it might be beneficial on an individual level for providing pain relief [16].

Insertional Achilles tendinopathy

Patients with insertional Achilles tendinopathy often experience pain with the compression of the heel, regardless of whether their symptoms are due to insertional tendinopathy, retrocalcaneal or superficial bursitis. Furthermore, when the ankle moves into dorsiflexion there is compression of the retrocalcaneal bursa, and possibly also of the anterior tendon fibres, between the Achilles tendon and the calcaneus, which might cause further symptoms and damage [10, 13, 20]. The modification of the patients' shoes to limit the heel counter compression as well as increasing the heel-to-toe gradient is therefore often recommended [30, 32, 59, 80, 86]. Furthermore, a heel lift is often placed in the shoe with the purpose of placing the ankle in a slightly plantar flexed position to alleviate some of the pull and compression of the Achilles tendon insertion on the calcaneus and bursae [30, 32, 59, 80, 86]. There is limited guidance in the literature, but we recommend that the heel lift height should be based on symptomatic response, with progressively increasing height if there is no response initially. Both the heel lift and shoe modifications are thought to decrease the patient's symptoms by reducing compression at the Achilles insertion, which may facilitate healing as compression is often considered an aetiological factor in insertional tendon pathology [20]. Since tendon healing is slow, the heel lift can be worn for several weeks. Another argument for the possible benefit of a heel lift holds that by placing the ankle in greater plantarflexion a more uniform loading of the Achilles tendon at the insertion site might be achieved [47]. There are, however, no studies that have evaluated the effectiveness or compared the use of these modifications with other treatments. On the other hand, there is no reason to believe that these treatments would have an adverse effect and, if the patients feel symptomatic relief, there is no reason not to recommend them.

Correction of biomechanical factors with orthotics

Intrinsic risk factors for Achilles tendon injury are often described as ab-normalities in the ankle or sub-talar joint range of motion and increased foot pronation [44, 59]. In the literature, there are only a few studies that have evaluated whether abnormal lower extremity mechanics and malalignment are risk factors for developing Achilles tendon injury, and none of these studies have looked at patients with pure insertional Achilles tendinopathy [38, 53, 57, 90]. In these studies, conflicting results have been found, such as that either increased or decreased dorsiflexion or an increased or decreased sub-talar joint range of motion will increase the risk of injury [38, 53]. A greater degree of foot pronation has also been linked to the occurrence of Achilles tendinopathy in some studies [57] but not in others [58]. The underlying mechanism linking biomechanical malalignment and injury may involve changes in the loading of the tendon at the insertion due to restricted movement in the sub-talar or talocrural joints or increased compression of the tendon and bursa at the insertion due to either reduced or increased pronation. However, there are no studies that have evaluated the effect of orthotics in patients with only insertional tendinopathy. For patients with Achilles tendinopathy, there is some limited evidence as regards the effectiveness of orthotics [24, 28, 56]. Of interest is that one study, on patients with Achilles tendinopathy, found that orthotics intended to limit the amount of eversion during running actually caused increased eversion compared to the absence of orthotics; however, the patients reported an improvement in symptoms [24], so the benefit may relate to a change in kinetics rather than kinematics. The evidence for the use of orthotics for injury in the Achilles region is limited, and this underscores the importance of orthotic prescription by an expert if biomechanical abnormalities are found and in following-up on their effectiveness.

Ultrasound

The use of therapeutic ultrasound has been found to enhance tendon healing in animal studies [25, 33]. There has also been a few clinical studies showing positive results [69], but ultrasound alone has been shown to be inferior to eccentric exercise in Achilles tendinopathy [17]. This highlights that it may only be appropriate to use ultrasound as an adjunct to other loading. Furthermore, systematic reviews and meta-analyses have failed to show that active ultra-sound is more effective than placebo [14, 69].

Low-level laser therapy

A systematic review evaluating the effect of low-level laser therapy (LLLT) on tendinopathy generally indicated a favourable outcome with this treatment [88]. They found four studies that evaluated the effect on Achilles tendinopathy, but none of these included patients with pain or symptoms from the insertion. Another systematic review evaluating physical therapies for Achilles tendinopathy found evidence for the benefit of using LLLT in combination with exercise [84]. One difficulty with comparing studies using LLLT is the use of various dosages. In general, this treatment has been combined with eccentric exercise and has been found to be more beneficial then eccentric exercise alone [83]. Recently-published clinical guidelines [88] have recommended, based on moderate evidence, that clinicians should consider the use of LLLT to decrease pain and stiffness in patients with Achilles tendinopathy.

Treatments aimed at decreasing pain and inflammation

Chronic Achilles tendinopathy has been shown not to be inflammatory and, therefore, the use of anti-inflammatory medications or modalities are questionable but may have a role in reducing tenocyte cellular response that may be associated with pain mechanisms [23]. Paratendinitis might occur in conjunction with mid-portion tendinopathy and could also partly explain symptomatic relief with treatments aimed at decreasing inflammation. Since insertional Achilles tendinopathy includes two inflammatory conditions (retrocalcaneal and superficial calcaneal bursitis), treatments aimed at decreasing inflammation might be warranted for these diagnoses. Here, the use of cryotherapy, anti-inflammatory medications and iontophoresis might be useful. However, there have been no studies that have evaluated the effectiveness of any of these treatment methods in this specific patient group. Ice is often used at the end of treatment in physical therapy, and the patients are often recommended to use cryotherapy at home to limit inflammation and pain. In the clinic, patients often report decreased pain with the use of cryotherapy, but further studies are needed to determine its effectiveness as a treatment. Iontophoresis was shown to have a positive effect on acute Achilles tendinopathy in a randomized double-blinded study, but here insertional injuries were excluded [60]. The majority of the above-described treatments appear to be geared towards limiting the inflammatory process and providing symptomatic relief. Limiting symptoms might be of particular importance so that the patient can tolerate and progress faster with other treatments, such as exercise.

Manual therapy

In the clinical setting, manual techniques such as joint mobilization and soft tissue massage are used by physical therapists. Sub-talar joint mobilizations are clinically recommended if decreases in the sub-talar joint range of motion exist. There is some evidence that restriction in the sub-talar joint range of motion is a risk factor for Achilles tendinopathy; however, whether this pertains to insertional problems as well is not known [38, 44, 53]. Deep friction massage has been proposed to aid in the recovery of mid-portion tendinopathy [16], but may have a negative effect with insertional problems if the bursae are inflamed. No randomized controlled-treatment studies exist that evaluate the effect of joint mobilization and/or soft tissue massage in this patient population.

Rehabilitation – exercise

When reviewing the literature regarding exercise as treatment for Achilles tendinopathy, there appears to be some confusion over strengthening and stretching exercises. Eccentric strengthening exercises have been shown in several studies to be effective for Achilles tendinopathy [7, 65, 71, 79]. However, in some studies this has been referred to as 'eccentric stretching' instead [30, 80]. Since strengthening and stretching exercises are performed differently and have different purposes, we will review their use and effectiveness separately.

Stretching

The stretching of the calf musculature is often a standard treatment recommendation for patients with pain and symptoms from and around the Achilles tendon. The purpose of stretching is to increase muscle-tendon length, reduce stiffness and increase the joint range of motion. Despite this general recommendation, there is only one study found in the literature that has evaluated the effectiveness of stretching compared with eccentric exercise in patients with Achilles tendon injury [63]. In this study, a broad inclusion criteria was used and patients with both mid-portion and insertional tendinopathy were included. Only 16% (7/45) had pain from the insertion. This study concluded that both groups improved, however, with no significant differences between the treatments. Moreover, they found that the patients with insertional Achilles tendinopathy showed less improvement. It is interesting to note that no measure of ankle range of motion was performed. Often, stretching is recommended for improving the range of motion; however, there is rarely any description or objective measure regarding whether this patient group has a deficit in range of motion. Instead, Achilles tendinopathy has been associated with both increased and decreased dorsiflexion range of motion [38, 53]. The tendinopathic tendon has also been found to have decreased stiffness, despite patients' complaints of a sensation of stiffness [18]. In addition, it is not known whether achieving greater dorsiflexion actually improves the symptoms in insertional tendinopathy. These patients instead have pain when placing the ankle in full dorsiflexion, presumably due to the compression of the bursae and the tendon onto the calcaneus. Furthermore, the anterior fibres of the tendon often comprise the damaged area, and these fibres were previously presumed to be more loaded in dorsiflexion. However, Lymanand co-workers [47] instead found the opposite. Using a cadaveric model, they found a differential strain distribution in the distal Achilles tendon. Moving the ankle from plantarflexion to dorsiflexion caused an increased stress in the posterior fibres but not in the anterior fibres. Stretching into dorsiflexion might, therefore, cause the compression of the anterior fibres, which might be counterproductive in patients with insertional Achilles tendinopathy. Moreover, it has been reported that ankle dorsiflexion range of motion was only increased by approximately one degree with stretching [72]. The improvement might also simply be due to increased stretch tolerance rather than increased compliance and/or lengthening of the muscle-tendon complex [52].

The question of whether stretching in this patient population relieves symptoms and can be considered as an effective intervention needs to be further investigated. The recommendation is that a thorough evaluation needs to be performed to determine whether there is a range of motion deficit that might be addressed with stretching. When prescribing stretching as a treatment, pain in the Achilles insertion during and after the treatment needs to be monitored, given the potential for compression in dorsiflexion.

Strengthening exercises

The effects of exercise training in the management of Achilles tendinopathy is promising, and the current consensus appears to be that all patients should be treated with an exercise programme for three to six months [1, 4, 7, 11, 35, 50, 62, 71, 79]. Muscular strength, power, endurance, flexibility and motor control are important in physical performance, and exercises aimed to improve these factors are therefore often prescribed in rehabilitation and injury prevention programmes for tendon injuries [21, 31, 81]. Moreover, patients with Achilles tendinopathy have impaired muscle function, such as decreased concentric and eccentric strength, muscular endurance and jumping ability, on their injured side [77]. Impaired muscle function has also been implicated as an aetiological factor for Achilles tendinopathy [8, 29, 36, 54]. Weakness of the plantar flexors could also allow for excessive dorsiflexion, which might then cause irritation at the insertional site of the Achilles tendon. Since the calf muscle is active both concentrically and eccentrically during walking, running and jumping, it might be important to strengthen it both in a concentric and eccentric manner.

Exercise is also recommended as a complement to other modalities of management, including surgery, sclerosing injections and medication [2, 60, 66, 67, 74, 85]. Eccentric strength training is particularly effective in improving muscle function and/or aiding in the healing process of the tendon [7, 27, 65, 71, 79]. There are, however, various rationales for different types of exercises, even though the main focus has been on the effects of eccentric training. Explanations for successful treatment with exercise include the improvement of muscular strength and lower leg function [9, 21, 62, 79, 82], repetitive stretching causing increased tensile strength [3, 7, 9], the mechanical insult of pain-producing nerves [3, 64], blocking circulation to the tendon [3, 6, 64], mechanotransduction for enhancing tendon healing [9, 12, 41, 68], improving the homogeneity of the passive structures, and the modulation of the neurological stretch response [9]. A recent systematic review found evidence for improved strength and jump performance but conflicting evidence for improved imaging outcomes (e.g., normalized structure and reduced anteroposterior diameter), alongside improved clinical outcomes following loading interventions in Achilles tendinopathy patients [55]. Many of the other proposed mechanisms have not been investigated, so the mechanisms for action of loading are largely uninvestigated but may not involve improved tendon structure. Poorer outcomes in the insertional tendinopathy group may be explained by the compression of the enthesis and increased pathology/symptoms [20].

Exactly what type of exercise – the intensity (load) – and how often it should be performed to achieve the best outcome for patients with Achilles tendinopathy is unclear. We review some of the exercise programmes proposed in the literature, their efficacy, and how they are used in clinical practice.

The eccentric exercise programme

In 1984, Curwin and Stanish [22] proposed an eccentric exercise programme to treat tendinitis (at that time, painful tendon injury was assumed to be due to the inflammation of the tendon). The rationale for their treatment programme was their clinical finding that, in many of the athletes with 'tendinitis', eccentric loading was somehow involved. In addition, they found that tendon pain could be reproduced in the clinic by loading the tendon eccentrically. Their view was that greater force production during eccentric activation caused a greater load in the tendon, which was thought to promote healing, improve muscle function and reduce pain and symptoms. To increase the load on the tendon, the programme focused on three areas: increasing the length of the tendon by stretching, increasing the load of the tendon by using eccentric exercise and adding external weights, and increasing the speed of muscle activation to increase the load of the tendon and thereby be more sports-specific.

The exercise was allowed to cause some pain, but the intensity was recommended to be at such level that only the last set of ten repetitions should cause some pain or discomfort. Stanish and co-workers [82] reported in 1986 that, in 200 patients who had followed their proposed eccentric exercise programme for six weeks, 44% had complete relief and 43% had a marked decrease in symptoms at the 16 month follow-up. Clement and co-workers [19] reported that 67% of 109 runners with Achilles tendinitis had an excellent result, with a mean recovery time of five weeks with an exercise programme that appears similar to the one described above. Neither of these studies were, however, randomized trials, and in the second study the patients also received other treatments aimed at controlling their inflammation, pain and biomechanical parameters.

An eccentric-only exercise programme

In 1998, Alfredsson and co-workers [7] published a non-randomized study using a protocol with just eccentric heel-rises with the knee straight or else bent. The treatment programme (Table 1) was also supposed to be painful and, if the exercises could be performed without experiencing any minor pain or discomfort, the patients were instructed to increase the load by adding weights in a back-pack.

Exercise	Number of Exercises	Progression
Heel-drop – knee straight Standing on edge of step. Start by standing on the toes and lower the heel all the way down. Go back up onto the toes by using the other leg.	3 sets of 15 repetitions, 2 times a day, 7 days a week for 12 weeks.	Do exercises even if painful and perform until they become pain-free. Add load until exercises are painful again.
Heel-drop – knee bent Standing on edge of step. Start by standing on the toes and lower the heel all the way down. Go back up onto the toes by using the other leg.	3 sets of 15 repetitions, 2 times a day, 7 days a week for 12 weeks.	Do exercises even if painful and perform until they become pain-free. Add load until exercises are painful again.

Table 1. Eccentric-only exercise protocol.

In the initial study [7, 15] patients on the waiting list for surgery were included, and after 12 weeks they were all reported to be satisfied and back at their pre-injury levels. Since then, this eccentric exercise programme has been evaluated in several studies [26, 50, 63, 70, 71, 75]. Most studies that have evaluated eccentric exercise as a treatment for Achilles tendinopathy report beneficial results; however, it is difficult to compare the various studies due to methodological differences [40, 92]. A five year follow-up of this exercise protocol found that there was a significant improvement between one and five years following the initiation of the exercises; however, 48% of the patients had received one or more alternative treatments [89]. The eccentric exercise programme has the patient standing on a step and promotes loading on a step while the ankle is moved into full dorsiflexion [7]. Since problems in the Achilles tendon insertion are a part of a complex syndrome, where the compression of the bursae and tendon onto the calcaneus at full dorsiflexion causes symptoms, performing an exercise that promotes excessive dorsiflexion might instead exacerbate the symptoms and inflammation. Therefore, performing the eccentric exercises, while limiting the amount of dorsiflexion, was proposed for chronic insertional Achilles tendinopathy and evaluated in a pilot study [34]. In this study, there was a 67% success rate as compared with 32% in the original eccentric exercise programme [26, 34].

A comprehensive treatment protocol

Since the early 1990s, Silbernagel and co-workers [76, 78, 79] have used a comprehensive treatment protocol (Table 2) for patients with Achilles tendinopathy. This protocol is based on the proposal by Curwin and Stanish [22] such that the load of the tendon is increased by both increasing the external weight and increasing the speed of movement. The protocol includes both concentric and eccentric exercises of the calf musculature (Figure 2). The reason for this is that both concentric and eccentric activations are included in all physical activities and that patients with Achilles tendinopathy have both concentric and eccentric strength deficits [77]. The exercise programme, complemented with a pain-monitoring model (described below), was tested in two randomized controlled trials and led to significant improvements in patients with mid-portion Achilles tendinopathy [78, 79]. In a five year follow-up of this treatment protocol, it was found that 80% of the patients were fully recovered and only one patient had received alternative treatment [76]. For patients with insertional Achilles tendinopathy, the same treatment protocol is recommended (with the exception that patients will not progress to standing on the edge of a step).

Phase 1: Weeks 1-2
Patient status: Pain and difficulty with all activities; difficulty performing ten one-legged heel-rises.
Goal: Begin to exercise; understanding the nature of their injury and of pain monitoring model.
Treatment programme: Perform exercises every day. • Pain monitoring model information and advice on exercise activity. • Circulation exercises (moving foot up/down). • Two-legged heel-rises standing on the floor (3x10-15). • One-legged heel-rises standing on the floor (3x10). • Sitting heel-rises (3x10). • Eccentric heel-rises standing on the floor (3x10).
Phase 2: Weeks 2-5 **(if insertional pain continues while standing on the floor)**
Patient status: Pain with exercise; morning stiffness; pain when performing heel-rises.
Goal: Begin strengthening.

Phase 2: Weeks 2-5 *(continued)*

Treatment programme: Perform exercises every day.
- Two-legged heel-rises standing on edge of step (3x15).
- One-legged heel-rises standing on edge of step (3x15).
- Sitting heel-rises (3x15).
- Eccentric heel-rises standing on edge of step (3x15).
- Quick rebounding heel-rises (3x20).

Phase 3: Weeks 3-12
(or longer if needed)
(if insertional pain continues standing on the floor)

Patient status: Handle the phase two exercise programme; no pain distally in tendon insertion; possibly decreased or increased morning stiffness.

Goal: Heavier strength training; increase or start running and/or jumping activity.

Treatment programme: Perform exercises every day and with a heavier load, 2-3 times per week.
- One-legged heel-rises standing on edge of step with added weight (3x15).
- Sitting heel-rises (3x15).
- Eccentric heel-rises standing on edge of step with added weight (3x15).
- Quick rebounding heel-rises (3x20).
- Plyometrics training.

Phase 4: Weeks 12-6 months
(or longer if needed)
(if insertional pain continues standing on the floor)

Patient status: Minimal symptoms; absence of morning stiffness every day; can participate in sports without difficulty.

Goal: Maintenance exercise; no symptoms.

Treatment programme: Perform exercises 2-3 times per week.
- One-legged heel-rises standing on edge of step with added weight (3x15).
- Eccentric heel-rises standing on edge of step with added weight (3x15).
- Quick rebounding heel-rises (3x20).

Table 2. Comprehensive treatment protocol.

Pain-monitoring model

The exercise programme used in the comprehensive treatment protocol for Achilles tendinopathy allowed the patient to experience pain during and after exercise. By using a pain-monitoring model (Figure 3), patients can be guided as to how to deal with the pain. Curwin and Stanish [22] described that some pain and discomfort is allowed, and proposed to increase the load as soon as the exercise was pain-free. The clinical experience is that patients are often afraid to perform physical activities that cause pain in the Achilles tendon from fear of further injury or a total Achilles tendon rupture. It was also found in one study that the degree of fear of movement (kinesiophobia) correlated with the recovery of heel-rise in endurance in patients with mid-portion Achilles tendinopathy [76]. This fear may prevent patients from loading the Achilles tendon sufficiently to cause meaningful adaptive positive changes in the tendon. The pain-monitoring model is used to facilitate the patients' understanding of the amount of pain allowed during and after exercise. The model was initially developed by Thomeé and presented in a randomized controlled trial in 1997 for patients with patello-femoral pain syndrome [87]. The pain-monitoring model is a very useful tool, which also helps the clinician and patient to determine how the exercise programme should progress.

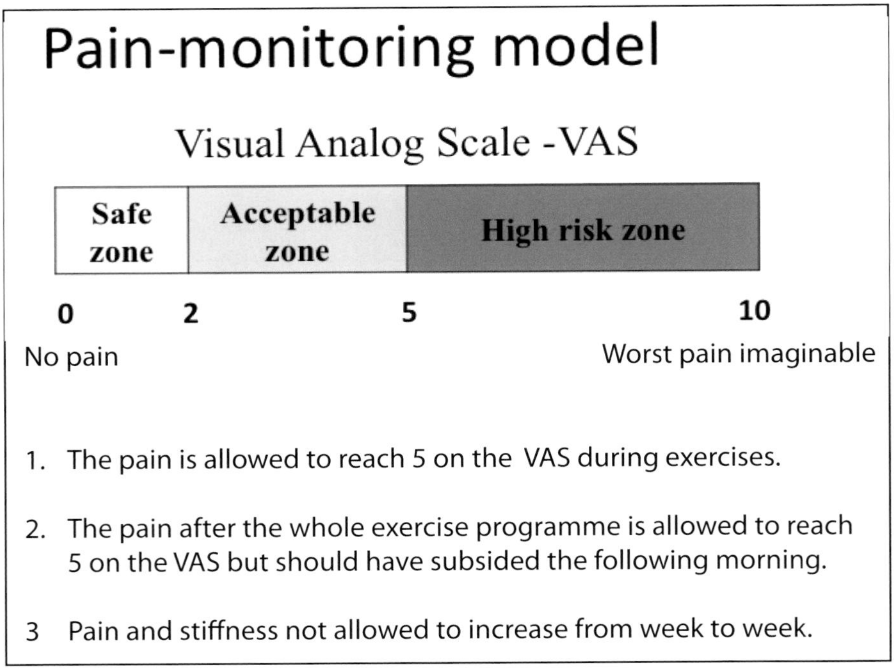

Pain-monitoring model

Visual Analog Scale -VAS

Safe zone	Acceptable zone	High risk zone

0   2   5   10

No pain   Worst pain imaginable

1. The pain is allowed to reach 5 on the VAS during exercises.

2. The pain after the whole exercise programme is allowed to reach 5 on the VAS but should have subsided the following morning.

3 Pain and stiffness not allowed to increase from week to week.

Figure 1. Pain-monitoring model.

Eccentric exercise compared with concentric exercise

Despite the numerous studies on eccentric exercise programmes, only two trials compared eccentric training with concentric training in patients with Achilles tendinopathy [50, 62]. In both these studies, the group that received eccentric treatment had a significantly greater improvement compared to the concentric group. The concentric treatment groups, however, also saw significant improvements. In these two studies, the eccentric and concentric exercise groups were not comparable as regards the load or training volumes [46, 50, 62]. A recent systematic review of studies comparing loading programmes in Achilles tendinopathy identified equivalent evidence for eccentric only exercises and the comprehensive treatment protocol discussed [55]. Clinically, isolating the eccentric component initially may not be indicated in patients who have a clear concentric deficit and, in these cases, the comprehensive programme may be more suitable.

Interestingly, Rees and co-workers [68] compared concentric and eccentric loading in the Achilles tendon and found no differences in peak tendon force or tendon length between the two exercises. They did find, however, a high-frequency oscillation in the tendon force with eccentric loading that was not found with concentric loading. The importance of the oscillation for tendon healing is not known. Thus, there is a need for further studies on the mechanism of the effect of eccentric training, as well as studies comparing eccentric training with other exercise protocols. However, it is commonly assumed that it is safe to conclude that eccentric-concentric combined exercise, if heavily loaded, can have a positive effect on patients with Achilles tendinopathy, and most certainly will not have a negative effect.

Summary of exercise as treatment

A systematic review by Kingma and co-workers [40] on eccentric overload training in patients with Achilles tendinopathy included nine studies [5, 7, 26, 50, 62, 71, 75, 79, 82] (three randomized controlled trials and six controlled trials). In six [5, 7, 26, 50, 71, 75] of those studies, only eccentric training was used; in the other three [62, 79, 82], the programme combined eccentric training with other interventions, such as stretching and ice. The durations of the exercise programmes were six or 12 weeks. Kingma and co-workers [40] concluded that the effect of eccentric exercise appeared promising, but no definite conclusions could be drawn due to methodological shortcomings. In a recent systematic review [51] on non-surgical treatment for mid-portion Achilles tendinopathy, five prospective randomized trials were identified where eccentric exercise was compared with controls [50, 56, 62, 70, 79]. Four of these trials showed a statistically significant improvement in pain scores in the eccentric groups compared with the control groups, whereas one trial showed no significant difference. In summary, they reported that 60% to 90% of patients reported a significant improvement in patient satisfaction and decreased pain with eccentric exercise. They concluded that there is currently more evidence in support of eccentric exercise than other interventions, such as extracorporeal shockwave therapy, local steroid therapy, sclerosing injections, deproteinized haemodialysate and topical glyceryl nitrate application. Another recent systematic review also came to similar conclusions [84].

The general consensus in the literature appears to be that most patients with insertional Achilles Tendinopathy will recover with non-surgical treatment, but the prognosis may be poorer than for mid-portion Achilles tendinopathy [10]. The success rate is reported to be between 75% and 95% [19, 45, 59, 91]. On the other hand, Nicholson and co-workers. reported that only 53% recovered without surgery [61]. They also found that the degree of damage and changes on the MRI predicted success with non-surgical treatment. In studies on surgical treatment, the usual view is that surgery was decided upon after failed non-surgical treatment. The length of the non-surgical treatment prior to performing surgery ranges from 6-12 weeks to a year [15, 48, 93].

Other aspects that might affect the outcome of exercise as treatment

As stated before, the natural history of Achilles tendinopathy is not fully known. There are also a variety of responses to exercise treatment in different studies, where the reported success rate ranges from approximately 60% to 90% [40, 49]. The wide variations found both in research and in the clinic might be due to the diversity of the patient population, whereas the exercise programmes used are normally very standardized. It can also be seen, when comparing various research studies, that there is a range of follow-up times [40, 51]. Since a tendon takes up to a year to improve, it might not be feasible to expect that 12 weeks of rehabilitation is enough, and the patient might continue to improve during this time. Studies have shown a continued improvement over time up to a year [71, 78, 79]. The individual patient's activity level, health status, previous injuries and attitude towards exercise might very well influence the outcome of the rehabilitation. Furthermore, the research indicates that a tendon's response to mechanical loading varies with age and gender. Further studies are needed to determine the effect of exercise, and in future it might be important to evaluate different subgroups separately and perform long-term follow-ups to receive answers as regards how to develop and implement exercise as treatment successfully.

It is also of great importance to remember that a thorough evaluation is crucial in order to design the exercise programme with the aim of improving individual impairments. It might not only be impairments around the foot and ankle that are relevant to the injury. The strength and function of the proximal joints and structures, such as the hip and trunk (the proximal kinetic chain), can also affect ankle and foot loading during walking and running and, hence, the load at the Achilles insertion. If such underlying causes of proximal kinematic abnormalities (such as poor core stability, dysfunctional motor patterning and a weak gluteus medius muscle) exist, they need to be identified and addressed within the rehabilitation programme.

Conclusion

Mid-portion Achilles tendinopathy

Patients with Achilles tendinopathy should receive rehabilitation exercises as their initial treatment. To experience a favourable outcome from exercise, the exercises are allowed to cause pain and should be performed daily. The use of a pain-monitoring model aids the clinician and patient in the balance between overloading and loading sufficiently to achieve a positive response to exercises. The exercise programme should consist of eccentric exercises, but also exercises such as concentric strengthening and others, to address possible functional deficits. The exercise programme needs to continue for at least 12 weeks, but more often needs to be continued for up to a year. It might also be beneficial to combine the exercise treatment with other treatments, such as laser therapy and the use of orthotics. Further research is needed to determine what combinations of treatments have the best results and for whom they are beneficial.

Insertional Achilles tendinopathy

It appears to be a consensus that the majority of patients with insertional Achilles tendinopathy will recover fully with non-surgical treatment. Interestingly, there are only a few studies that evaluate the effects of such treatments. Historically, these patients have been referred to physical therapy where the impairments and injury have been addressed with strengthening and stretching exercises, modalities for minimizing pain and inflammation, and manual techniques for improving any limitations in joint movement. However, based on the literature exercise along with shockwave therapy has the greatest evidence of effectiveness. We recommend performing a thorough evaluation of each individual patient and treating the impairments found. A strengthening programme that includes eccentric exercise for the calf musculature should be prescribed to all patients and performed for at least 12 weeks. It is important to point out that excessive dorsiflexion during the exercise might limit the success of the treatment, possibly due to the compression of the tendon and bursa onto the calcaneus. Having the patients stand on the floor instead of on a step when performing calf muscle exercises is therefore recommended.

References

1. Alfredson H. Chronic midportion Achilles tendinopathy: an update on research and treatment. Clin Sports Med. 2003;22:727-41.
2. Alfredson H. The chronic painful Achilles and patellar tendon: research on basic biology and treatment. Scand J Med Sci Sports. 2005;15:252-9.
3. Alfredson H, Cook J. A treatment algorithm for managing Achilles tendinopathy: new treatment options. Br J Sports Med. 2007;41:211-6.
4. Alfredson H, Lorentzon R. Chronic Achilles tendinosis: recommendations for treatment and prevention. Sports Med. 2000;29:135-46.
5. Alfredson H, Lorentzon R. Intratendinous glutamate levels and eccentric training in chronic Achilles tendinosis: a prospective study using microdialysis technique. Knee Surg Sports Traumatol Arthrosc. 2003;11:196-9.
6. Alfredson H, Öhberg L, Forsgren S. Is vasculo-neural ingrowth the cause of pain in chronic Achilles tendinosis? An investigation using ultrasonography and colour Doppler, immunohistochemistry, and diagnostic injections. Knee Surg Sports Traumatol Arthrosc. 2003;11:334-8.
7. Alfredson H, Pietilä T, Jonsson P, Lorentzon R. Heavy-load eccentric calf muscle training for the treatment of chronic Achilles tendinosis. Am J Sports Med. 1998;26:360-6.
8. Alfredson H, Pietilä T, Öhberg L, Lorentzon R. Achilles tendinosis and calf muscle strength. The effect of short-term immobilization after surgical treatment. Am J Sports Med. 1998;26:166-71.
9. Allison GT, Purdam C. Eccentric loading for Achilles tendinopathy–strengthening or stretching? Br J Sports Med. 2009;43:276-9.
10. Almekinders LC, Weinhold PS, Maffulli N. Compression etiology in tendinopathy. Clin Sports Med. 2003;22:703-10.
11. Angermann P, Hovgaard D. Chronic Achilles tendinopathy in athletic individuals: results of nonsurgical treatment. Foot Ankle Int. 1999;20:304-6.
12. Aspenberg P. Stimulation of tendon repair: mechanical loading, GDFs and platelets. A mini-review. Int Orthop. 2007;31:783-9.
13. Benjamin M, Moriggl B, Brenner E, Emery P, McGonagle D, Redman S. The "enthesis organ" concept: why enthesopathies may not present as focal insertional disorders. Arthritis and rheumatism. 2004;50:3306-13.
14. Brosseau L, Casimiro L, Robinson V, Milne S, Shea B, Judd M, Wells G, Tugwell P. Therapeutic ultrasound for treating patellofemoral pain syndrome. Cochrane database of systematic reviews (Online). 2001:CD003375.
15. Calder JD, Saxby TS. Surgical treatment of insertional Achilles tendinosis. Foot Ankle Int. 2003;24:119-21.
16. Carcia CR, Martin RL, Houck J, Wukich DK. Achilles pain, stiffness, and muscle power deficits: achilles tendinitis. J Orthop Sports Phys Ther. 2010;40:A1-26.
17. Chester R, Costa ML, Shepstone L, Cooper A, Donell ST. Eccentric calf muscle training compared with therapeutic ultrasound for chronic Achilles tendon pain--a pilot study. Man Ther. 2008;13:484-91.
18. Child S, Bryant AL, Clark RA, Crossley KM. Mechanical properties of the achilles tendon aponeurosis are altered in athletes with achilles tendinopathy. Am J Sports Med. 2010;38:1885-93.
19. Clement DB, Taunton JE, Smart GW. Achilles tendinitis and peritendinitis: etiology and treatment. Am J Sports Med. 1984;12:179-84.
20. Cook JL, Purdam C. Is compressive load a factor in the development of tendinopathy? Br J Sports Med. 2012;46:163-8.
21. Cook JL, Purdam CR. Rehabilitation of lower limb tendinopathies. Clin Sports Med. 2003;22:777-89.
22. Curwin S. Tendinitis : its etiology and treatment. Lexington, Mass.: Collamore Press; 1984.
23. Danielson P. Reviving the "biochemical" hypothesis for tendinopathy: new findings suggest the involvement of locally produced signal substances. Br J Sports Med. 2009;43:265-8.
24. Donoghue OA, Harrison AJ, Laxton P, Jones RK. Orthotic control of rear foot and lower limb motion during running in participants with chronic Achilles tendon injury. Sports Biomech. 2008;7:194-205.
25. Enwemeka CS. The effects of therapeutic ultrasound on tendon healing. A biomechanical study. Am J Phys Med Rehabil. 1989;68:283-7.
26. Fahlström M, Jonsson P, Lorentzon R, Alfredson H. Chronic Achilles tendon pain treated with eccentric calf-muscle training. Knee Surg Sports Traumatol Arthrosc. 2003;11:327-33.
27. Fyfe I, Stanish WD. The use of eccentric training and stretching in the treatment and prevention of tendon injuries. Clin Sports Med. 1992;11:601-24.
28. Gross ML, Davlin LB, Evanski PM. Effectiveness of orthotic shoe inserts in the long-distance runner. Am J Sports Med. 1991;19:409-12.

29. Haglund-Åkerlind Y, Eriksson E. Range of motion, muscle torque and training habits in runners with and without Achilles tendon problems. Knee Surg Sports Traumatol Arthrosc. 1993;1:195-9.
30. Heckman DS, Gluck GS, Parekh SG. Tendon disorders of the foot and ankle, part 2: achilles tendon disorders. Am J Sports Med. 2009;37:1223-34.
31. Hess GP, Cappiello WL, Poole RM, Hunter SC. Prevention and treatment of overuse tendon injuries. Sports Med. 1989;8:371-84.
32. Irwin TA. Current concepts review: insertional achilles tendinopathy. Foot Ankle Int. 2010;31:933-9.
33. Jackson BA, Schwane JA, Starcher BC. Effect of ultrasound therapy on the repair of Achilles tendon injuries in rats. Med Sci Sports Exerc. 1991;23:171-6.
34. Jonsson P, Alfredson H, Sunding K, Fahlstrom M, Cook J. New regimen for eccentric calf-muscle training in patients with chronic insertional Achilles tendinopathy: results of a pilot study. Br J Sports Med. 2008;42:746-9.
35. Kader D, Saxena A, Movin T, Maffulli N. Achilles tendinopathy: some aspects of basic science and clinical management. Br J Sports Med. 2002;36:239-49.
36. Kannus P. Etiology and pathophysiology of chronic tendon disorders in sports. Scand J Med Sci Sports. 1997;7:78-85.
37. Kannus P, Jozsa L, Natri A, Järvinen M. Effects of training, immobilization and remobilization on tendons. Scand J Med Sci Sports. 1997;7:67-71.
38. Kaufman KR, Brodine SK, Shaffer RA, Johnson CW, Cullison TR. The effect of foot structure and range of motion on musculoskeletal overuse injuries. Am J Sports Med. 1999;27:585-93.
39. Kearney R, Costa ML. Insertional achilles tendinopathy management: a systematic review. Foot Ankle Int. 2010;31:689-94.
40. Kingma JJ, de Knikker R, Wittink HM, Takken T. Eccentric overload training in patients with chronic Achilles tendinopathy: a systematic review. Br J Sports Med. 2007;41:e3.
41. Kjaer M. Role of extracellular matrix in adaptation of tendon and skeletal muscle to mechanical loading. Physiol Rev. 2004;84:649-98.
42. Kountouris A, Cook J. Rehabilitation of Achilles and patellar tendinopathies. Best practice & research Clinical rheumatology. 2007;21:295-316.
43. Krishna Sayana M, Maffulli N. Insertional Achilles tendinopathy. Foot Ankle Clin. 2005;10:309-20.
44. Kvist M. Achilles tendon injuries in athletes. Ann Chir Gynaecol. 1991;80:188-201.
45. Kvist M. Achilles tendon injuries in athletes. Sports Med. 1994;18:173-201.
46. Langberg H, Kongsgaard M. Eccentric training in tendinopathy--more questions than answers. Scand J Med Sci Sports. 2008;18:541-2.
47. Lyman J, Weinhold PS, Almekinders LC. Strain behavior of the distal achilles tendon: implications for insertional achilles tendinopathy. Am J Sports Med. 2004;32:457-61.
48. Maffulli N, Testa V, Capasso G, Sullo A. Calcific insertional Achilles tendinopathy: reattachment with bone anchors. Am J Sports Med. 2004;32:174-82.
49. Maffulli N, Walley G, Sayana MK, Longo UG, Denaro V. Eccentric calf muscle training in athletic patients with Achilles tendinopathy. Disabil Rehabil. 2008;30:1677-84.
50. Mafi N, Lorentzon R, Alfredson H. Superior short-term results with eccentric calf muscle training compared to concentric training in a randomized prospective multicenter study on patients with chronic Achilles tendinosis. Knee Surg Sports Traumatol Arthrosc. 2001;9:42-7.
51. Magnussen RA, Dunn WR, Thomson AB. Nonoperative treatment of midportion Achilles tendinopathy: a systematic review. Clin J Sport Med. 2009;19:54-64.
52. Magnusson SP, Aagard P, Simonsen E, Bojsen-Moller F. A biomechanical evaluation of cyclic and static stretch in human skeletal muscle. Int J Sports Med. 1998;19:310-6.
53. Mahieu NN, Witvrouw E, Stevens V, Van Tiggelen D, Roget P. Intrinsic risk factors for the development of achilles tendon overuse injury: a prospective study. Am J Sports Med. 2006;34:226-35.
54. Mahieu NN, Witvrouw E, Stevens V, Van Tiggelen D, Roget P. Intrinsic Risk Factors for the Development of Achilles Tendon Overuse Injury: A Prospective Study. Am J Sports Med. 2005.
55. Malliaras P, Barton CJ, Reeves ND, Langberg H. Achilles and patellar tendinopathy loading programmes: a systematic review comparing clinical outcomes and identifying potential mechanisms for effectiveness. Sports Med. 2013;43:267-86.
56. Mayer F, Hirschmuller A, Muller S, Schuberth M, Baur H. Effects of short-term treatment strategies over 4 weeks in Achilles tendinopathy. Br J Sports Med. 2007;41:e6.
57. McCrory JL, Martin DF, Lowery RB, Cannon DW, Curl WW, Read HM, Jr., Hunter DM, Craven T, Messier SP. Etiologic factors associated with Achilles tendinitis in runners. Med Sci Sports Exerc. 1999;31:1374-81.
58. Munteanu SE, Barton CJ. Lower limb biomechanics during running in individuals with achilles tendinopathy: a systematic review. Journal of foot and ankle research. 2011;4:15.
59. Myerson MS, McGarvey W. Disorders of the Achilles tendon insertion and Achilles tendinitis. Instr Course Lect. 1999;48:211-8.

60. Neeter C, Thomeé R, Silbernagel KG, Thomeé P, Karlsson J. Iontophoresis with or without dexamethazone in the treatment of acute Achilles tendon pain. Scand J Med Sci Sports. 2003;13:376-82.
61. Nicholson CW, Berlet GC, Lee TH. Prediction of the success of nonoperative treatment of insertional Achilles tendinosis based on MRI. Foot Ankle Int. 2007;28:472-7.
62. Niesen-Vertommen S, Taunton J, Clement D, Mosher R. The effect of eccentric versus concentric exercise in the management of Achilles tendonitis. Clin J Sport Med. 1992;2:109-13.
63. Norregaard J, Larsen CC, Bieler T, Langberg H. Eccentric exercise in treatment of Achilles tendinopathy. Scand J Med Sci Sports. 2007;17:133-8.
64. Öhberg L, Alfredson H. Effects on neovascularisation behind the good results with eccentric training in chronic mid-portion Achilles tendinosis? Knee Surg Sports Traumatol Arthrosc. 2004;12:465-70.
65. Öhberg L, Lorentzon R, Alfredson H. Eccentric training in patients with chronic Achilles tendinosis: normalised tendon structure and decreased thickness at follow up. Br J Sports Med. 2004;38:8-11; discussion
66. Paavola M, Kannus P, Orava S, Pasanen M, Järvinen M. Surgical treatment for chronic Achilles tendinopathy: a prospective seven month follow up study. Br J Sports Med. 2002;36:178-82.
67. Paavola M, Orava S, Leppilahti J, Kannus P, Järvinen M. Chronic Achilles tendon overuse injury: complications after surgical treatment. An analysis of 432 consecutive patients. Am J Sports Med. 2000;28:77-82.
68. Rees JD, Lichtwark GA, Wolman RL, Wilson AM. The mechanism for efficacy of eccentric loading in Achilles tendon injury; an in vivo study in humans. Rheumatology (Oxford, England). 2008.
69. Robertson VJ, Baker KG. A review of therapeutic ultrasound: effectiveness studies. Phys Ther. 2001;81:1339-50.
70. Rompe JD, Nafe B, Furia JP, Maffulli N. Eccentric loading, shock-wave treatment, or a wait-and-see policy for tendinopathy of the main body of tendo Achillis: a randomized controlled trial. Am J Sports Med. 2007;35:374-83.
71. Roos EM, Engström M, Lagerquist A, Söderberg B. Clinical improvement after 6 weeks of eccentric exercise in patients with mid-portion Achilles tendinopathy -- a randomized trial with 1-year follow-up. Scand J Med Sci Sports. 2004;14:286-95.
72. Rosenbaum D, Hennig EM. The influence of stretching and warm-up exercises on Achilles tendon reflex activity. J Sports Sci. 1995;13:481-90.
73. Rowe V, Hemmings S, Barton C, Malliaras P, Maffulli N, Morrissey D. Conservative management of midportion Achilles tendinopathy: a mixed methods study, integrating systematic review and clinical reasoning. Sports Med. 2012;42:941-67.
74. Schepsis AA, Wagner C, Leach RE. Surgical management of Achilles tendon overuse injuries. A long-term follow-up study. Am J Sports Med. 1994;22:611-9.
75. Shalabi A, Kristoffersen-Wilberg M, Svensson L, Aspelin P, Movin T. Eccentric training of the gastrocnemius-soleus complex in chronic Achilles tendinopathy results in decreased tendon volume and intratendinous signal as evaluated by MRI. Am J Sports Med. 2004;32:1286-96.
76. Silbernagel KG, Brorsson A, Lundberg M. The majority of patients with Achilles tendinopathy recover fully when treated with exercise alone: a 5-year follow-up. Am J Sports Med. 2011;39:607-13.
77. Silbernagel KG, Gustavsson A, Thomee R, Karlsson J. Evaluation of lower leg function in patients with Achilles tendinopathy. Knee Surg Sports Traumatol Arthrosc. 2006;14:1207-17.
78. Silbernagel KG, Thomee R, Eriksson BI, Karlsson J. Continued sports activity, using a pain-monitoring model, during rehabilitation in patients with Achilles tendinopathy: a randomized controlled study. Am J Sports Med. 2007;35:897-906.
79. Silbernagel KG, Thomeé R, Thomeé P, Karlsson J. Eccentric overload training for patients with chronic Achilles tendon pain--a randomised controlled study with reliability testing of the evaluation methods. Scand J Med Sci Sports. 2001;11:197-206.
80. Solan M, Davies M. Management of insertional tendinopathy of the Achilles tendon. Foot Ankle Clin. 2007;12:597-615, vi.
81. Stanish WD, Curwin S, Mandell S. Tendinitis: its etiology and treatment. New York: Oxford University Press; 2000.
82. Stanish WD, Rubinovich RM, Curwin S. Eccentric exercise in chronic tendinitis. Clin Orthop Relat Res. 1986;65-8.
83. Stergioulas A, Stergioula M, Aarskog R, Lopes-Martins RA, Bjordal JM. Effects of low-level laser therapy and eccentric exercises in the treatment of recreational athletes with chronic achilles tendinopathy. Am J Sports Med. 2008;36:881-7.
84. Sussmilch-Leitch SP, Collins NJ, Bialocerkowski AE, Warden SJ, Crossley KM. Physical therapies for Achilles tendinopathy: systematic review and meta-analysis. Journal of foot and ankle research. 2012;5:15.

85. Testa V, Capasso G, Benazzo F, Maffulli N. Management of Achilles tendinopathy by ultrasound-guided percutaneous tenotomy. Med Sci Sports Exerc. 2002;34:573-80.

86. Thomas JL, Christensen JC, Kravitz SR, Mendicino RW, Schuberth JM, Vanore JV, Weil LS, Sr., Zlotoff HJ, Bouche R, Baker J. The diagnosis and treatment of heel pain: a clinical practice guideline-revision 2010. J Foot Ankle Surg. 2010;49:S1-19.

87. Thomeé R. A comprehensive treatment approach for patellofemoral pain syndrome in young women. Phys Ther. 1997;77:1690-703.

88. Tumilty S, Munn J, McDonough S, Hurley DA, Basford JR, Baxter GD. Low level laser treatment of tendinopathy: a systematic review with meta-analysis. Photomed Laser Surg. 2010;28:3-16.

89. van der Plas A, de Jonge S, de Vos RJ, van der Heide HJ, Verhaar JA, Weir A, Tol JL. A 5-year follow-up study of Alfredson's heel-drop exercise programme in chronic midportion Achilles tendinopathy. Br J Sports Med. 2012;46:214-8.

90. Van Ginckel A, Thijs Y, Hesar NG, Mahieu N, De Clercq D, Roosen P, Witvrouw E. Intrinsic gait-related risk factors for Achilles tendinopathy in novice runners: a prospective study. Gait Posture. 2009;29:387-91.

91. Wagner E, Gould JS, Kneidel M, Fleisig GS, Fowler R. Technique and results of Achilles tendon detachment and reconstruction for insertional Achilles tendinosis. Foot Ankle Int. 2006;27:677-84.

92. Woodley BL, Newsham-West RJ, Baxter GD. Chronic tendinopathy: effectiveness of eccentric exercise. Br J Sports Med. 2007;41:188-98; discussion 99.

93. Yodlowski ML, Scheller AD, Jr., Minos L. Surgical treatment of Achilles tendinitis by decompression of the retrocalcaneal bursa and the superior calcaneal tuberosity. Am J Sports Med. 2002;30:318-21.

"There's no easy way out. If there were, I would have bought it. And believe me, it would be one of my favourite things!"

Oprah Winfrey

Chapter 10

Rehabilitation Following Achilles Tendon Rupture

Karin Grävare Silbernagel, Annelie Brorsson, Jón Karlsson

Take Home Message

- *Early mobilization and weight-bearing are beneficial for both surgically- and non-surgically-treated patients.*

- *The progression in rehabilitation should be based both on the time since injury and the recovery of functional milestones.*

- *It is very common that patients heal with an elongated tendon and, therefore, will not recover to the same heel-rise height.*

- *There are two ways to increase the load of the tendon: increase the external load or increase the speed of loading.*

Introduction

When discussing what treatments to recommend following an Achilles tendon rupture, the focus has mostly been on whether the injury should be treated surgically or non-surgically. In several systematic reviews [3, 11, 12, 15, 17, 39, 45,] it has been found that surgically-treated patients have a lower risk of re-rupture but a greater risk of other complications, such as wound complications, infections and sural nerve injury. In more recent years, there has been a move towards early

151

mobilization with the use of functional brace instead of cast immobilization. It has been found that the risk for re-rupture has decreased with the use of earlier mobilization protocols and that this is beneficial for both surgically- and non-surgically-treated patients [22, 42]. In two recent studies [27, 46] that compared identical early mobilization protocols for both surgically- and non-surgically-treated patients, the results indicate no significant differences in the rate of re-rupture between the groups. The rates of re-rupture were, for the surgically-treated groups, 4% in one of the studies [27] and 2.8% in the other [46], and for the non-surgically-treated groups it was 12% [27] and 4.2% respectively [46]. In general, it can be concluded that the re-rupture risk is very low with both treatment options so long as early mobilization is utilized.

There is, however, still the issue whereby the majority of patients will have long-term deficits in terms of strength and function, and these deficits appear to become permanent in many cases [16, 31]. Gait abnormalities have been found 24 months after injury [8] and patients report having difficulties with running and jumping. The recovery also takes a year or longer, with fear of re-injury being one reason for not returning to sports [24, 31]. Of interest is also that there are large variations between patients regardless of treatment. Some patients have full recovery in functional tests whereas others have only limited recovery when comparing the injured side to the uninjured side [27]. The reason for this is still not well-known.

The purpose of rehabilitation

The aim of rehabilitation following injury is to address and treat any impairment in lower extremity function and structure, limitations in activity and restrictions in participation. However, in order to improve current treatment protocols for both early and late rehabilitation, it is important to understand the anatomic and functional reasons for these deficits and also understand how exercise affects tendon loading.

Muscular weakness

Following an Achilles tendon rupture, injury and immobilization cause hypotrophy of the calf musculature and other muscles around the ankle [24]. The strength testing of the calf musculature has found deficits of approximately 10-30% [16]. Calf muscle endurance is also often measured using a heel-rise test [21, 36]. With this test, it has been found that patients had a mean deficit of 30% six months after injury and, at 12 months, this deficit was approximately 20% [36]. This calf muscle deficit has been shown to correlate to the degree of tendon elongation [26, 37]. The heel-rise height also appears to be of relevance for function [26, 37]. A recent study [5] also looked at what factors were associated with the delayed recovery of calf muscle endurance at one year. This study found that being male, having pain at rest at three months or having lower function at six months correlated to the delayed recovery of calf muscle endurance at one year. Another recent study [30] looking at the short-term recovery of heel-rise capability found that only 50% of the patients had recovered the ability to perform at least one heel-rise three months after injury. In that study, there were also no differences between patients treated surgically or non-surgically. However, the patients who had recovered the ability to perform a heel-rise were more often male and were significantly younger. Patients who could perform a heel-rise also had less patient-reported symptoms.

Tendon elongation

The tendon goes through a biphasic elongation during the healing process [25, 29]. Similar elongation has been shown in tendons treated both with and without surgery [34]. Both calf muscle weakness and heel-rise height deficits have been proposed to be caused by tendon elongation [26, 37]. One study found a significant correlation between the degree of tendon elongation and the amount of reduction in heel-rise height on the injured side compared to the healthy side [37]. Furthermore, it has been shown that tendon elongation limits the ability to generate plantar flexion force [26]. Gait abnormalities in patients with an Achilles tendon rupture have also been correlated to the occurrence of tendon elongation [38]. A lesser degree of tendon elongation has also been found to correlate with better clinical outcomes [13]. The avoidance of tendon elongation is probably of major importance in terms of the recovery of function.

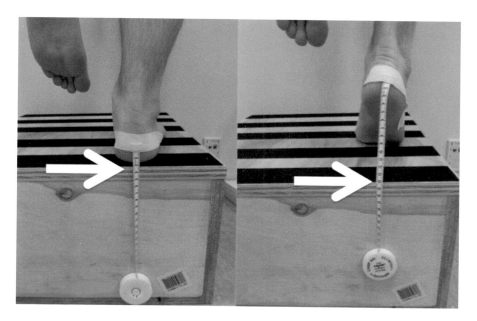

Figure 1. A simple clinical test for evaluating the maximal heel-rise height using a tape measure.

Are functional deficits due to difficulty with muscle activation or tendon elongation?

In a pilot study [41] an attempt was made to bring clarity to the question of whether the functional deficits seen were due to neuromuscular recruitment issues combined with tendon elongation or else mainly just tendon elongation. A comparison was made between healthy individuals and patients with Achilles tendon rupture. In all the patients, the injured Achilles tendon was longer than the non-injured side. There were no side-to-side differences in tendon lengths in the healthy subjects. It was shown that during gait there was an increased muscle activity of the gastrocnemius on the side that was injured compared with the healthy side. The triceps surae muscles' activation was also correlated to the elongation of the Achilles tendon. This suggests that the measured muscle weakness is not due to the inability of the muscle to contract but rather is caused by the anatomical changes of the tendon. Increased muscle activity might be required to account for taking up the slack of the longer tendon.

The importance of rehabilitation exercises

It can be considered common knowledge that, in order to regain muscle strength, the muscle needs to be progressively exposed to increased load. The rehabilitation following an Achilles tendon rupture therefore focuses on strength exercises for all the muscles around the ankle, with major focus on the calf muscle. The tendon also benefits from being exposed to loading during the healing process [2, 18]. Increased physical activity in an animal study resulted in a larger and stronger callus in a shorter time [1]. Furthermore, a higher degree of physical activity has been associated with more mature tissue repair in another animal study [6]. In humans, early loading has also been found to improve tendon structure [2, 18]. Kangas and co-workers [13] found that early motion resulted in a lesser degree of tendon elongation compared with immobilization in patients with an Achilles tendon rupture.

In the translation of animal and basic science research to the rehabilitation programme, there is a fear of overloading the tendon during the early phase. The focus is, of course, to get the patient better, but both the physical therapists' and the patients' fears of re-rupture might have a negative impact on the dosage of loading. One study also found a significant negative correlation between kinesiophobia (fear of movement) and patient-reported symptoms three months after injury [30]. Having knowledge of how exercise and activity load the tendon is, therefore, important in order to being able to prescribe appropriate and safe exercises during all stages of healing.

How do the specifics of the exercises affect the tendon?

A high load on the Achilles tendon occurs in activities during which the so-called 'stretch-shortening cycle' (SSC) is utilized [9, 20]. The SSC is a combination of an eccentric muscle action (with the lengthening of the muscle and tendon), followed by an immediate concentric muscle action (a shortening of the muscle-tendon complex) [4, 10, 19]. The faster the loading during activities that use the SSC, the greater the load on the Achilles tendon.

In vivo measurements of Achilles tendon load during various types of activities have been performed using a buckle-type transducer by Komi and co-workers [20]. They showed that the forces in the Achilles tendon varied considerably between individuals. Taken together, they found that during running the Achilles tendon was loaded up to 12 times the body weight, but that the actual load was dependent on the speed of running. They also measured a force of approximately 3.5 times the body weight during walking, whereas during cycling the load was close to the body weight.

To design an exercise programme that progressively increases the load of the tendon, it is important to understand that there are two ways to manipulate the load on the tendon, either by changing the external load or by changing the speed of loading (Figure 2).

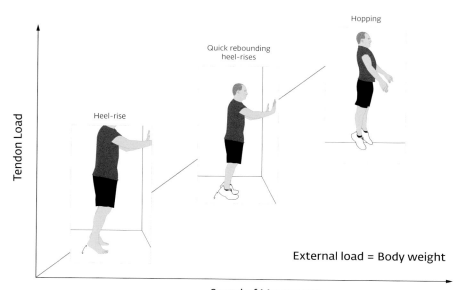

Figure 2. One way to increase the load by utilizing the speed of loading is by moving from a slow, double-leg heel-rise to a quick, rebounding heel-rise, and finally hopping (a rhythmic vertical jumping motion like as with a jumping rope). During hopping the tendon, is loaded by up to five times the body weight as compared to half the body weight during a slow double leg heel-rise [9].

Review over current clinical protocols

Rehabilitation generally starts at around 6-8 weeks after injury, when the cast or functional bracing is removed. Often, there is a very general description to slowly progress the load with exercise during rehabilitation. In most studies, the patients are allowed to walk when the brace is removed around week 6-8 after the injury [15, 24, 27, 46]. If walking is allowed, then bilateral standing heel-rises should be tolerated well as long as the speed of movement is slow and controlled. Interestingly, often both the patient and the physical therapist express a fear of having the tendon re-rupture, and this often slows down the rehabilitation. It is therefore common to focus on unloaded range of motion exercises early on, but instead the mechanical loading of the tendon is important for healing. In the last decade, there has been a move towards early mobilization [14, 23, 40, 43]. This usually means using a functional brace that allows weight-bearing. Heel-lifts are used in the functional brace to keep the ankle in plantar flexion. Most protocols keep the ankle at around at least 20-25° of plantar flexion for the first two weeks, followed by a decrease of 5-10° per week with the goal of having the ankle in at least 0° of plantar flexion by the time the functional brace is removed. Despite defining this type of protocol for early mobilization, there is very little mobilization and loading of the tendon; rather, it implies that the patient becomes more mobile.

Rehabilitation phases

Rehabilitation can be divided into four different phases following an Achilles tendon rupture.

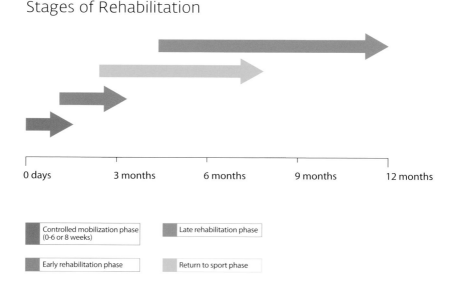

Figure 3. Stages of rehabilitation.

The problem with dividing the rehabilitation into phases is that the phases historically have been described in terms of time. However, as described earlier there are large variations in recovery and – as mentioned before – one study 30 found that only half of the patients were able to perform a single leg heel-rise at three months after injury. Hence, there are very distinct differences in physical ability, and this should guide how to progress each individual patient. Progression from one rehabilitation phase to another should, therefore, be based both on the time since injury and the recovery of functional milestones.

The controlled mobilization phase: weeks 0-8

Most recent studies allow weight-bearing through the heel in a functional brace, either immediately or after the first two weeks [7, 27, 46]. The ankle position is usually controlled by placing heel-lifts in the brace. Most of the protocols do not describe any specific exercise to provide for the loading of the tendon during this early phase.

Two recent studies have utilized identical protocols with functional braces during this phase for both surgical and non-surgical treatment [27, 46]. Nilsson-Helander and co-workers [27] used a cast for two weeks and then a brace that allowed early mobility but where weight-bearing was not allowed until week 6. The weight-bearing was allowed when the position of the brace allowed for the foot to be flat on the ground. Active range of motion (AROM) was allowed after the first two weeks, but the amount of dorsiflexion was controlled by the brace. During weeks 2-4, the dorsiflexion was limited to -30°, while for weeks 4-6 it was limited to -10° and for weeks 6-8 it was limited to +10°. This protocol was tolerated well by both groups and there were no significant differences in functional outcomes between the groups.

Willits and co-workers [46] followed a similar protocol for the first two weeks. For the following two weeks (weeks 2-4), Willits and co-workers [46] allowed AROM of plantar flexion and dorsiflexion to neutral, inversion and eversion below neutral, and protected weight-bearing with crutches. The same exercises were allowed for weeks 4-6 and, at this stage, full weight-bearing was allowed. During weeks 6-8, slow stretch into dorsiflexion was allowed. The protocol also states that graduated exercises were allowed, but it is not clear what specific exercises were used. This study weaned the subject off the boot during weeks 8-12. Furthermore, this treatment protocol was tolerated well by both surgically- and non-surgically-treated patients.

In one recently completed study [32] the surgically-treated group was allowed to bear weight and begin isometric submaximal plantar flexion in the brace immediately. After two weeks light resistance training – with the use of a resistance band for the ankle and calf muscle along with sitting heel-rises – was initiated. The goal was to increase the load of the tendon so as to promote healing and minimize muscle hypotrophy. The main limitation was in restricting the amount of dorsiflexion. This limitation was 15° of plantar flexion during weeks

2-4, 10° of plantar flexion during weeks 4-5 and 0° of plantar flexion during weeks 5-6. The brace was discontinued after six weeks. The surgically-treated group did not have any re-rupture. In this study, the non-surgically-treated group was allowed immediate weight-bearing and used the brace for eight weeks with no specific exercise instructions while wearing the brace. In this group, there were five re-ruptures. At three months, 50% of the patients were able to perform one-legged heel-rises and there was no significant difference between the surgically and non-surgically-treated patients. The next logical step is to see whether this early rehabilitation protocol is also possible for non-surgically-treated patients, and whether this results in less tendon elongation and better improvements over the long-term.

Taken together, most studies appear to include more or less immobilization in weeks 0-2. Afterwards, some lighter range of motion activity and/or isometric loading of plantar flexion may be allowed through weeks 6-8. Some then discontinue with the brace at week 6 and others at week 8, with large variations among physicians and practices. In general, the move to early mobilization has been beneficial in reducing re-rupture rates and improving functional outcomes[17]. However, the amount of loading on the tendon is still very limited at this early phase, and if the results from animal studies can be translated to humans it appears that a greater amount of loading during this phase would be beneficial. Since the tendon elongation appears to be one major factor limiting the recovery of full function, it might be important to limit the amount of stretching of the ankle into dorsiflexion during this phase. More studies are therefore needed to evaluate the degree of tendon elongation following an Achilles tendon rupture.

The early rehabilitation phase: 6-11 weeks

This phase can be considered to start when the patients are allowed to walk without a brace. Since walking has been shown to load the tendon with approximately 3.5 times the body weight [20], it can be considered safe to start the double-leg heel-rise exercise as long as the speed of movement is slow and controlled. The main goal of this phase is to start the strengthening of the calf musculature. The triceps surae is important both for stability during standing and for control and propulsion during walking. This is also the phase with the greatest risk of re-rupture [24]. If the risk of re-rupture is because the tendon is weak or due to the weak muscle's inability to control the loading of the tendon is unknown. Since the patients often have limited activity with their calf muscles, many of them also have problems with the swelling of the lower leg.

The aim of rehabilitation during this stage is also to treat any other strength, range of motion, balance or gait deficits of the injured leg (Table 1). The main goal of this phase is to achieve a unilateral heel-rise, full active ankle range of motion, walk without a limp and have normal a push-off during gait. One clinical guideline is: if the patient can achieve at least five single leg heel-rises, of about 90% of available height, then they can progress to increasing the load of the tendon by increasing the speed of loading and progress to bilateral hops and gentle jogging in place.

The stretching of the Achilles tendon is normally not recommended at this stage, since tendon elongation is one of the main issues following a rupture. Full ankle dorsiflexion range of motion is, on the other hand, important to regain. To protect the Achilles tendon, you can work on the dorsiflexion range of motion with the knee bent to limit the two joint gastrocnemius muscles being stretched across the knee joint.

Early Rehabilitation Phase (6-11 weeks)
Visit for physical therapy 2-3 times a week and home exercises daily

Exercises programme:

– Exercise bike
– Ankle range of motion
– Ankle strengthening using a resistance band or cable machine
– Sitting heel-rise with external load (25-50% of body weight)
– Standing heel-rise progressing from two legs to one legs
– Gait training
– Balance exercises
– Leg presses
– Leg extensions
– Leg curls
– Foot exercises

If the patient meets the criteria of five single leg heel-rises at 90% of height, then start:

– Bilateral rebounding heel-rises
– Bilateral hops in place
– Gentle jogging in place

Table 1. General rehabilitation programmes during the early rehabilitation phase.

The late rehabilitation phase: weeks 12-15

This phase starts when the milestone of performing at least one unilateral heel-rise is achieved or – at the latest – around week 15 if unable to meet the heel-rising criteria. The idea is that starting to increase activities despite not having achieved the heel-rise milestone is safe after 15 weeks and – perhaps – these exercises might actually help in achieving the strength milestone. The goal of this phase is to slowly progress to running and jumping (Table 2). The exercises for the Achilles tendon and calf musculature are increased by increasing the external load and/or increasing the speed of the load (fast rebounding exercises) (Figure 2). At this time, the patients can progress from a two leg jump to a one leg jump. It is therefore important to continuously perform functional evaluations so as to determine when to start the running and jumping programme. If the tendon is elongated, the patient cannot be expected to achieve an equal height of heel-rise. This is, therefore, an unrealistic goal. Instead, it is better to evaluate the number of repetitions that the patient is able to perform and compare them to the uninjured side. Having the patient perform the heel-rise from 10° of dorsiflexion allows for the better recruitment of the calf muscle compared to 0°, if the tendon is elongated.

Criteria for starting a running progression programme
Must be 12 weeks post injury and able to achieve five unilateral heel-rises at 90% of available height
If the patient is not able to perform the heel-rise criteria at weeks 14-15, he/she can begin the running progression if they are able to raise at least 70% of their bodyweight during a single heel-rise.

Table 2. Criteria for starting a running progression programme.

During this early phase, it is recommended to leave three days between running activities to allow for the muscles and Achilles tendon to recover. However, it should be remembered to continue to evaluate functionality and symptoms and to adjust accordingly for each individual patient.

The return to sports phase

Current recommendations for returning to sport are mostly time-based. The expected return to running is between 12-16 weeks, depending on the type of treatment (surgery versus no surgery, and early mobilization in a functional brace or not) [44]. Patients treated with surgery and early mobilization are considered to be able to start running at week 12, whereas those treated non-surgically and with immobilization are expected to start running after 16 weeks. Since studies have found no differences in function between those treated with and without surgery, there might not be any reason for suggesting different times for returning to sports based on this variable [27, 46]. There are, on the other hand, large variations between individual patients, and this strongly implies that it is important to use both the timeframe and functional milestone criteria when recommending a return to sports. A test battery has been used for many years to evaluate function in these patients [27, 28, 31, 35]. This test battery and other combinations of tests to evaluate strength, muscle endurance and jumping ability can be recommended for performance prior to a return to sports. After other injuries – such as ACL injury – it is often recommended that the patient achieve 90% of the function of the non-injured side. These same criteria can be used for this patient group as well. The only variable that might not recover to that level is the heel-rise height, since it has been found that patients who have an elongated tendon will not recover to the same heel-rise height [37].

Is it safe to return to running and jumping?

A recent case study [38] reported both pre- and post-injury running kinematics in a patient with an Achilles tendon rupture. This study showed that the patient had increased ankle dorsiflexion and rear-foot abduction after injury when compared with pre-injury data. This patient also had an elongated tendon when compared to the uninjured side. The patient returned, however, back to her normal running routine and reported only minor limitations with running. Whether there is an increased risk of other injuries due to running with these altered mechanics is currently not known. In a study of professional football players with Achilles tendon ruptures, it was found that 32% did not return to football and that those who did had an average reduction of 50% in performance level [33]. Further long-term studies are needed to determine whether these changes are common and whether they predispose the patients to other injuries.

Conclusion

Taken as a whole, it is time to focus the treatment on having the patients achieving full function instead of just avoiding re-rupture. Since some patients are recovering fully, there appears to be the potential for most patients to have similar recovery. The rehabilitation performed at each stage is important for helping the patients achieve full function. The current research indicates that previous treatments might have been too conservative, especially in the early-phase (i.e., the first weeks after the injury). Future research is needed to determine the ideal loading conditions during the controlled mobilization phase, with the goal being to prevent long-term deficits such as tendon elongation.

References

1. Andersson T, Eliasson P, Aspenberg P. Tissue memory in healing tendons: short loading episodes stimulate healing. J Appl Physiol. 2009;107:417-21.
2. Aspenberg P. Stimulation of tendon repair: mechanical loading, GDFs and platelets. A mini-review. Int Orthop. 2007;31:783-9.
3. Bhandari M, Guyatt GH, Siddiqui F, Morrow F, Busse J, Leighton RK, Sprague S, Schemitsch EH. Treatment of acute Achilles tendon ruptures: a systematic overview and metaanalysis. Clin Orthop Relat Res. 2002:190-200.
4. Bosco C, Tarkka I, Komi PV. Effect of elastic energy and myoelectrical potentiation of triceps surae during stretch-shortening cycle exercise. Int J Sports Med. 1982;3:137-40.
5. Bostick GP, Jomha NM, Suchak AA, Beaupre LA. Factors associated with calf muscle endurance recovery 1 year after achilles tendon rupture repair. J Orthop Sports Phys Ther. 2010;40:345-51.
6. Bring DK, Reno C, Renstrom P, Salo P, Hart DA, Ackermann PW. Joint immobilization reduces the expression of sensory neuropeptide receptors and impairs healing after tendon rupture in a rat model. J Orthop Res. 2009;27:274-80.
7. Costa ML, MacMillan K, Halliday D, Chester R, Shepstone L, Robinson AH, Donell ST. Randomised controlled trials of immediate weight-bearing mobilisation for rupture of the tendo Achillis. J Bone Joint Surg Br. 2006;88:69-77.
8. Don R, Ranavolo A, Cacchio A, Serrao M, Costabile F, Iachelli M, Camerota F, Frascarelli M, Santilli V. Relationship between recovery of calf-muscle biomechanical properties and gait pattern following surgery for achilles tendon rupture. Clin Biomech (Bristol, Avon). 2007;22:211-20.
9. Fukashiro S, Komi PV, Järvinen M, Miyashita M. In vivo Achilles tendon loading during jumping in humans. Eur J Appl Physiol Occup Physiol. 1995;71:453-8.
10. Ishikawa M, Komi PV. Effects of different dropping intensities on fascicle and tendinous tissue behavior during stretch-shortening cycle exercise. J Appl Physiol. 2004;96:848-52.
11. Jiang N, Wang B, Chen A, Dong F, Yu B. Operative versus nonoperative treatment for acute Achilles tendon rupture: a meta-analysis based on current evidence. Int Orthop. 2012;36:765-73.
12. Jones MP, Khan RJ, Carey Smith RL. Surgical interventions for treating acute achilles tendon rupture: key findings from a recent cochrane review. J Bone Joint Surg Am. 2012;94:e88.
13. Kangas J, Pajala A, Ohtonen P, Leppilahti J. Achilles tendon elongation after rupture repair: a randomized comparison of 2 postoperative regimens. Am J Sports Med. 2007;35:59-64.
14. Kangas J, Pajala A, Siira P, Hamalainen M, Leppilahti J. Early functional treatment versus early immobilization in tension of the musculotendinous unit after Achilles rupture repair: a prospective, randomized, clinical study. The Journal of trauma. 2003;54:1171-80.
15. Khan RJ, Carey Smith RL. Surgical interventions for treating acute Achilles tendon ruptures. Cochrane database of systematic reviews (Online). 2010:CD003674.
16. Khan RJ, Fick D, Brammar TJ, Crawford J, Parker MJ. Interventions for treating acute Achilles tendon ruptures. Cochrane database of systematic reviews (Online). 2004:CD003674.
17. Khan RJ, Fick D, Keogh A, Crawford J, Brammar T, Parker M. Treatment of acute achilles tendon ruptures. A meta-analysis of randomized, controlled trials. J Bone Joint Surg Am. 2005;87:2202-10.
18. Kjaer M, Langberg H, Miller BF, Boushel R, Crameri R, Koskinen S, Heinemeier K, Olesen JL, Dossing S, Hansen M, Pedersen SG, Rennie MJ, Magnusson P. Metabolic activity and collagen turnover in human tendon in response to physical activity. J Musculoskelet Neuronal Interact. 2005;5:41-52.
19. Komi PV. Stretch-shortening cycle: a powerful model to study normal and fatigued muscle. J Biomech. 2000;33:1197-206.
20. Komi PV, Fukashiro S, Järvinen M. Biomechanical loading of Achilles tendon during normal locomotion. Clin Sports Med. 1992;11:521-31.
21. Lunsford BR, Perry J. The standing heel-rise test for ankle plantar flexion: criterion for normal. Phys Ther. 1995;75:694-8.
22. Maffulli N, Tallon C, Wong J, Lim KP, Bleakney R. Early weightbearing and ankle mobilization after open repair of acute midsubstance tears of the achilles tendon. Am J Sports Med. 2003;31:692-700.
23. Metz R, Verleisdonk EJ, van der Heijden GJ, Clevers GJ, Hammacher ER, Verhofstad MH, van der Werken C. Acute Achilles tendon rupture: minimally invasive surgery versus nonoperative treatment with immediate full weightbearing--a randomized controlled trial. Am J Sports Med. 2008;36:1688-94.
24. Möller M, Movin T, Granhed H, Lind K, Faxen E, Karlsson J. Acute rupture of tendon Achillis. A prospective randomised study of comparison between surgical and non-surgical treatment. J Bone Joint Surg Br. 2001;83:843-8.
25. Mortensen NH, Saether J, Steinke MS, Staehr H, Mikkelsen SS. Separation of tendon ends after Achilles tendon repair: a prospective, randomized, multicenter study. Orthopedics. 1992;15:899-903.

26. Mullaney MJ, McHugh MP, Tyler TF, Nicholas SJ, Lee SJ. Weakness in end-range plantar flexion after Achilles tendon repair. Am J Sports Med. 2006;34:1120-5.

27. Nilsson-Helander K, Silbernagel KG, Thomee R, Faxen E, Olsson N, Eriksson BI, Karlsson J. Acute achilles tendon rupture: a randomized, controlled study comparing surgical and nonsurgical treatments using validated outcome measures. Am J Sports Med. 2010;38:2186-93.

28. Nilsson-Helander K, Sward L, Silbernagel KG, Thomee R, Eriksson BI, Karlsson J. A new surgical method to treat chronic ruptures and reruptures of the Achilles tendon. Knee Surg Sports Traumatol Arthrosc. 2008;16:614-20.

29. Nystrom B, Holmlund D. Separation of tendon ends after suture of achilles tendon. Acta Orthop Scand. 1983;54:620-1.

30. Olsson N, Karlsson J, Eriksson BI, Brorsson A, Lundberg M, Silbernagel KG. Ability to perform a single heel-rise is significantly related to patient-reported outcome after Achilles tendon rupture. Scand J Med Sci Sports. 2012. (epub ahead of print)

31. Olsson N, Nilsson-Helander K, Karlsson J, Eriksson BI, Thomee R, Faxen E, Silbernagel KG. Major functional deficits persist 2 years after acute Achilles tendon rupture. Knee Surg Sports Traumatol Arthrosc. 2011;19:1385-93.

32. Olsson N, Silbernagel KG, Eriksson BI, Sansone M, Brorsson A, Nilsson-Helander K, Karlsson J. Stable surgical repair with accelerated rehabilitation versus nonsurgical treatment for acute achilles tendon ruptures: a randomized controlled study. Am J Sports Med. 2013;41:2867-76.

33. Parekh SG, Wray WH, 3rd, Brimmo O, Sennett BJ, Wapner KL. Epidemiology and outcomes of Achilles tendon ruptures in the National Football League. Foot Ankle Spec. 2009;2:283-6.

34. Schepull T, Kvist J, Aspenberg P. Early E-modulus of healing Achilles tendons correlates with late function: similar results with or without surgery. Scand J Med Sci Sports. 2012;22:18-23.

35. Silbernagel KG, Gustavsson A, Thomee R, Karlsson J. Evaluation of lower leg function in patients with Achilles tendinopathy. Knee Surg Sports Traumatol Arthrosc. 2006;14:1207-17.

36. Silbernagel KG, Nilsson-Helander K, Thomee R, Eriksson BI, Karlsson J. A new measurement of heel-rise endurance with the ability to detect functional deficits in patients with Achilles tendon rupture. Knee Surg Sports Traumatol Arthrosc. 2010;18:258-64.

37. Silbernagel KG, Steele R, Manal K. Deficits in heel-rise height and achilles tendon elongation occur in patients recovering from an achilles tendon rupture. Am J Sports Med. 2012;40:1564-71.

38. Silbernagel KG, Willy R, Davis I. Preinjury and postinjury running analysis along with measurements of strength and tendon length in a patient with a surgically repaired Achilles tendon rupture. J Orthop Sports Phys Ther. 2012;42:521-9.

39. Soroceanu A, Sidhwa F, Aarabi S, Kaufman A, Glazebrook M. Surgical versus nonsurgical treatment of acute Achilles tendon rupture: a meta-analysis of randomized trials. J Bone Joint Surg Am. 2012;94:2136-43.

40. Suchak AA, Bostick GP, Beaupre LA, Durand DC, Jomha NM. The influence of early weight-bearing compared with non-weight-bearing after surgical repair of the Achilles tendon. J Bone Joint Surg Am. 2008;90:1876-83.

41. Suydam SM, Buchanan TS, Manal K, Silbernagel KG. Compensatory muscle activation caused by tendon lengthening post-Achilles tendon rupture. Knee Surg Sports Traumatol Arthrosc. 2013. (epub ahead of print)

42. Twaddle BC, Poon P. Early motion for Achilles tendon ruptures: is surgery important? A randomized, prospective study. Am J Sports Med. 2007;35:2033-8.

43. van der Eng DM, Schepers T, Schep NW, Goslings JC. Rerupture Rate after Early Weightbearing in Operative Versus Conservative Treatment of Achilles Tendon Ruptures: A Meta-Analysis. J Foot Ankle Surg. 2013. (epub ahead of print)

44. van Sterkenburg MN, van Dijk CN, Donley BG. Guidelines for sport resumption. In: van Dijk CN, Karlsson J, Maffulli N, Thermann H, editors. Achilles tendon rupture Current concepts: DJO Publications. p. 108-23.

45. Wilkins R, Bisson LJ. Operative versus nonoperative management of acute Achilles tendon ruptures: a quantitative systematic review of randomized controlled trials. Am J Sports Med. 2012;40:2154-60.

46. Willits K, Amendola A, Bryant D, Mohtadi NG, Giffin JR, Fowler P, Kean CO, Kirkley A. Operative versus nonoperative treatment of acute Achilles tendon ruptures: a multicenter randomized trial using accelerated functional rehabilitation. J Bone Joint Surg Am. 2010;92:2767-75.

*"But I must have the confidence
and I must be worthy of the great".*

Ernest Hemingway

Chapter 11

Extracorporeal Shock Wave Therapy

John P. Furia, Jan D. Rompe

Take Home Message

• *ESWT, insofar as it is used to treat Achilles tendinopathy, is effective, easy to perform and associated with a quick return to work and sport.*

• *ESWT, insofar as it is used to treat Achilles tendinopathy, is safe and well tolerated.*

• *The favourable results from ESWT are stable at extended follow-up.*

Introduction

Achilles tendinopathy is a frustrating condition with a prevalence of approximately 11% in the general population [2, 41-42, 58]. Achilles tendinopathy is the most common tendinopathy that occurs in runners and was identified in 56% of a group of high performance middle-aged runners [21]. There are two types of Achilles tendinopathy, insertional tendinopathy occurs at the bone-tendon junction, and mid-portion tendinopathy is located more proximally [34]. Each condition still can afflict both active and sedentary segments of the population. The precise aetiology remains unclear.

Physiological risk factors include hyperpronation, varus deformity of the forefoot, leg length discrepancy, advanced age and limited mobility of the sub-talar joint [1, 8, 22, 33, 35-36]. Overly intensive alteration in physical training, such as what occurs with increased interval training, excessive hill training, and increased mileage, are also associated with this condition [8, 35, 42, 55]. Other risk factors include poor technique, fatigue and increased mechanical overload [3-4, 8, 23, 35, 42, 54, 57].

Traditional non-surgical treatment consists of relative rest, activity modification, anti-inflammatory medications, various forms of physical therapy, heel-lifts, taping, heavy-load eccentric and concentric calf muscle training, and orthotics [4, 8, 17-22, 32, 35, 41-42, 59]. The optimal type of non-surgical treatment is unclear. There is little evidence to support the use of any one particular therapy for this condition.

Surgery is reserved for chronic cases. Options include the open excision of the degenerative tendon with or without paratendon stripping, the creation of multiple longitudinal tenotomies, and debridement [17, 32, 41, 55, 65-66, 69]. Success rates vary from series to series [17, 32, 41, 51, 65-66, 69] and the rate of complications, particularly complications related to wound healing, can be high [41-42].

Extracorporeal shockwave therapy (ESWT) has been shown to be an effective treatment for various musculoskeletal disorders, including plantar fasciopathy, shoulder calcific tendinopathy, lateral epicondylitis, greater trochanteric pain syndrome, medial tibial stress reaction, patella tendinopathy, and non-union of fractures of bones [5-6, 10, 12-14, 38-39, 46, 48-49, 52-53, 67-68, 72]. Investigators have also demonstrated that ESWT is a safe and highly effective treatment for both insertional and mid-portion Achilles tendinopathy [11, 24, 45, 50]. The aim of this chapter is to explain the rationale, justify the use, and summarize the clinical results, of using ESWT as a treatment for Achilles tendinopathy.

ESWT: basic principles

Physics

In physics, a shockwave is defined as an acoustic pressure wave, one characterized by a high peak pressure (up to 500 bar), a fast initial rise time of less than 10 ns, a short lifecycle (less than 10 ms), and a broad frequency spectrum (16–20 MHz) [15, 37, 56].

There are many types of shockwave generators designed specifically for musculoskeletal applications. Depending on the device, electromagnetic-, electrohydraulic-, piezoelectric- or electro-pneumatic-derived energy is transformed into a shockwave [15, 37, 56]. Each device concentrates and focuses the shockwaves so that the cumulative wave-energy can be applied in a sufficient quantity to stimulate a tissue response [15, 37].

Such 'focused' shockwaves are transmitted to a relatively small area (the 'focus') and can be targeted in a precise manner so that the maximum energy is several centimetres below the skin [15, 37]. The depth of penetration can be manipulated by varying the intensity of the treatment, allowing for the clinician to treat both superficial and relatively deep structures.

So called 'radial' shockwaves are produced by smaller, less expensive and more widely-available office-based devices. 'Radial' shockwaves transfer their maximum energy more superficially, at or just below the skin surface, and distribute the energy radially into the treated tissues [52]. The biological response produced by these pneumatic devices and the older, electro hydraulic, electromagnetic and piezoelectric devices is similar and the physical properties of a shockwave are the same regardless of the method.

For clinical use, the shockwaves are applied directly to tissues using the shockwave generator's targeting device. The waves are dispersed from the application site and then can be absorbed, reflected or dissipated, depending upon the properties of the particular tissue [15, 37].

Shockwaves have both a direct and indirect effect on treated tissues [37, 56]. Energy from absorbed shockwaves results in tensile forces. The tensile forces produce a biological response (i.e., a growth factor release, inflammatory factor inhibition, enhanced neutrophil activity, increased cytokine-mediated vascularity and enhanced angiogenesis) in the treated tissues. This accounts for the direct effect [37, 56].

Shockwaves may also have an indirect effect on treated tissues. One of the well-recognized physical phenomena associated with the application of shockwaves is the production of so-called cavitation bubbles in the treated tissues [15, 37]. These small bubbles are a source of potential energy. The repetitive application of shockwaves stimulates the bubbles to expand, contract, collide and ultimately collapse, thereby releasing additional energy in the treated tissues [15, 37]. This additional energy also stimulates a biological response, the so-called 'indirect effect' [15, 37].

Parameters

The musculoskeletal adaptations that result from shockwave application are parameter-specific [31, 41, 62]. Not all protocols are effective and a protocol that is effective for one indication may not be effective for another. ESWT is generally very safe. However, in animal models, very excessive SW energy has resulted in cellular damage [31, 62]. For these reasons, it is important to understand how the various shockwave-specific parameters can be adjusted to produce the desired response.

Before considering specific treatment parameters, however, it is first necessary to distinguish between high-energy (>0.2mJ/mm2) and low-energy (<0.2mJ/mm2) therapy. High-energy ESWT usually consists of one or two treatment sessions, each of which is typically performed in an operating room or an ambulatory surgical centre setting with the use of some form of anaesthesia. High-energy treatments are usually used when treating deeper structures, tend to be more painful than low-energy treatments, and are commonly used to treat disorders of bone.

Low-energy ESWT is typically - although not always - performed in a greater number of sessions [2, 42, 58, 60-61]. Low-energy treatments are often used for more superficial structures, require minimal or no anaesthesia, and are commonly used when treating tendinopathies, fasciopathies and more superficially-located bones. Both high-energy and low-energy procedures have yielded excellent clinical results. There is a scarcity of comparative data and what little exists is conflicting [15].

The critical treatment parameters include the total amount of energy per treatment, the number of shocks per session, the frequency of shocks, the energy per shock, the number of treatments, and the interval of time between treatments. Each can be manipulated to modulate the clinical response.

The term 'energy flux density' (EFD) refers to the amount of delivered energy in an area of tissue at a given point in time [15, 37]. The EFD is a standard method of quantifying the total energy delivered in a treatment session. The EFD is simply the product of the energy per shock and the number of shocks, and is expressed in unit mJ/mm^2.

High and low-energy sessions can yield an equivalent EFD. For example, an high-energy session utilizing an energy level of 0.3 mJ/mm2 and 1,000 shocks and a low-energy session using 0.1 mJ/mm^2 and 3,000 shocks each yield an equivalent EFD of 300 mJ/mm^2.

The number of shocks, the interval of time between shocks, the number of treatments and the interval of time between treatments are additional parameters that can determine the therapeutic response [31, 37, 62]. Like energy, the parameters are easily manipulated and this, in part, explains why the protocols used to treat the same condition can vary significantly.

ESWT: biological response

Recent histological, biochemical and immunological basic science studies have greatly advanced our understanding as to how shockwaves effect treated tissues [25-31, 63-64, 70-71, 73-75]. These effects include enhanced neo-vascularity, accelerated growth factor release, selective neural inhibition, stem cell recruitment, and the inhibition of molecules that have a role in inflammation [25-31, 63-64, 70-71, 73-75]. Neural inhibition, enhanced neo-vascularity and increased growth factor release are probably the most important effects on the Achilles tendon, and will therefore be the focus of this section.

ESWT has both a central and peripheral effect on nerve activity. Regarding the central effect, Maier and co-workers, using a rabbit model, demonstrated that ESWT resulted in a significant decrease in substance P six weeks following treatment [28]. In the periphery, ESWT leads to the selective dysfunction of sensory unmyelinated nerve fibres without affecting larger motor neurons [40, 51]. The application of shockwaves results in the liberation of neuropeptides, such as calcitonin gene-related peptides (CGRPs), resulting in a local 'neurogenic inflammation' that prevents sensory nerve re-innervation in the treated area. It has been hypothesized that this inhibition of re-innervation contributes to long-term pain reduction.

ESWT up-regulates the expression of proteins and growth factors that are critical for angiogenesis. Wang and co-workers have reported on the effect of low-energy ESWT on neovascularization at the tendon–bone junction in rabbits [76]. Bone-tendon junctions treated with low-energy ESWT had a higher number of neo-vessels and angiogenesis-related markers, including endothelial nitric oxide synthase, vessel endothelial growth factor (VEGF) and proliferating cell nuclear antigen, when compared to untreated controls [76]. Of note, VEGF is an important mitogenic factor for vascular endothelial cells, and endothelial cell proliferation is a critical aspect of angiogenesis [76].

Chen and co-workers demonstrated that low-energy ESWT promotes the healing of collagenase-induced Achilles tendinopathy in rats by inducing the transforming growth factor beta 1 (TGF-b1) and the insulin-like growth factor-I (IGF-I). Both TGF-b1 and IGF-I can have anabolic effects on diseased tissues [7-8].

To summarize, ESWT appears to produce its effects on the Achilles tendon by up-regulating those proteins critical for angiogenesis, selectively inhibiting afferent nerve fibres, and accentuating the release of growth factors important in tendon healing. Additional studies are necessary to sort out the relative importance of each of these effects.

ESWT: clinical applications

Indications and contraindications

The indications for using ESWT as a treatment for Achilles tendinopathy include the failure of traditional non-surgical therapies, the chronicity of symptoms, a persistence greater than 4-6 months, and an absence of an absolute contraindication. Absolute contraindications include active infection, malignancy, pregnancy, advanced peripheral neuropathy, skeletal immaturity and unresolved fractures. Relative contraindications include, severe alterations in biomechanics and untreated or poorly-controlled systemic inflammatory arthropathies.

Procedure

The procedure is similar for both high and low-energy treatments. The patient is positioned in either the prone or lateral decubitus position. The area of intended treatment is prepared with ultrasound gel. The targeting device of the shockwave generator is coupled to the skin. Depending on the shockwave generator, shockwaves are delivered in either a lateral to medial direction, tangential to the Achilles tendon, or else posterior to anterior, in line with the Achilles tendon (Figure 1).

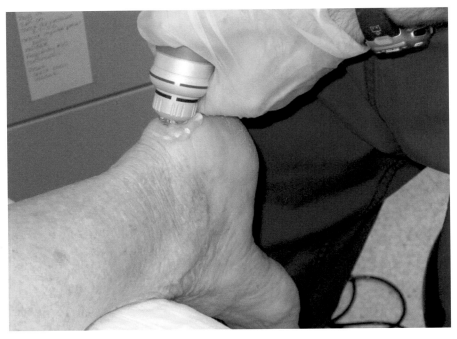

Figure 1. Shockwaves applied posterior to anterior, in line with the Achilles tendon.

Shockwaves are focused on the area of maximal tenderness, either at the bone-tendon junction or in an area usually located approximately 4-6 cm proximal to the tendon insertion.

The ankle is repetitively dorsiflexed, plantar flexed, inverted and everted throughout the procedure, to ensure that the entire insertion of the Achilles tendon as well as the surrounding tissue are treated. To confirm adequate depth of penetration, the examiner feels for the shockwave vibrations along the margins of the treated tissue (Figure 2).

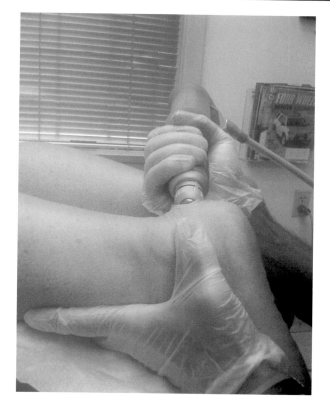

Figure 2. To confirm accurate targeting and adequate depth of penetration, the examiner feels for the shockwave vibrations along the margins of the treated tissue.

Protocols

Protocols vary from centre to centre. High-energy protocols typically involve a single treatment of 3,000-4,000 shocks, with a total energy flux density of 600-800 mJ/mm ^{2}. Low-energy protocols often – but not always – utilize multiple treatments of 2,000 shocks with a total energy flux density of 360 mJ/mm ^{2}. The frequency of shockwave delivery ranges from 4-10 shocks/second.

Post-treatment care

Patients are allowed to be weight-bearing – as tolerated – and do not require immobilization. Patients who work in a sedentary occupation can usually return to work within 24 hours post-treatment. Low-impact activities, such as cycling, weight training and swimming are allowed immediately. A return to higher impact activities, such as running, is made on a case-by-case basis, but usually within 4-6 weeks post-treatment.

Clinical results

Lohrer and co-workers reported significant pain reduction and increased functionality in patients with Achilles tendinopathy who were treated with radial ESWT [24]. There was no control group, however. In a smaller trial consisting of 39 patients, Peers reported his experience using low-energy ESWT for the treatment of patients with chronic Achilles tendinopathy [43]. At early follow-up (12 weeks), the 20 treated patients had significantly improved visual analogue scores (VASs) when compared with an untreated control group. A 77% success rate was reported. Perlick and co-workers. compared ESWT with surgery as a treatment for both forms of Achilles tendinopathy [44]. At one year follow-up, there was a statistically significant reduction in VASs in both groups: from 73 to 38, and from 70 to 28 in the ESWT and operative group, respectively. However, the data was not stratified among the two types of Achilles tendinopathy. Fridman and co-workers reported their experience using high-energy ESWT to treat 23 patients with either non-insertional Achilles tendinopathy, insertional Achilles tendinopathy, or both [9]. They noted that 87% of the treated patients were improved and would have the procedure again.

The good results reported in these preliminary, studies stimulated others to perform more rigorous trials. Rasmussen and co-workers performed a double-blind, placebo-controlled trial in which patients with chronic Achilles tendinopathy were randomized to receive either active ESWT or sham ESWT as a supplement to eccentric strengthening and stretching over four weeks [45]. At short-term (12 week) follow-up, the mean American Foot and Ankle Society Score (AOFAS) increased from 74 (SD 12) to 81 (SD 16) in the placebo group, and from 70 (SD 6.8) to 81 (SD 16) in the intervention group. The authors concluded that ESWT was an effective supplement for the treatment of chronic Achilles tendinopathy, but unfortunately - as in the Perlick trial - the data was not stratified among the two types of Achilles tendinopathy [45].

Using a more rigorous inclusion criteria, Furia evaluated the effects of high-energy ESWT on a consecutive series of patients with chronic insertional Achilles tendinopathy that had not responded to non-surgical management [11]. 35 patients with chronic insertional Achilles tendinopathy were treated with a single-dose high-energy ESWT (ESWT group: 3,000 shocks, 0.21 mJ/mm^2, total energy flux density of 604 mJ/mm^2). 33 patients with chronic insertional Achilles tendinopathy were not treated with ESWT, but instead were treated with additional forms of non-surgical therapy (the control group).

One month, three months, and 12 months after treatment, the degree of improvement in the VASs for the treated patients was greater for the ESWT group than for the controls. The number of patients with excellent or good Roles and Maudsley scores (i.e., successful results) 12 months following treatment was statistically greater in the ESWT group compared with the control group. Overall, the percentage of excellent or good results using the Roles and Maudsley scores at 12 months following the procedure for the ESWT and control groups were 82.9% and 39.4%, respectively.

In a subsequent randomized controlled trial, Rompe and co-workers compared eccentric loading with ESWT as a treatment for chronic insertional Achilles tendinopathy [50]. 50 patients with chronic recalcitrant insertional Achilles tendinopathy who had failed treatment with traditional non-surgical measures received either an eccentric strengthening programme (Group 1, 25 patients) or a repetitive low-energy ESWT (Group 2, 25 patients). Primary follow-up was at four months, and afterwards the patients were allowed to cross over. The last follow-up evaluation was at one year after completion of the initial treatment. The patients were assessed for pain, function and activity by a validated questionnaire, namely the Victorian Institute of Sport Assessment-Achilles (VISA-A) questionnaire.

At four months from the baseline, the mean VISA-A score had increased in both groups, from 53 to 63 points in Group 1, and from 53 to 80 points in Group 2. The mean pain rating decreased from seven to five points in Group 1 and from seven to three points in Group 2. Seven patients (28%) in Group 1 and 16 patients (64%) in Group 2 reported that they were completely recovered or much improved.

For all the outcome measures, the group that received ESWT showed significantly more favourable results than the group treated with eccentric loading. At four months, 18 of the 25 patients in Group 1 had opted to cross over, as did eight of the 25 patients in Group 2. The favourable results after shockwave therapy at four months were stable at the one year follow-up evaluation.

The authors concluded that eccentric loading showed inferior results when compared to low-energy ESWT in patients with chronic recalcitrant insertional Achilles tendinopathy.

As regards chronic mid-portion Achilles tendinopathy, Rasmussen and co-workers, using a traditional low-energy protocol, identified significant improvement in functional scores in ESWT-treated patients when compared to a placebo [45]. Adverse effects were minimal and the good results were stable at short-term follow-up.

Conclusion

ESWT is a safe and effective treatment for both insertional and mid-portion Achilles tendinopathy. The procedure is well tolerated, easy to perform, and is associated with a quick return to work and sport. Further refinements in shockwave generators and less expensive devices should result in the wider application of this promising technology.

References

1. Alfredson H, Pietila T, Jonsson P, Lorentzon R. Heavy load eccentric calf muscle training for the treatment of chronic Achilles tendinosis. Am J Sports Med. 1998; 26: 360-366.
2. Alfredson H, Lorentzon R. Chronic Achilles tendinosis. Recommendations for treatment and prevention. Sports Medicine. 2000; 29(2): 135-146.
3. Almekinders LC. Tendinitis and other chronic tendinopathies. J Am Acad Orthop Surg. 1998; 6: 157-164.
4. Baxter DE, Zingas C. The foot in running. J Am Acad Ort. 1995; 3: 136-145.
5. Brys, P, Bellemans J, Peers, KH, Lysens H, Roeland J. Cross-sectional outcome analysis of athletes with chronic patellar tendinopathy treated surgically and by Extracorporeal Shock Wave Therapy. Clin J Sports Med. 2003: 13; 79-83.
6. Buch M, Knorr U, Fleming L, Amendola A, Bachmann C, Theodore G, Zingas C. Shock wave therapy for the treatment of chronic plantar fasciitis. Orthopade 2002; 31(7): 637-644. 7 Chen
7. YJ, Wang CJ, Yang KD Extracorporeal shock waves promote healing collagenase-induced Achilles tendinitis and increase TGF-beta1 and IGF-I expression. J Orthop Res. 2004; 22: 854–861.
8. Clement DB, Taunton JE, Smart GW. Achilles tendonitis and peritendinitis: etiology and treatment. Am J Sports Med 1984; 12: 179-184.
9. Fridman R, Cain JD, Weil L, Weil L Sr. Extracorporeal shockwave therapy for the treatment of Achilles Tendinopathies. J Am Podiatric Med Association. 2008; 98: 466-468.
10. Furia JP. Safety and efficacy of extracorporeal shock wave therapy for chronic lateral epicondylitis. Am J Orthop. 2005; 24:13-19.
11. Furia JP. High energy ESWT as a treatment for chronic insertional Achilles tendinopathy. Am J Sports Med. 2006; 34: 733-740.
12. Furia JP, Rompe JD, Maffulli N. Low-energy extracorporeal shock wave therapy as a treatment for greater trochanteric pain syndrome. J Am Sports Med. 2009; 37(9) :1806-1813.
13. Furia JP, Juliano PJ, Wade A, Schaden W, Mitterymayer R. Shock wave therapy as a treatment for nonunion of the proximal fifth metatarsal metaphyseal (Jones) fracture. J Bone Joint Surg Am. 2010; 92: 846-854.
14. Gerdesmeyer L, Wagenpfeil S, Haake M, Maier M, Loew M, Wortier K, Lampe R, Seil R, Handle G, Gassel S, Rompe JD. Extracorporeal shock wave therapy for the treatment of chronic calcifying tendonitis of the rotator cuff: a randomized controlled trial. JAMA. 2003;290:2573-2580.
15. Gerdesmeyer L, Henne M, Gobel M, Diehl P. Physical principles and generation of shockwaves. In Extracorporeal Shock Wave Therapy: Technologies, Basics, Clinical Results. Data Trace Media, Towson, MD 2007, pp. 11-20.
16. Hemmingway E. The Old Man and the Sea. Charles Scribner's Sons Publisher, New York, New York, 1952, pp. 1-127.
17. Jakobsen TJ, Petersen L, Haarbo J, Munch M, Larsen PB. Tenoxicam vs placebo in the treatment of tendonitis, periostititis, and sprains. Current Therapeutic Research. 1989; 45(2): 213-220.
18. James SL, Bates BT, Osternig LR. Injuries to runners. Am J Sports Med.1978; 6: 40-50.
19. Jones DC, James SL: Overuse injuries of the lower extremity: Shin splints, iliotibial band friction syndrome, and exertional compartment syndromes. Clin Sports Med. 1987; 6: 273-290.
20. Jones DC: Achilles tendon problems in runners. AAOS Instructional Course Lectures 1998;47:419-427.
21. Knoblock K, Yoon U, Vogt PM. Acute and overuse injuries correlated to training in masters running athletes. Foot and Ankl Int. 2008; 29: 671-676.
22. Kvist M. Achilles tendon injuries in athletes. Ann Chir Gynaecol. 1991; 80: 188-201.
23. Leadbetter WB. Cell-matrix response in tendon injury. Clin Sports Med. 1992; 11: 533-578.
24. Lorher H, Schöll J, Arentz S. Achilles tendinopathy and patellar tendinopathy. Results of radial shockwave therapy in patients with unsuccessfully treated tendinoses [in German]. Sportverletz Sportschaden. 2002; 16: 108-114.
25. Ma HZ, Zeng BF, Li XL. Upregulation of VEGF in subchondral bone of necrotic femoral heads in rabbits with use of extracorporeal shock waves. Calcif Tissue Int. 2007;81: 124-131.
26. Ma HZ, Zeng BF, Li XL, Chai YM. Temporal and spatial expression of BMP-2 in sub-chondral bone of necrotic femoral heads in rabbits by use of extracorporeal shock waves. Acta Orthop. 2008; 79: 98-105.
27. Maier M, Milz S, Tischer T. Influence of extracorporeal shock-wave application on normal bone in an animal model in vivo. Scintigraphy, MRI and histopathology. J Bone Joint Surg Br. 2002; 84(4): 592-599.
28. Maier M, Averbeck B, Milz S, et al. Substance P and prostaglandin E2 release after shock wave application to the rabbit femur. Clin Orthop Relat Res. 2003; 406: 237-245.
29. Maier M, Hausdorf J, Tischer T, Milz S, Weiler C, Refior HJ, Schmitz C. New bone formation by extracorporeal shock waves. Dependence of induction on energy flux density. Orthopade. 2004; 33(12): 1401-10.

30. Martini L, Giavaresi G, Fini M, et al. Effect of extracorporeal shock wave therapy on osteoblastlike cells. Clin Orthop Relat Res. 2003; 413: 269-280.

31. Martini L, Fini M, Giavaresi G, et al. Primary osteoblasts response to shock wave therapy using different parameters. Artif Cells Blood Substit Immobil Biotechnol.2003; 31(4): 449-466.

32. Maquirrian J, Ayerza M, Costa-Paz M, Muscolo L. Endoscopic surgery in chronic Achilles tendinopathies: A preliminary report. Arthroscopy. 2002; 18: 298-303.

33. McCrory JL, Martin DF, Lowery RB, Cannon DW, Curl WW, Read HM Jr, Hunter Dm, Craven T, Messier SP. Etiologic factors associated with Achilles tendonitis in runners. Med Sci Sports Exerc. 1999; 31: 1374-1381.

34. McLauchlan GJ, Handoll HG. Interventions for treating acute and chronic Achilles tendonitis. The Cochrane Database of Systematic Reviews. The Cochrane Library 2004; 4: 1-35.

35. Myerson M, McGarvey W. Disorders of the Achilles insertion and Achilles tendonitis. AAOS Instructional Course Lectures. 1999; 48: 211-218.

36. Nigg BM. The role of impact forces and foot pronation: a new paradigm. Clin J Sports Med. 2001; 11: 2-9.

37. Ogden JA, Toth-Kischkat A, Schultheiss R. Principles of shock wave therapy. Clin Orthop Relat Res. 2001; 387: 8-17.

38. Ogden JA, Alvarez RG, Levitt R, Marlow M. Shock wave therapy for chronic plantar fasciitis. Clin Orthop Relat Res. 2001; 387: 47-59.

39. Ogden JA, Alvarez RG, Levitt RL, Johnson JE, Marlow ME. Electrohydraulic high-energy shock-wave treatment for chronic plantar fasciitis. J Bone Joint Surg Am. 2004; 86A: 2216-2228.

40. Ohtori S, Inoue G, Mannoji C, et al. Shock wave application to rat skin induces degeneration and reinnervation of sensory nerve fibers. Neurosci Lett. 2001; 315: 57-60.

41. Paavola M, Orava S, Leppilanti P, Kannus P, Jazzen M. Chronic Achilles tendon overuse injury: complications after surgical treatment. Am J Sports Med. 2000; 28: 77-82.

42. Paavola M, Kannus P, Jarvinen TA, Khan K, Jozsa L, Jarvinen M. Current concepts review: Achilles tendinopathy. J Bone Joint Surg Am. 2002; 84: 2062-2076.

43. Peers K. Extracorporeal Shock Wave Therapy in Chronic Achilles and Patellar Tendinopathy. Leuven, Belgium: Leuven University Press; 2003: 61-75.

44. Perlick L, Schiffmann R, Kraft CN, Wallny T, Diedrich O. Extracorporeal shock wave treatment of the Achilles tendinitis: experimental and preliminary clinical results [in German]. Z Orthop Ihre Grenzgeb. 2002; 140: 275-280.

45. Rassmussen S, Christensen M, Mathiesen, I, Simonsen O. Shockwave therapy for chronic Achilles tendinopathy - a double-blind, randomized clinical trial of efficacy. Acta Orthop. 2008; 79: 249–256.

46. Rompe JD, Hopf C. Kullmer K, Heine J, Burger R. Analgesic effects of extracorporeal shock wave therapy chronic tennis elbow. J Bone and Joint Surg Br. 1996; 78: 233-237.

47. Rompe JD, Kirkpatrick CJ, Kullmer K, Schwitalle M, Krischek O. Dose-related effects of shock waves on rabbit tendo Achillis. A sonographic and histological study. J Bone Joint Surg Br. 1998; 80: 546-552.

48. Rompe JD, Schoellner C, Nafe B. Evaluation of low-energy extracorporeal shock wave treatment for treatment of chronic plantar fasciitis. J Bone Joint Surg Am. 2002; 84: 335-341.

49. Rompe JD, Decking J, Schoellner C, Theis C. Repetitive low-energy shock wave treatment for chronic lateral epicondylitis in tennis players. Am Journal of Sports Med. 2004; 32: 734-743.

50. Rompe JD, Furia JP, Maffulli N. Eccentric loading compared with shock wave treatment for chronic insertional Achilles tendinopathy. J Bone Joint Surg Am. 2008; 90: 52-61.

51. Rompe JD, Furia JP, Maffulli N. Mid-portion Achilles tendinopathy-current options for treatment. Disability and Rehabilitation. 2008; 30(20-22): 1666-1676.

52. Rompe, JD, Cacchio A, Segal N, Furia JP, Maffulli, N. Home stretching, local corticosteroid injection or radial shockwave application for greater trochanteric pain syndrome. Am J Sports. 2009: 37; 1981-1990.

53. Rompe JD, Cacchio A, Furia JP, Maffulli N. Low-energy extracorporeal shock wave therapy as a treatment for medial tibial stress syndrome. Am J Sports Med. 2010; 38: 125-132.

54. Saltzman CL, Tearse DS. Achilles tendon injuries. J of the American Academy of Orthopaedic Surgeons. 1998; 6: 316-325.

55. Schepsis AA, Jones H, Haas AL. Achilles tendon disorders in athletes. Am J of Sports Med. 2002; 30: 287-304.

56. Schleberger R, Delius M, Dahmen GP. Orthopedic Extracorporeal shock wave therapy (ESWT): method analysis and suggestion of a prospective study design-consensus report. In Chaussy C, Eisenberger F, Jocham D, Wilbert D (eds.). High-energy Shock Waves in Medicine. Stuttgart, Thieme, 108-111, 1997.

57. Sharma P, Maffulli N. Current concepts review tendon injury and tendinopathy: healing and repair. J Bone Joint Surg Am. 2005; 87: 187-2002.

58. Soma CA, Mandelbaum BR. Achilles tendon disorders. Clin Sports Med. 1994; 13(4): 811-823.

59. Sorosky B, Press J, Plastaras C, Rittenburg J. The practical management of Achilles tendinopathy. Clin J Sport Med. 2004; 14: 40-44.

60. Speed CA, Nichols D, Wies J, et al. Extracorporeal shock wave therapy for plantar fasciitis. A double-blind, randomized, controlled trial. J Orthop Res. 2003; 21: 937-940.

61. Speed CA, Nichols D, Wies J, et al. Extracorporeal shock wave therapy for lateral epicondylitis - a double-blind, randomized, controlled trial. J Orthop Res. 2002; 20: 895-898.

62. Sukol DM, Johannes DJ, Pierik JM, Van Eijck W, Kristelljn JE. The effect of high-energy shock waves focused on cortical bone: an in vitro study. J of Surgical Res. 1993; 54: 46-51.

63. Takahashi N, Wada Y, Ohtori S, Saisu T, Moriya H. Application of shock waves to rat skin decreases calcitonin gene-related peptide immunoreactivity in dorsal root ganglion neurons. Auton Neurosci. 2003; 107: 81-84.

64. Takahashi N, Ohtori S, Saisu T, Moriya H, Wada Y. Second application of low-energy shock waves has a cumulative effect on free nerve endings. Clin Orthop Relat Res. 2006; 443: 315-319.

65. Tallon C, Coleman BD, Khan KM, Maffulli N. Outcome of surgery for chronic Achilles tendinopathy. Am J Sports Med. 2001; 29: 315-320.

66. Testa V, Capasso G, Benazzo F, Maffulli N. Management of Achilles tendinopathy by ultrasound-guided percutaneous tenotomy. Med Sci Sports Exer. 2001; 34:573-580.

67. Theodore GH, Buch M, Amendola A, Bachman C, Fleming LL, Zingas C. Extracorporeal shock wave therapy for the treatment of plantar fasciitis. Foot and Ankle Int. 2004; 25: 290-297.

68. Valchanou VD, Michailov P. High-energy shock wave in the treatment of delayed and nonunion of fractures. Int Orthop. 1991; 15: 181-184.

69. Vulpiani MC, Guzzini M, Ferretti A. Operative treatment of chronic Achilles tendinopathy. International Orthopaedics (SICOT). 2003; 27: 307-310.

70. Wang FS, Yang KD, Chen RF, et al. Extracorporeal shock wave promotes growth and differentiation of bone-marrow stromal cells towards osteoprogenitors associated with induction of TGF-beta1. J Bone Joint Surg Br. 2002; 84(3): 457-461.

71. Wang FS, Yang KD, Kuo YR, et al. Temporal and spatial expression of bone morphogenetic proteins in extracorporeal shock wave-promoted healing of segmental defect. Bone. 2003; 32(4): 387-396.

72. Wang CJ, Yang KD, Wang FS: Shock wave therapy for calcific tendonitis of the shoulder. Am Journal of Sports Med. 2003; 31: 425-430.

73. Wang CJ, Wang FS, Yang KD, Weng LH, Hsu CC, Huang CS, Yang LC. Shock wave therapy induces neovascularization at the tendon-bone junction. A study in rabbits. J Orthop Res. 2003; 21: 984-989.

74. Wang CJ, Yang KD, Wang FS, Hsu CC, Chen HH. Shock wave treatment shows dose-dependent enhancement of bone mass and bone strength after fracture of the femur. Bone. 2004; 34: 225-230.

75. Wang CJ, Huang HY, Pal CH. Shock wave-enhanced neovascularisation at the tendon-bone junction: an experiment in dogs. J Foot Ankle Surg. 2004; 41: 16-22.

76. Wang CJ, Wang FS, Yang KD, Weng LH, Sun YC, Yang YJ. The effect of shock wave treatment at the tendon-bone interface - an histomorphological and biomechanical study in rabbits. J Orthop Res. 2005; 23: 274-280.

Chapter 12

Autologous Blood and Platelet-Rich Plasma

Umile G. Longo, John G. Kennedy, Niall A. Smyth,
Johannes L. Tol, Nicola Maffulli

Take Home Message

- *Biomechanical and histological studies at both the in vitro- and in vivo-level suggest a potential beneficial effect of using platelet-rich plasma and autologous blood in Achilles tendon pathology.*

- *Unfortunately, despite good biomechanical and histological results and the worldwide use of autologous blood and platelet-rich plasma injections for the management of tendon injuries, the few well conducted randomized controlled trials have shown no significant clinical advantage over other, well-tested non-surgical modalities.*

Introduction

Growth factors are an exciting prospect in the management of tendinopathy because of their ability to stimulate healing in musculoskeletal tissues [42].

Autologous blood injection for tendinopathy is a relatively new treatment modality, which aims to directly deliver growth factors contained in blood to the injury site to act as humoral mediators and biological catalysts in the healing cascade promoting tissue repair and regeneration[42]. The procedure has been recognized by the National Institute for Health and Clinical Excellence (NICE) of the English National Health Service, although the latest (January 2009) guidelines state that, currently, there is insufficient evidence for its routine use outside the setting of audits and research[42].

Platelet-rich plasma (PRP) therapy is an autologous blood product produced by the centrifugation of whole blood, yielding a concentration of platelets greater than baseline levels. Its potential in treating tendon pathology has been gathering ever greater interest as a source of the local application of the bioactive molecules involved in the healing process[2, 81]. 'PRP', however, is an overarching term that describes many autologous platelet-rich blood products that differ in their composition[27].

There is significant basic science evidence to support the use of blood products - in particular PRP - for use in tendinopathies, with several clinical case series supporting this. However, there are few randomized controlled trials investigating these products, and of the few there are, the evidence is not yet compelling that these treatments should be employed for routine use in treating tendon pathology[25].

Autologous blood injection

Injection of autologous blood has been used for the management of tendino-pathy[28] to provide cellular and humoral mediators to induce healing in areas where the healing response has failed. The use of autologous blood injection is thought to lead to tendon healing through collagen regeneration and the stimulation of a well-ordered angiogenic response. It is hypothesized that transforming growth factor-β and the basic fibroblast growth factor carried in the blood will allow them to act as humoral mediators to induce the healing cascade[37, 87]. Although the results of laboratory studies are encouraging, they have only been performed on healthy tendons or surgically-induced lesions, given the lack of a good experimental model for tendinopathy. At present, it is unclear whether these results can be extrapolated to tendinopathic tendons. So-called 'needling' of the tendon has been described in conjunction with the use of autologous blood. In this respect, however, the results of autologous blood administration are confounded by the concomitant needling[87].

Autologous blood injections have been used in tendinopathy of the extensor carpi radialis brevis[20, 28, 78, 95,] the patellar tendon[38] and the Achilles tendon[84]. However, a recent systematic review of these studies concluded that there were no advantages in using autologous blood products in patients with tendinopathies[24]. In a recent randomized controlled trial[84], 33 patients (18 women, 15 men) with a mean age of 50 years representing 40 patients with Achilles tendinopathy of a mean duration of 11 months were randomized to a blind peritendinous autologous blood injection added to standard treatment (eccentric loading exercises) or to standard treatment alone (eccentric loading exercises) for 12 weeks. Improvements in VISA-A of 7.7 units and 8.7 units were observed in the treatment and control groups, respectively, at six weeks relative to the baseline, with no clear effect from the blood injection. At 12 weeks, the VISA-A score improved to 18.9 units in the treatment group, revealing a blood injection effect of 9.6 units, relative to a comparatively unchanged condition in the controls. Predictors of response to treatment were unremarkable, and a 21% rate of post-injection flare was the only noteworthy side-effect.

PRP

Despite its apparent clinical popularity and a steadily increasing number of clinical studies, there is still only limited understanding of the role of the cellular and extra-cellular elements, the optimal concentrations of platelets, and the timing and effect of leucocytes. Several commercial systems are currently available to produce a 'platelet-rich plasma' or a 'platelet gel' from autologous blood. These systems involve spinning autologous blood in a centrifuge to form a dense, suturable fibrin matrix or injectable fluid that can be easily placed directly at the tendon repair site. The rationale for using PRP-derived growth factors for enhancing wound healing has been proposed since the early 1980s [45]. During this decade, orthopaedic surgeons began to use PRP, especially to augment bone grafts, even though to date no definitive evidence is available for its use to improve bone healing [32]. The use of PRP to improve tendon healing has been advocated only relatively recently [74, 75, 89]. The specific elements of PRP have not been uniformly defined, although an understanding of tendon healing [24, 61] is critical in optimizing PRP formulation and application therapies [51, 65].

PRP therapies: biology

Tendon healing involves different phases [50] that involve multiple cell types and several signalling networks [2]. Platelets play a role in all of these events as they release many biochemical mediators [48, 64]. Platelets adhere avidly at sites of vascular injury, become activated, and release intracellular stores. Each platelet contains dense granules, lysosomes and about 80 α-granules. The α-granules are heterogeneous, and recent proteomic studies have identified more than 300 proteins, which are released in a selective manner upon activation [71]. Some of these molecules represent classical growth factors considered responsible for the beneficial effects of PRP, such as platelet-derived growth factors (PDGFs), transforming growth factors (TGFs), fibroblastic growth factors (FGFs), endothelial growth factors (EGFs), hepatocyte growth factor (HGFs), connective tissue growth factors (CTGFs) and vascular endothelial growth factors (VEGFs). TGF-β has been shown to be increased in the subacromial bursa at the time of surgery for rotator cuff repair as compared with samples from patients with shoulder instability [88]. TGF-β is also believed to enhance collagen deposition, and has been associated with fibrotic healing [15, 86]. These findings regarding the individual bioactive components of PRP support the potential role of its use in the management of tendon pathology. The biological mechanism of other biochemical mediators needs to be better understood.

Additional examples of bioactive molecules seldom mentioned in studies of PRPs include chemokine CXCL7 and platelet factor-4 (PF4 or CXCL4) in innate immune response, thrombospondin-1 (TSP-1) in angiogenesis, and urokinase plasminogen activator (uPA) in cell migration. CXCL7 (β-thromboglobulin or neutrophil-activating peptide-2 (NAP-2) is a strong chemoattractant and activator of neutrophils [31]. PF4 prevents monocyte apoptosis and promotes macrophage differentiation. It induces a unique macrophage transcriptome, with molecular similarities to both the pro- and anti-inflammatory activation patterns [33].

There may be a dual role to PRP in tendon inflammation. Platelets act as modulators thanks to the secretion of high levels of chemokines that control the influx of leukocytes and monocytes in the injured tissue [44]. Moreover, PRP may terminate inflammation as various growth factors, such as HGF, VEGF and TGF-b, restore non-inflammatory cells' phenotypes [7, 10, 21].

Platelets are also known to influence angiogenesis. Alpha-granules contain both pro- and anti-angiogenic proteins. Angiogenic activators include platelet-derived growth factors (PDGF AB and C), TGF-b1, VEGF, HGF and other soluble cytokines (namely, IL-8, angiopoietin CXCL12 and metalloproteinases (MMPs) -1, -2 and -9) [81]. Inhibitors of angiogenesis include thrombospondin-1 (TSP-1) 36, angiostatin, endostatin, fibronectin and tissue inhibitors of metalloproteinases (TIMPs -1 to -4) [80]. The mechanisms of platelet-regulated angiogenesis are not fully understood. An agonist-specific release may be responsible for the differential secretion of pro- and anti-angiogenic stores [16, 100] and, therefore, environment plays an important role. Vascular permeability is also increased by small molecules stored in dense granules, such as histamine, noradrenaline, dopamine and serotonin.

PRP may also influence cell migration, matrix remodelling, cell proliferation and gene expression. Human tenocyte cultures treated with PRP have demonstrated the increased proliferation and production of VEGF and HGF [3, 4]. A high number of resident and precursor cells allow a proportional synthesis of matrix proteins. Moreover, HGF has an antifibrotic effect. Platelets also contain fibrinolytic factors and their inhibitors, such as uPA and plasminogen activator inhibitor type-1 (PAI-1). Platelets also contain MMPs in an inactive form, the activity of which is regulated by the molecular microenvironment. The effect of PRP on gene expression has also been investigated. In a culture of tendon-derived stem cells, Zhang and Wang reported that PRP upregulated tenocyte-related genes, including COL1 and tenascin C. This potentially indicates that PRP promotes tenocyte proliferation by stimulating undifferentiated cells in the tendon [105]. With regard to matrix remodelling, tendons cultured with PRP demonstrated a decrease in the type-3 to type-1 collagen ratio [73, 91]. This could - potentially - improve tendon structure, as the overproduction of type-3 collagen can result in a structurally inferior tendon [39].

PRP therapy composition

Commercial PRP therapies include different categories and concentrations with varying biological effects and potential uses. However, some parameters are essential for the proper classification of platelet concentrates [27]. They include preparation kits and centrifuges, the content of platelets and leukocytes, and fibrin networks. The duration and complexity of the procedure, the cost of the device and preparation kits are all relevant in daily practice, considering the repetitive use of these techniques [27]. The final volume of usable concentrate, and the adequate collection and preservation of platelets and leucocytes, determine the pharmacological effects of the product [27]. The fibrinogen concentration and polymerization type define the material characteristics of the concentrate [18, 79, 99]. Depending on these pharmacological and material characteristics, platelet concentrates can be classified into four categories: leucocyte-poor or pure platelet-rich plasma (P-PRP), leucocyte- and platelet-rich plasma (L-PRP), leucocyte-poor or pure platelet-rich fibrin (P-PRF), leucocyte- and platelet-rich fibrin (L-PRF).

The main difference between the L-PRP and the P-PRP types of platelet concentrates is their leucocyte content. Studies on leucocytes in PRP confirmed their anti-infectious action [17, 77] and immune regulation role [26, 29]. Leukocytes in PRP attract more neutrophils from the blood stream. Additionally, neutrophils produce chemotactically active CXCL7, which is also secreted by platelets [31]. Thus, the process of neutrophils' influx and activation is amplified, with possible clinical implications. Moreover, leucocytes produce VEGF, which may play a role in the promotion of angiogenesis [103]. Recently, L-PRP has been demonstrated to stimulate anabolism and the remodelling of tendons [91], and it has been successfully used for the treatment of tendinopathy [74]. No negative effects - including uncontrolled immune reaction or impairment - of PRP have been reported [30]. However, compelling evidence for the preferential use of leukocyte PRP is still lacking. Some doubts arise from a priori observations on the potential of neutrophils in exacerbating tissue damage [6, 40].

A fibrin matrix provides a support scaffold for platelets and leucocytes, fibrinogen concentration being the principle contributor to the density of the biological adjunct [79]. A high-density fibrin network can be considered equivalent to a biomaterial [18]. The ratio between fibrinogen and thrombin concentration is responsible for fibrin polymerization and its biochemical architecture [79]. Slow physiological fibrin polymerization produces a flexible fibrin network able to support cytokine enmeshment and cellular migration [99]. Most growth factors and cytokines are released during fibrin formation/retraction. The kinetics of this process is crucial in signalling and cellular functions: cellular responses can be influenced by acute or gradual increases in extracellular factors.

181

In vitro and animal studies

In vitro studies have focused on the potential of PRP in stimulating cell proliferation. Different cell types have been studied, including osteoblasts [19, 98], fibroblasts [46], tenocytes [3], chondrocytes [1], periodontal ligament cells [82] and bone mesenchymal stem cells (BMSCs) [54]. However, there are some contrasting observations regarding this topic [14, 92]. PRP's ability to induce cellular differentiation is also controversial. The stimulation of osteoblastic differentiation has been reported in some studies [19, 34, 98], while others have demonstrated an inhibitory effect [14, 93]. In a recent systematic review by Baksh and co-workers [9] analysing the basic scientific evidence regarding PRP and tendon models, the authors reported that nine studies had assessed the effect of PRP on tenocyte proliferation. Of these, eight reported a significant increase in cell proliferation in the presence of PRP [3, 7, 12, 23, 39, 97, 102, 104]. Collagen production has also been assessed by in vitro studies examining the effect of PRP in tendon models, with the majority of studies concluding that PRP increases collagen synthesis [73, 91, 102].

The in vivo evidence regarding the effect of PRP in tendon models has proven promising. The majority of the studies have performed a histological assessment of tendons following PRP treatment for acute lesions or surgically-transected tendons. The findings of these studies include earlier tendon healing with the increased organization of fibroblasts and collagen bundles [11, 56, 60]. However, not all animal studies have found a significant difference between the PRP-treated tendons and the controls [41, 94]. Increased angiogenesis and cell numbers have also been observed at the histological level and on ultrasonography imaging [3, 5, 11, 57, 58, 105]. Bosch and co-workers reported an increase in blood flow and angiogenesis, assessed using Doppler ultrasonography and Factor VIII immunostaining, in lesions created in the flexor digitorum profundus tendons in an equine model [11]. Increased tendon regeneration and strength have also been reported following PRP injection [8, 101]. Spang and co-workers demonstrated in a rat patella model that PRP increased the load to failure of tendon repairs augmented with PRP when compared to a control [94]. The increased mechanical strength of PRP-treated tendon repairs has been further reported in additional studies [11, 59]. PRP also improves tendon defect healing by the overexpression of IGF-1 and by altering the expression of TGF-beta1 [52, 53, 57, 58].

In vivo tendon research is not without its limitations. As an example, multiple studies assess the effect of PRP on surgically-created acute lesions. However, from a clinical perspective, chronic tendon pathology is more common [66-70]. Creating chronic tendinopathy using an animal model is more challenging. However, examples of this have been documented in the literature [49, 55].

Clinical studies

To date, few clinical studies have been performed in assessing the application of PRP for Achilles tendon ruptures and tendinopathy [90]. With regard to tendon ruptures, Sánchez and co-workers [89] reported their results using a platelet-rich fibrin matrix as an adjunct to Achilles tendon repair in a case-control study of 12 athletic patients. The authors reported that the group treated with a platelet-rich fibrin matrix recovered their range of motion and resumed regular training activities seven weeks earlier than the control group. However, these results are in contrast to a study by Schepull and co-workers, in which the authors performed a single-blinded randomized trial on 30 patients with an Achilles tendon rupture. At one year follow-up, no significant differences were evident between the PRP and control groups in relation to the heel raise index and the mechanical variables. The PRP-treated group probably had a clinically relevant lower score on the validated Achilles Tendon Total Rupture Score (ATRS). The cause of this potentially detrimental effect is unknown.

The effect of PRP when used for the management for chronic Achilles tendinopathy has also received limited clinical investigation. Owens and co-workers[83] reported their outcomes in ten patients who had an Achilles intra-tendinous PRP injection as an alternative to surgical treatment. At a mean follow-up of 13.9 months, one patient had progressed to open surgical debridement of the tendon. In addition, of the six patients who underwent a MRI investigation before and after the PRP injection, there were no statistically significant differences in the degree of tendinopathy. Monto[76], in a 30 patient case series, concluded that PRP improved clinical outcomes in 93% of patients who had previously failed non-surgical treatment. In contrast to the previous study, however, the author described how 93% of patients exhibited a resolution of their pre-treatment imaging abnormalities at six months following treatment, as assessed by MRI and ultrasonography. To date, there is only one Level I study regarding the use of PRP for chronic Achilles tendino-pathy. De Vos and co-workers[25] performed a stratified, block-randomized, double-blind, placebo-controlled trial at a single centre on 54 patients with Achilles tendinopathy undergoing exercises (usual care) combined with either a PRP injection (PRP group) or a saline injection (placebo group). At 24 weeks follow-up, in patients with chronic Achilles tendinopathy who were treated with eccentric exercises, a PRP injection compared with a saline injection did not result in superior VISA-A scores[23], nor superior ultrasonographic improvement[22]. Moreover, at one year follow-up the PRP group showed no clinical or ultrasonographic superiority compared with the saline injection[22]. The results of this study may have been confounded by the eccentric Achilles tendon loading protocol and by the type of leukocyte-rich PRP used. However, to date this is the only randomized control trial on which to base clinical guidelines.

Discussion

Understanding of the biological mechanisms and the basis of the therapeutic effects of PRP is intimately connected with a knowledge of the biology of healing processes. Healing involves a multitude of molecules and interactions responsible for complex environmental stimuli and mechanisms that are not yet completely understood.

PRP allows for a focused administration of growth factors previously identified as crucial in normal bone-to-tendon and tendon-to-tendon healing. The simultaneous administration of several biochemical molecules may provide an appropriate healing environment, mimicking and potentiating what happens in vivo where growth factors work in concert. However, not all PRP biochemical mediators have been investigated, and further studies are needed to define their biological mechanisms [68].

PRP products differ in terms of leukocyte and platelet concentrations, as well as their fibrin networks. The biology of the composition of each PRP product needs to be better studied, and successful formulation needs to be defined. The type of PRP product should be considered when comparing results from different studies. Even the same PRP and application protocol may produce different concentrations of growth factors, and results vary at both the intra- and inter-personal level [13, 72].

In vitro studies are limited by the use of several PRP products. Moreover, the immunogenicity of platelet concentrates may influence experiments on animal cell lines [34, 93] and commercialized cell lineages [43, 92], while primary cultures of human cells [14, 35, 98] should be considered as the gold standard. The results of the basic scientific evidence regarding PRP are promising; however, the outcomes do not necessarily translate to clinically relevant benefits in humans [85, 96]. The results of clinical studies assessing the use of PRP in patients with Achilles tendon pathology are mixed, indicating a need for further investigation. Even though a number of important questions remain regarding the biological mechanisms of PRP, patient-oriented research can be performed thanks to the safety of these products.

Conclusion

Achilles tendinopathy is a common orthopaedic condition leading to pain and functional impairment. Despite its frequency and related disability, the aetiology and pathogenesis of this condition is still debated. Basic scientific studies have shown the potential of PRP in tendon pathology, but up to now this beneficial effect has not been reproduced in high-level clinical studies [62, 63, 68]. Further elucidation of the molecular mechanism of healing would be helpful in identifying the critical steps to target. Many molecules determining the beneficial effect of PRP have been described, but others need to be studied [47]. The successful formulations and applications of PRP also need to be defined, as well as a standardized description of PRP to be used in pre-clinical and clinical studies in order to allow for a comparison of results. In vitro studies need to be performed on cultures of human tenocytes from tendinopathic tendons, and animal studies should concentrate on tendinopathy models. To date, the clinical results of PRP for tendon pathology are mixed, with available studies being qualitatively different. Adequately powered randomized controlled trials are necessary to further elucidate the role of PRP in tendon pathology. To compare results, it is important that methods are adequately described, including optimal PRP compositions and concentrations, volumes and buffering/activation, application techniques, timing, rehabilitation protocols, and validated clinical outcome measures.

184

References

1. Akeda K, An HS, Okuma M, et al. Platelet-rich plasma stimulates porcine articular chondrocyte proliferation and matrix biosynthesis. Osteoarthritis Cartilage. 2006;14(12):1272-1280.

2. Andia I, Sanchez M, Maffulli N. Tendon healing and platelet-rich plasma therapies. Expert Opin Biol Ther. 10(10):1415-1426.

3. Anitua E, Andia I, Sanchez M, et al. Autologous preparations rich in growth factors promote proliferation and induce VEGF and HGF production by human tendon cells in culture. J Orthop Res. 2005;23(2):281-286.

4. Anitua E, Sanchez M, Nurden AT, et al. Reciprocal actions of platelet-secreted TGF-beta1 on the production of VEGF and HGF by human tendon cells. Plast Reconstr Surg. 2007;119(3):950-959.

5. Anitua E, Sanchez M, Nurden AT, et al. Autologous fibrin matrices: a potential source of biological mediators that modulate tendon cell activities. J Biomed Mater Res A. 2006;77(2):285-293.

6. Anitua E, Sanchez M, Nurden AT, et al. Platelet-released growth factors enhance the secretion of hyaluronic acid and induce hepatocyte growth factor production by synovial fibroblasts from arthritic patients. Rheumatology (Oxford). 2007;46(12):1769-1772.

7. Anitua E, Sanchez M, Zalduendo MM, et al. Fibroblastic response to treatment with different preparations rich in growth factors. Cell Prolif. 2009;42(2):162-170.

8. Aspenberg P, Virchenko O. Platelet concentrate injection improves Achilles tendon repair in rats. Acta Orthop Scand. 2004;75(1):93-99.

9. Baksh N, Hannon CP, Murawski CD, Smyth NA, Kennedy JG. Platelet-rich plasma in tendon models: a systematic review of basic science literature. Arthroscopy. 2013.

10. Bendinelli P, Matteucci E, Dogliotti G, et al. Molecular basis of anti-inflammatory action of platelet-rich plasma on human chondrocytes: mechanisms of NF-kappaB inhibition via HGF. J Cell Physiol. 225(3):757-766.

11. Bosch G, Moleman M, Barneveld A, van Weeren PR, van Schie HT. The effect of platelet-rich plasma on the neovascularization of surgically created equine superficial digital flexor tendon lesions. Scand J Med Sci Sports. 21(4):554-561.

12. Carofino B, Chowaniec DM, McCarthy MB, et al. Corticosteroids and local anesthetics decrease positive effects of platelet-rich plasma: an in vitro study on human tendon cells. Arthroscopy. 2012;28(5):711-719.

13. Castillo TN, Pouliot MA, Kim HJ, Dragoo JL. Comparison of growth factor and platelet concentration from commercial platelet-rich plasma separation systems. Am J Sports Med. 2011;39(2):266-271.

14. Cenni E, Ciapetti G, Pagani S, Perut F, Giunti A, Baldini N. Effects of activated platelet concentrates on human primary cultures of fibroblasts and osteoblasts. J Periodontol. 2005;76(3):323-328.

15. Chan KM, Fu SC, Wong YP, Hui WC, Cheuk YC, Wong MW. Expression of transforming growth factor beta isoforms and their roles in tendon healing. Wound Repair Regen. 2008;16(3):399-407.

16. Chatterjee M, Huang Z, Zhang W, et al. Distinct platelet packaging, release, and surface expression of proangiogenic and antiangiogenic factors on different platelet stimuli. Blood. 117(14):3907-3911.

17. Cieslik-Bielecka A, Gazdzik TS, Bielecki TM, Cieslik T. Why the platelet-rich gel has antimicrobial activity? Oral Surg Oral Med Oral Pathol Oral Radiol Endod. 2007;103(3):303-305; author reply 305-306.

18. Clark RA. Fibrin and wound healing. Ann N Y Acad Sci. 2001;936:355-367.

19. Clausen C, Hermund NU, Donatsky O, Nielsen H, Osther K. Homologous activated platelets stimulate differentiation and proliferation of primary human bone cells. Cells Tissues Organs. 2006;184(2):68-75.

20. Connell DA, Ali KE, Ahmad M, Lambert S, Corbett S, Curtis M. Ultrasound-guided autologous blood injection for tennis elbow. Skeletal Radiol. 2006;35(6):371-377.

21. Coudriet GM, He J, Trucco M, Mars WM, Piganelli JD. Hepatocyte growth factor modulates interleukin-6 production in bone marrow derived macrophages: implications for inflammatory mediated diseases. PLoS One. 5(11):e15384.

22. de Jonge S, de Vos RJ, Weir A, et al. One-year follow-up of platelet-rich plasma treatment in chronic Achilles tendinopathy: a double-blind randomized placebo-controlled trial. Am J Sports Med. 2011;39(8):1623-1629.

23. de Mos M, van der Windt AE, Jahr H, et al. Can platelet-rich plasma enhance tendon repair? A cell culture study. Am J Sports Med. 2008;36(6):1171-1178.

24. de Vos RJ, van Veldhoven PL, Moen MH, Weir A, Tol JL, Maffulli N. Autologous growth factor injections in chronic tendinopathy: a systematic review. Br Med Bull.

25. de Vos RJ, Weir A, van Schie HT, et al. Platelet-rich plasma injection for chronic Achilles tendinopathy: a randomized controlled trial. Jama. 2010;303(2):144-149.

26. Dohan DM, Choukroun J, Diss A, et al. Platelet-rich fibrin (PRF): a second-generation platelet concentrate. Part III: leucocyte activation: a new feature for platelet concentrates? Oral Surg Oral Med Oral Pathol Oral Radiol Endod. 2006;101(3):e51-55.

27. Dohan Ehrenfest DM, Rasmusson L, Albrektsson T. Classification of platelet concentrates: from pure platelet-rich plasma (P-PRP) to leucocyte- and platelet-rich fibrin (L-PRF). Trends Biotechnol. 2009;27(3):158-167.

28. Edwards SG, Calandruccio JH. Autologous blood injections for refractory lateral epicondylitis. J Hand Surg Am. 2003;28(2):272-278.

29. El-Sharkawy H, Kantarci A, Deady J, et al. Platelet-rich plasma: growth factors and pro- and anti-inflammatory properties. J Periodontol. 2007;78(4):661-669.

30. Everts PA, Devilee RJ, Brown Mahoney C, et al. Exogenous application of platelet-leukocyte gel during open subacromial decompression contributes to improved patient outcome. A prospective randomized double-blind study. Eur Surg Res. 2008;40(2):203-210.

31. Flad HD, Brandt E. Platelet-derived chemokines: pathophysiology and therapeutic aspects. Cell Mol Life Sci. 67(14):2363-2386.

32. Forriol F, Longo UG, Concejo C, Ripalda P, Maffulli N, Denaro V. Platelet-rich plasma, rhOP-1 (rhBMP-7) and frozen rib allograft for the reconstruction of bony mandibular defects in sheep. A pilot experimental study. Injury. 2009;40 Suppl 3:S44-49.

33. Gleissner CA, Shaked I, Little KM, Ley K. CXC chemokine ligand 4 induces a unique transcriptome in monocyte-derived macrophages. J Immunol. 184(9):4810-4818.

34. Goto H, Matsuyama T, Miyamoto M, Yonamine Y, Izumi Y. Platelet-rich plasma/osteoblasts complex induces bone formation via osteoblastic differentiation following subcutaneous transplantation. J Periodontal Res. 2006;41(5):455-462.

35. Graziani F, Ivanovski S, Cei S, Ducci F, Tonetti M, Gabriele M. The in vitro effect of different PRP concentrations on osteoblasts and fibroblasts. Clin Oral Implants Res. 2006;17(2):212-219.

36. Isenberg JS, Frazier WA, Roberts DD. Thrombospondin-1: a physiological regulator of nitric oxide signaling. Cell Mol Life Sci. 2008;65(5):728-742.

37. Iwasaki M, Nakahara H, Nakata K, Nakase T, Kimura T, Ono K. Regulation of proliferation and osteochondrogenic differentiation of periosteum-derived cells by transforming growth factor-beta and basic fibroblast growth factor. J Bone Joint Surg Am. 1995;77(4):543-554.

38. James SL, Ali K, Pocock C, et al. Ultrasound guided dry needling and autologous blood injection for patellar tendinosis. Br J Sports Med. 2007;41(8):518-521.

39. Jo CH, Kim JE, Yoon KS, Shin S. Platelet-rich plasma stimulates cell proliferation and enhances matrix gene expression and synthesis in tenocytes from human rotator cuff tendons with degenerative tears. Am J Sports Med. 2012;40(5):1035-1045.

40. John T, Lodka D, Kohl B, et al. Effect of pro-inflammatory and immunoregulatory cytokines on human tenocytes. J Orthop Res. 28(8):1071-1077.

41. Kajikawa Y, Morihara T, Sakamoto H, et al. Platelet-rich plasma enhances the initial mobilization of circulation-derived cells for tendon healing. J Cell Physiol. 2008;215(3):837-845.

42. Kampa RJ, Connell DA. Treatment of tendinopathy: is there a role for autologous whole blood and platelet rich plasma injection? Int J Clin Pract. 2010;64(13):1813-1823.

43. Kawase T, Okuda K, Wolff LF, Yoshie H. Platelet-rich plasma-derived fibrin clot formation stimulates collagen synthesis in periodontal ligament and osteoblastic cells in vitro. J Periodontol. 2003;74(6):858-864.

44. Kim MH, Curry FR, Simon SI. Dynamics of neutrophil extravasation and vascular permeability are uncoupled during aseptic cutaneous wounding. Am J Physiol Cell Physiol. 2009;296(4):C848-856.

45. Knighton DR, Hunt TK, Thakral KK, Goodson WH, 3rd. Role of platelets and fibrin in the healing sequence: an in vivo study of angiogenesis and collagen synthesis. Ann Surg. 1982;196(4):379-388.

46. Krasna M, Domanovic D, Tomsic A, Svajger U, Jeras M. Platelet gel stimulates proliferation of human dermal fibroblasts in vitro. Acta Dermatovenerol Alp Panonica Adriat. 2007;16(3):105-110.

47. Lippi G, Longo UG, Maffulli N. Genetics and sports. Br Med Bull. 2010;93:27-47.

48. Longo UG, Berton A, Khan WS, Maffulli N, Denaro V. Histopathology of rotator cuff tears. Sports Med Arthrosc. 2011;19(3):227-236.

49. Longo UG, Forriol F, Campi S, Maffulli N, Denaro V. Animal models for translational research on shoulder pathologies: from bench to bedside. Sports Med Arthrosc. 2011;19(3):184-193.

50. Longo UG, Lamberti A, Maffulli N, Denaro V. Tissue engineered biological augmentation for tendon healing: a systematic review. Br Med Bull. 2011;98:31-59.

51. Longo UG, Oliva F, Olivia F, Denaro V, Maffulli N. Oxygen species and overuse tendinopathy in athletes. Disabil Rehabil. 2008;30(20-22):1563-1571.

52. Longo UG, Ronga M, Maffulli N. Achilles tendinopathy. Sports Med Arthrosc. 2009;17(2):112-126.

53. Longo UG, Ronga M, Maffulli N. Acute ruptures of the Achilles tendon. Sports Med Arthrosc. 2009;17(2):127-138.

54. Lucarelli E, Beccheroni A, Donati D, et al. Platelet-derived growth factors enhance proliferation of human stromal stem cells. Biomaterials. 2003;24(18):3095-3100.

55. Lui PP, Maffulli N, Rolf C, Smith RK. What are the validated animal models for tendinopathy? Scand J Med Sci Sports. 2011;21(1):3-17.

56. Lyras D, Kazakos K, Verettas D, et al. Immunohistochemical study of angiogenesis after local administration of platelet-rich plasma in a patellar tendon defect. Int Orthop. 2010;34(1):143-148.

57. Lyras DN, Kazakos K, Agrogiannis G, et al. Experimental study of tendon healing early phase: is IGF-1 expression influenced by platelet rich plasma gel? Orthop Traumatol Surg Res. 96(4):381-387.

58. Lyras DN, Kazakos K, Tryfonidis M, et al. Temporal and spatial expression of TGF-beta1 in an Achilles tendon section model after application of platelet-rich plasma. Foot Ankle Surg. 16(3):137-141.

59. Lyras DN, Kazakos K, Verettas D, et al. The effect of platelet-rich plasma gel in the early phase of patellar tendon healing. Arch Orthop Trauma Surg. 2009;129(11):1577-1582.

60. Lyras DN, Kazakos K, Verettas D, et al. The influence of platelet-rich plasma on angiogenesis during the early phase of tendon healing. Foot Ankle Int. 2009;30(11):1101-1106.

61. M-Dan O, Mann G, Maffulli N. Platelet-rich plasma: any substance into it? Br J Sports Med. 2010 Jul;44(9):618-9.

62. Maffulli N, Longo UG. Conservative management for tendinopathy: is there enough scientific evidence? Rheumatology (Oxford). 2008;47(4):390-391.

63. Maffulli N, Longo UG. How do eccentric exercises work in tendinopathy? Rheumatology (Oxford). 2008;47(10):1444-1445.

64. Maffulli N, Longo UG, Berton A, Loppini M, Denaro V. Biological factors in the pathogenesis of rotator cuff tears. Sports Med Arthrosc. 2011;19(3):194-201.

65. Maffulli N, Longo UG, Denaro V. Novel approaches for the management of tendinopathy. J Bone Joint Surg Am. 2010;92(15):2604-2613.

66. Maffulli N, Longo UG, Gougoulias N, Caine D, Denaro V. Sport injuries: a review of outcomes. Br Med Bull. 2011;97:47-80.

67. Maffulli N, Longo UG, Gougoulias N, Loppini M, Denaro V. Long-term health outcomes of youth sports injuries. Br J Sports Med. 2010;44(1):21-25.

68. Maffulli N, Longo UG, Loppini M, Denaro V. Current treatment options for tendinopathy. Expert Opin Pharmacother. 2010;11(13):2177-2186.

69. Maffulli N, Longo UG, Spiezia F, Denaro V. Sports injuries in young athletes: long-term outcome and prevention strategies. Phys Sportsmed. 2010;38(2):29-34.

70. Maffulli N, Wong J, Almekinders LC. Types and epidemiology of tendinopathy. Clin Sports Med. 2003;22(4):675-692.

71. Maynard DM, Heijnen HF, Gahl WA, Gunay-Aygun M. The alpha-granule proteome: novel proteins in normal and ghost granules in gray platelet syndrome. J Thromb Haemost. 8(8):1786-1796.

72. Mazzocca AD, McCarthy MB, Chowaniec DM, et al. Platelet-rich plasma differs according to preparation method and human variability. J Bone Joint Surg Am. 2012;94(4):308-316.

73. McCarrel T, Fortier L. Temporal growth factor release from platelet-rich plasma, trehalose lyophilized platelets, and bone marrow aspirate and their effect on tendon and ligament gene expression. J Orthop Res. 2009;27(8):1033-1042.

74. Mishra A, Pavelko T. Treatment of chronic elbow tendinosis with buffered platelet-rich plasma. Am J Sports Med. 2006;34(11):1774-1778.

75. Mishra A, Woodall J, Jr., Vieira A. Treatment of tendon and muscle using platelet-rich plasma. Clin Sports Med. 2009;28(1):113-125.

76. Monto RR. Platelet rich plasma treatment for chronic Achilles tendinosis. Foot Ankle Int. 2012;33(5):379-385.

77. Moojen DJ, Everts PA, Schure RM, et al. Antimicrobial activity of platelet-leukocyte gel against Staphylococcus aureus. J Orthop Res. 2008;26(3):404-410.

78. Moon YL, Jo SH, Song CH, Park G, Lee HJ, Jang SJ. Autologous bone marrow plasma injection after arthroscopic debridement for elbow tendinosis. Ann Acad Med Singapore. 2008;37(7):559-563.

79. Mosesson MW, Siebenlist KR, Meh DA. The structure and biological features of fibrinogen and fibrin. Ann N Y Acad Sci. 2001;936:11-30.

80. Nurden AT. Platelets, inflammation and tissue regeneration. Thromb Haemost. 105 Suppl 1:S13-33.

81. Nurden AT, Nurden P, Sanchez M, Andia I, Anitua E. Platelets and wound healing. Front Biosci. 2008;13:3532-3548.

82. Okuda K, Kawase T, Momose M, et al. Platelet-rich plasma contains high levels of platelet-derived growth factor and transforming growth factor-beta and modulates the proliferation of periodontally related cells in vitro. J Periodontol. 2003;74(6):849-857.

83. Owens RF, Ginnetti J, Conti SF, Latona C. Clinical and magnetic resonance imaging outcomes following platelet rich plasma injection for chronic midsubstance Achilles tendinopathy. Foot Ankle Int. 2011;32(11):1032-1039.

84. Pearson J, Rowlands D, Highet R. Autologous blood injection to treat Achilles tendinopathy? A randomized controlled trial. J Sport Rehabil. 2012;21(3):218-224.

85. Plachokova AS, Nikolidakis D, Mulder J, Jansen JA, Creugers NH. Effect of platelet-rich plasma on bone regeneration in dentistry: a systematic review. Clin Oral Implants Res. 2008;19(6):539-545.

86. Pryce BA, Watson SS, Murchison ND, Staverosky JA, Dunker N, Schweitzer R. Recruitment and maintenance of tendon progenitors by TGFbeta signaling are essential for tendon formation. Development. 2009;136(8):1351-1361.

87. Rabago D, Best TM, Zgierska AE, Zeisig E, Ryan M, Crane D. A systematic review of four injection therapies for lateral epicondylosis: prolotherapy, polidocanol, whole blood and platelet-rich plasma. Br J Sports Med. 2009;43(7):471-481.

88. Sakai H, Fujita K, Sakai Y, Mizuno K. Immunolocalization of cytokines and growth factors in subacromial bursa of rotator cuff tear patients. Kobe J Med Sci. 2001;47(1):25-34.

89. Sanchez M, Anitua E, Azofra J, Andia I, Padilla S, Mujika I. Comparison of surgically repaired Achilles tendon tears using platelet-rich fibrin matrices. Am J Sports Med. 2007;35(2):245-251.

90. Schepull T, Kvist J, Norrman H, Trinks M, Berlin G, Aspenberg P. Autologous platelets have no effect on the healing of human Achilles tendon ruptures: a randomized single-blind study. Am J Sports Med. 2011;39(1):38-47.

91. Schnabel LV, Mohammed HO, Miller BJ, et al. Platelet rich plasma (PRP) enhances anabolic gene expression patterns in flexor digitorum superficialis tendons. J Orthop Res. 2007;25(2):230-240.

92. Slapnicka J, Fassmann A, Strasak L, Augustin P, Vanek J. Effects of activated and nonactivated platelet-rich plasma on proliferation of human osteoblasts in vitro. J Oral Maxillofac Surg. 2008;66(2):297-301.

93. Soffer E, Ouhayoun JP, Dosquet C, Meunier A, Anagnostou F. Effects of platelet lysates on select bone cell functions. Clin Oral Implants Res. 2004;15(5):581-588.

94. Spang JT, Tischer T, Salzmann GM, et al. Platelet concentrate vs. saline in a rat patellar tendon healing model. Knee Surg Sports Traumatol Arthrosc. 2011;19(3):495-502.

95. Suresh SP, Ali KE, Jones H, Connell DA. Medial epicondylitis: is ultrasound guided autologous blood injection an effective treatment? Br J Sports Med. 2006;40(11):935-939.

96. Thor A, Franke-Stenport V, Johansson CB, Rasmusson L. Early bone formation in human bone grafts treated with platelet-rich plasma: preliminary histomorphometric results. Int J Oral Maxillofac Surg. 2007;36(12):1164-1171.

97. Tohidnezhad M, Varoga D, Wruck CJ, et al. Platelet-released growth factors can accelerate tenocyte proliferation and activate the anti-oxidant response element. Histochem Cell Biol. 2011;135(5):453-460.

98. Uggeri J, Belletti S, Guizzardi S, et al. Dose-dependent effects of platelet gel releasate on activities of human osteoblasts. J Periodontol. 2007;78(10):1985-1991.

99. van Hinsbergh VW, Collen A, Koolwijk P. Role of fibrin matrix in angiogenesis. Ann N Y Acad Sci. 2001;936:426-437.

100. Villeneuve J, Block A, Le Bousse-Kerdiles MC, et al. Tissue inhibitors of matrix metalloproteinases in platelets and megakaryocytes: a novel organization for these secreted proteins. Exp Hematol. 2009;37(7):849-856.

101. Virchenko O, Aspenberg P. How can one platelet injection after tendon injury lead to a stronger tendon after 4 weeks? Interplay between early regeneration and mechanical stimulation. Acta Orthop. 2006;77(5):806-812.

102. Visser LC, Arnoczky SP, Caballero O, Egerbacher M. Platelet-rich fibrin constructs elute higher concentrations of transforming growth factor-β1 and increase tendon cell proliferation over time when compared to blood clots: a comparative in vitro analysis. Vet Surg. 2010;39(7):811-817.

103. Werther K, Christensen IJ, Nielsen HJ. Determination of vascular endothelial growth factor (VEGF) in circulating blood: significance of VEGF in various leucocytes and platelets. Scand J Clin Lab Invest. 2002;62(5):343-350.

104. Zhai W, Wang N, Qi Z, Gao Q, Yi L. Platelet-rich plasma reverses the inhibition of tenocytes and osteoblasts in tendon-bone healing. Orthopedics. 2012;35(4):e520-525.

105. Zhang J, Wang JH. Platelet-rich plasma releasate promotes differentiation of tendon stem cells into active tenocytes. Am J Sports Med. 38(12):2477-2486.

*"Injections are the best thing ever
invented for feeding doctors."*

Gabriel Garcia Marquez

CHAPTER 13

INJECTION TREATMENT IN PATIENTS WITH ACHILLES TENDINOPATHY

Ruben Zwiers, Maayke N. van Sterkenburg, C. Niek van Dijk

Take Home Message

• *Corticosteroid injections around the Achilles tendon are controversial, the lack of a significant effect, together with possible risks on rupture, is the reason why their use should not be recommended.*

• *Several injection treatments around the Achilles tendon are used, with variable results. Although most of them are probably not harmful, further research is needed for a more comprehensive analysis of the clinical results and definitive recommendations on injection therapy.*

Introduction

For many years, injection therapies have been used for the management of Achilles tendinopathy. Initially, injections were primarily used to manage the symptoms. However, novel injection strategies are increasingly described with disease-modifying or healing promotion potentials[46]. A recent systematic review of nine RCTs with conflicting methodologies have shown variable results. The authors concluded that the quality of the current evidence is low. More prospective randomized controlled trials are needed to make definite recommendations concerning invasive non-surgical treatment[20].

In this chapter, an overview is provided of injectable treatment options for chronic Achilles tendinopathy apart from autologous blood and platelet-rich plasma (Table 1).

Corticosteroids

Although corticosteroid injections are a commonly used treatment for chronic tendinopathies, the rationale for the use of anti-inflammatory injections in Achilles tendinopathy is debated [44]. Especially in chronic Achilles tendinopathy, the mechanism behind a positive effect remains unclear, since inflammation is absent in chronic tendinopathy. In particular, there might be other effects of corticosteroids that contribute to symptoms relief [37, 41, 44].

The injection of corticosteroids around weight-loaded tendons is associated with an increased risk of tendon ruptures [7, 14, 18, 21, 23, 29]. However, some prospective studies have not shown any direct adverse events after corticosteroid injections [16, 19, 39].

A systematic review by Magnussen and co-workers [28] showed three randomized controlled trials reporting on corticosteroid administration, two by injection and one by iontophoresis. One of the studies reported some benefit of the local steroids [19] where the other studies found no effect [16]. The location of the injections was guided by ultrasound in the study by Fredberg and co-workers, while Da Cruz and co-workers did not confirm correct injection placement. Magnussen and co-workers concluded that there is no significant evidence to draw any conclusions on the utility of local corticosteroid treatment in patients with mid-portion Achilles tendinopathy. Together with the risk of tendon rupture, the use of corticosteroid injections should not be recommended in patients with chronic Achilles tendinopathy.

The use of corticosteroid injections for bursitis is well-known. Some injection sites have been reasonably well studied (e.g., olecranon and prepatellar bursitis) [1], but only two studies evaluated the clinical results in patients with retrocalcaneal bursitis. Both describe one case in which corticosteroids were injected successfully using ultrasound guidance [13, 45].

High volume injections

Neovascularization and accompanying nerve in-growth occurs in patients with tendinopathy [2, 24]. This ingrowth of new vessels and associated nerves from the ventral side of the tendon may be a source of pain [35]. The hypothesized rationale behind high-volume injections was that they would produce local mechanical effects, causing neo-vessels to stretch, break or occlude [12]. By occluding and possibly breaking these vessels, the accompanying nerve supply would also be damaged, either by trauma or ischaemia, and therefore decrease the pain.

Preliminary studies have shown that a high volume injection with normal saline, local anaesthetic and corticosteroid, can significantly reduce pain and improve short- and long-term function in patients with Achilles tendinopathy [12, 22]. An ultrasound-guided high volume injection appears to be safe and relatively inexpensive, with the potential to offer an alternative non-surgical treatment option [22]. In other studies, hydrocortisone acetate was used in the high volume injections, primarily to prevent an acute mechanical inflammatory reaction produced by the large amount of fluid injected in the proximity of the tendon. A recent study used aprotinin instead of hydrocortisone acetate [27]. In this study, a significant improvement of the VISA-A score was found at one year follow-up. In addition, a relatively high rate of return to sport was reported in athletic patients with mid-portion Achilles tendinopathy, presenting with a definite area of neo-vascularity. No serious adverse events related to the injections were found.

Sclerosing agents (Polidocanol)

Sclerosing therapy for chronic Achilles tendinopathy is based on the hypothesis that the process of neovascularization in the damaged tendon is the source of the patient's pain [5, 34]. Some studies have implicated neovascularization as a possible pain generator in Achilles tendinopathy, possibly because the sensory nerves can be linked to the vessels [5, 34, 35]. These findings led to the hypothesis that the destruction of the vessels and nerves might lead to pain relief [4, 5, 15, 26, 32-34, 49].

A sclerosing agent, Polidocanol (not FDA approved), is injected under ultrasound- and colour Doppler-guidance into the neovascularization area outside the tendon. The reports of this treatment mostly include retrospective case series with relatively short follow-up [5, 6, 26, 32, 33, 48].

The largest and most recent series in these retrospective reports included 53 tendon injections in patients with mid-portion Achilles tendinopathy. Only 44% of the tendons were painless or minimally painful at six weeks following treatment. At 2.7 to 5.1 years follow-up, 53% of the treated tendons had undergone additional non-surgical or surgical treatment. The average number of needed injections was 2.7 [48].

The only prospective comparative studies involved small numbers of patients [5, 6, 49]. Injections of Polidocanol in ten patients (Group A) were compared with injections of Lidocaine in ten patients (Group B) with mid-portion Achilles tendinopathy [5]. At three months follow-up, five of the ten patients in the Polidocanol group were satisfied with their results, while none of the ten patients in group B reported any pain relief. Another report from the same group compared Polidocanol injections (ten patients) to the open revision of the neurovascular area outside the tendon (ten patients), also in patients with mid-portion Achilles tendinopathy [6]. At three months follow-up, eight of ten patients with surgery and six of nine patients (one patient was lost to follow-up) with injections reported good results; at 12 months follow-up, all ten patients with surgery and six of nine with injections reported good results.

Sclerotherapy often requires multiple injections to achieve pain relief. Therefore, another comparative study treated 52 tendons with sclerosing therapy in two different concentrations, aiming to determine whether higher concentrations would lead to fewer injections. At 14 months follow-up, 37 (71%) patients had good results, and after additional injections all 52 patients were considered satisfactory. However, higher concentrations did not reduce the number of injections needed [49].

Only one pilot study with a limited number of patients has been performed on insertional Achilles tendinopathy. Öhberg and co-workers prospectively analysed 11 patients, who were treated with repeated Polidocanol injections until symptoms disappeared or decreased. Up to five injections were administered [32]. Eight of the 11 patients were satisfied with the treatment. The mean VAS score during activity decreased from 84.5 mm before treatment to 14 mm in the successfully-treated patients and 58 mm in the three poor cases.

Although the FDA listed DVT, necrosis and ulceration at the treatment site and reversible cardiac arrest as known adverse events related to Polidocanol, Alfredson and co-workers reported only two complications that "possibly might be related" to sclerosing therapy in 150 Achilles tendons: one total Achilles tendon rupture and one partial rupture [3].

Additional data obtained from larger randomized comparative studies are needed before sclerosing therapy can be considered as a first-line management for Achilles tendinopathy.

Protease inhibitors (Aprotinin)

Once, Aprotinin was the most popular option of all the alternative substances available for injection [40]. For over 35 years, it has been used as an off-label injection for the management of tendinopathy [8, 10, 11, 42]. Aprotinin is a broad-spectrum protease (including matrix metalloproteinase (MMP)) inhibitor. Initially, it was indicated for use in open heart and liver surgery to reduce blood loss. Proponents of aprotinin in tendon disorders suggest that, by inhibiting the enzymes that break down or degrade tendons, the healing response may be promoted.

However, the clinical results of aprotinin injections have been conflicting. Aprotinin appears to be efficacious in patellar tendinopathy [11], whereas a prospective randomized controlled trial by Brown and co-workers failed to show any significant benefit over placebo in patients with Achilles tendino-pathy [9]. The same group of authors subsequently reported successful treatment of non-insertional Achilles tendinopathy in a non-randomized study [36].

The debate over the use of this drug is now purely academic, as it was temporarily withdrawn worldwide in 2007 after studies suggested that its use increased the risk of complications or death. This was confirmed by follow-up studies and it was entirely and permanently withdrawn in May 2008, except for very restricted research use.

Hyperosmolar dextrose

Dextrose is one of the osmotic classes of prolotherapy. Prolotherapy is based on the concept of creating irritation or injury to stimulate healing of a ligament. Hyperosmolar dextrose has been used as part of prolotherapy regimes for the treatment of chronic tendon pain since as early as the 1940s. The injected solution is said to initiate a local inflammatory response, causing fibroblast proliferation and subsequent collagen production, resulting in increased tendon strength (although the evidence for this is scant). Dextrose acts by causing an osmotic shock to cells leading to the release of pro-inflammatory substances. Several studies have shown increased ligament mass and thickness after repeated prolotherapy injections [17]. Using a modification of this technique, Maxwell and co-workers performed intratendinous injections of hyperosmolar dextrose under ultrasound guidance, targeting the abnormal anechoic and hypoechoic areas in the tendon. In their uncontrolled pilot study, they retrospectively analysed 33 patients with mid-portion and/or insertional Achilles tendinopathy. The mean VAS during daily activities decreased by 3.6 points at follow-up (12 months). The mean number of treatment sessions was four [30]. Ryan and co-workers retrospectively analysed 71 treated patients with Achilles tendinopathy, of which 22 suffered from insertional tendinopathy. The mean VAS during daily activities decreased significantly by 41.3 points in the insertional tendinopathy and 40.7 (on a 100 point VAS scale) at follow-up (28.6 months) [43]. A recent study by Yelland and co-workers randomized 43 patients with mid-portion Achilles tendinopathy to eccentric loading exercise, hyperosmolar dextrose or combined treatment. The VISA-A scores increased in all groups; however, at six weeks and 12 months follow-up, these increases were significantly less for eccentric loading exercise than for combined treatment. A combination with prolotherapy give more rapid improvements in symptoms than did eccentric loading exercise alone, but the long-term VISA-A scores were similar [50].

Other injections

Low-dose heparin has been used in the management of Achilles tendinopathies with the aim of limiting the formation of adhesions. However, there is some evidence that there is no beneficial effect [25], and it has even been suggested that heparin, in itself, can cause degenerative tendinopathy in rats [47].

Pförringer and co-workers performed a double-blind, placebo-controlled trial to assess the effect of deproteinized haemodialysate, a filtered extract from calf blood. There was a significant reduction of tendon diameter and a reduction of pain as regards activity. No adverse effects were observed, though the follow-up was short [38].

Injection Type	Substance	Type of Achilles Tendinopathy	Level of Evidence	+ /-	Conclusion
Corticosteroid injections	Triamcinolone Methylprednisolone	Mid-portion	Two RCTs, several case series	– Conflicting outcomes – Possible risk on ruptures	Use should not be recommended
High volume injections	Normal saline Hydrocortisone Aprotinin	Mid-portion	No RCTs, several case series	+ Promising results – Limited evidence	No definitive conclusion possible
Sclerosing agents	Polidocanol	Mid-portion	Three RCTs, several case series	+ Promising results in small RCTs – Small sample-size RCTs – Conflicting outcomes	No definitive conclusion possible
		Insertional	No RCT, one case series	+ Promising results – Very limited evidence	No definitive conclusion possible
Protease inhibitors	Aprotinin	Mid-portion	One RCT, some case series	– RCT has shown no benefit over placebo – Withdrawn after the suggestion of severe complications	No role in clinical practice
Prolotherapy	Hyperosmolar dextrose	Mid-portion	One RCT, some case series	+ Promising short-term results – Limited evidence	No definitive conclusion possible
		Insertional	No RCT, two case series	+ Promising results – Very limited evidence	No definitive conclusion possible
Anticoagulants	Low-dose heparin	Mid-portion	One RCT	– Small sample size – No difference in comparison with placebo	No definitive conclusion possible
Haemodialysate	Deproteinized haemodialysate from calf blood (Actovegin®)	Mid-portion	One RCT	+ Promising short-term results – Limited evidence	No definitive conclusion possible

Table 1. Overview of injectable treatment options for chronic Achilles tendinopathy.

194

Conclusion

There are multiple injection possibilities for treating Achilles tendinopathy. However, none of these options have been studied to such an extent that a definitive recommendation can be given as to their use. Corticosteroid injections around the Achilles tendon may cause considerable harm, and therefore are meant to be contraindicated. Due to the lack of scientific evidence, there appears to be no room for injection therapies for insertional Achilles tendon problems (including chronic retrocalcaneal bursitis) in daily clinical practice. For mid-portion Achilles tendinopathies, several different techniques show good results and, therefore, these options might be interesting for evaluation in more depth in an accurate clinical study setting.

References

1. Aaron DL, Patel A, Kayiaros S, Calfee R. Four common types of bursitis: diagnosis and management. J Am Acad Orthop Surg. 2011; 19(6): 359-367.
2. Alfredson H. Chronic midportion Achilles tendinopathy: an update on research and treatment. Clin J Sport Med. 2003; 22(4): 727-741.
3. Alfredson H. The chronic painful Achilles and patellar tendon: research on basic biology and treatment. Scand J Med Sci Sports. 2005; 15(4): 252.
4. Alfredson H, Lorentzon R. Sclerosing polidocanol injections of small vessels to treat the chronic painful tendon. Cardiovasc Hematol Agents Med Chem. 2007; 5(2): 97-100.
5. Alfredson H, Ohberg L. Sclerosing injections to areas of neo-vascularisation reduce pain in chronic Achilles tendinopathy: a double-blind randomised controlled trial. Knee Surg Sports Traumatol Arthrosc. 2005; 13(4): 338-344.
6. Alfredson H, Ohberg L, Zeisig E, Lorentzon R. Treatment of midportion Achilles tendinosis: similar clinical results with US and CD-guided surgery outside the tendon and sclerosing polidocanol injections. Knee Surg Sports Traumatol Arthrosc. 2007; 15(12): 1504-1509.
7. Astrom M. Partial rupture in chronic Achilles tendinopathy. A retrospective analysis of 342 cases. Acta Orthop Scand. 1998; 69(4): 404.
8. Aubin F, Javaudin L, Rochcongar P. Utilisation de laprotinine dans le traitement des tendinopathies d'Achille du sportif á propos de 62 cas traits au CHR de Rennes. Journal de Pharmacie Clinique. 1997; 16(4): 270-273.
9. Brown R, Orchard J, Kinchington M, Hooper A, Nalder G. Aprotinin in the management of Achilles tendinopathy: a randomised controlled trial. Br J Sports Med. 2006; 40(3): 275-279.
10. Capasso G, Maffulli N, Testa V, Sgambato A. Preliminary results with peritendinous protease inhibitor injections in the management of Achilles tendinitis. J Sports Traumatol Rel Res 1993;15: 37–43.
11. Capasso G, Testa V, Maffulli N, Bifulco G. Aprotinin, corticosteroids and normosaline in the management of patellar tendinopathy in athletes: a prospective randomized study. Sports Exercise and Injury. 1997; 3: 111-115.
12. Chan O, O'Dowd D, Padhiar N. High volume image guided injections in chronic Achilles tendinopathy. Disabil Rehabil. 2008; 30(20-22): 1697-1708.
13. Checa A, Chun W, Pappu R. Ultrasound-guided diagnostic and therapeutic approach to Retrocalcaneal Bursitis. J Rheumatol. 2011; 38(2): 391-392.
14. Chechick A, Amit Y, Israeli A, Horoszowski H. Recurrent rupture of the Achilles tendon induced by corticosteroid injection. Br J Sports Med. 1982; 16(2): 89-90.
15. Clementson M, Lorén I, Dahlberg L, Aström M. Sclerosing injections in midportion Achilles tendinopathy: a retrospective study of 25 patients. Knee surgery, sports traumatology, arthroscopy: official journal of the ESSKA. 2008; 16(9): 887.
16. DaCruz DJ, Geeson M, Allen MJ, Phair I. Achilles paratendonitis: an evaluation of steroid injection. Br J Sports Med. 1988; 22(2): 64-65.
17. Dagenais S, Yelland MJ, Del MC, Schoene ML. Prolotherapy injections for chronic low-back pain. Cochrane Database Syst Rev. 2007; (2): CD004059.
18. Ford LT, DeBender J. Tendon rupture after local steroid injection. Southern Medical Journal. 1979; 72(7): 827.
19. Fredberg U, Bolvig L, Pfeiffer-Jensen M, Clemmensen D, Jakobsen BW, Stengaard-Pedersen K. Ultrasonography as a tool for diagnosis, guidance of local steroid injection and, together with pressure algometry, monitoring of the treatment of athletes with chronic jumper's knee and Achilles tendinitis: a randomized, double-blind, placebo-controlled study. Scand J Rheumatol. 2004; 33(2): 94-101.
20. Gross CE, Hsu AR, Chahal J, Holmes GB. Injectable Treatments for Noninsertional Achilles Tendinosis: A Systematic Review. Foot Ankle Int. 2013; 34(5): 619-28)
21. Halpern AA, Horowitz BG, Nagel DA. Tendon ruptures associated with corticosteroid therapy. West J Med. 1977; 127(5): 378-382.
22. Humphrey J, Chan O, Crisp T et al. The short-term effects of high volume image guided injections in resistant non-insertional Achilles tendinopathy. J Sci Med Sport. 2010; 13(3): 295-298.
23. Kleinman M, Gross AE. Achilles tendon rupture following steroid injection. Report of three cases. J Bone Joint Surg Am. 1983; 65(9): 1345-1347.
24. Kristoffersen M, Ohberg L, Johnston C, Alfredson H. Neovascularisation in chronic tendon injuries detected with colour Doppler ultrasound in horse and man: implications for research and treatment. Knee Surg Sports Traumatol Arthrosc. 2005; 13(6): 505-508.
25. Larsen AI, Egfjord M, Jelsdorff HM. Low-dose heparin in the treatment of calcaneal peritendinitis. Scand J Rheumatol. 1987; 16(1): 47-51.

26. Lind B, Ohberg L, Alfredson H. Sclerosing polidocanol injections in mid-portion Achilles tendinosis: remaining good clinical results and decreased tendon thickness at 2-year follow-up. Knee Surg Sports Traumatol Arthrosc. 2006; 14(12): 1327-1332.

27. Maffulli N, Spiezia F, Longo UG, Denaro V, Maffulli GD. High volume image guided injections for the management of chronic tendinopathy of the main body of the Achilles tendon. Phys Ther Sport. 2012; 14(3)163-7.

28. Magnussen RA, Dunn WR, Thomson AB. Nonoperative treatment of midportion Achilles tendinopathy: a systematic review. Clin J Sport Med. 2009; 19(1): 54-64.

29. Mahler F, Fritschy D. Partial and complete ruptures of the Achilles tendon and local corticosteroid injections. Br J Sports Med. 1992; 26(1): 7-14.

30. Maxwell NJ, Ryan MB, Taunton JE, Gillies JH, Wong AD. Sonographically guided intratendinous injection of hyperosmolar dextrose to treat chronic tendinosis of the Achilles tendon: a pilot study. AJR Am J Roentgenol. 2007; 189(4): W215-W220.

31. McLauchlan GJ, Handoll HH. Interventions for treating acute and chronic Achilles tendinitis. Cochrane Database Syst Rev. 2001; (2): CD000232.

32. Ohberg L, Alfredson H. Sclerosing therapy in chronic Achilles tendon insertional pain-results of a pilot study. Knee Surg Sports Traumatol Arthrosc. 2003; 11(5): 339-343.

33. Ohberg L, Alfredson H. Ultrasound guided sclerosis of neovessels in painful chronic Achilles tendinosis: pilot study of a new treatment. Br J Sports Med. 2002; 36(3): 173-175.

34. Ohberg L, Lorentzon R, Alfredson H. Eccentric training in patients with chronic Achilles tendinosis: normalised tendon structure and decreased thickness at follow up. Br J Sports Med. 2004; 38(1): 8-11.

35. Ohberg L, Lorentzon R, Alfredson H. Neovascularization in Achilles tendons with painful tendinosis but not in normal tendons: an ultrasonographic investigation. Knee Surg Sports Traumatol Arthrosc. 2001; 9(4): 233-238.

36. Orchard J, Massey A, Brown R, Cardon-Dunbar Al, Hofmann J. Successful Management of Tendinopathy With Injections of the MMP-inhibitor Aprotinin. Clin Orthop Relat Res. 2008; 466(7): 1625.

37. Paavola M, Kannus P, Järvinen TA, Järvinen TL, Józsa L, Järvinen M. Treatment of tendon disorders. Is there a role for corticosteroid injection? Foot and Ankle Clinics. 2002; 7(3): 501.

38. Pförringer W, Pfister A, Kuntz GÄ. The treatment of Achilles paratendinitis: Results of a double-blind, placebo-controlled study with a deproteinized hemodialysate. Clin J Sport Med. 1994; 4(2): 92-99.

39. Read MT. Safe relief of rest pain that eases with activity in achillodynia by intrabursal or peritendinous steroid injection: the rupture rate was not increased by these steroid injections. Br J Sports Med. 1999; 33(2): 134.

40. Rees JD, Wilson AM, Wolman RL. Current concepts in the management of tendon disorders. Rheumatology. 2006; 45(5): 508.

41. Rees JD, Wolman RL, Wilson A. Eccentric exercises; why do they work, what are the problems and how can we improve them? Br J Sports Med. 2009; 43(4): 242-246.

42. Rochcongar P, Thoribe B, Le Beux P, Jan J. Tendinopathie calcanéenne et sport: place des injections d'aprotinine. Science and Sports. 2005; 20(5): 261-267.

43. Ryan M, Wong A, Taunton J. Favorable outcomes after sonographically guided intratendinous injection of hyperosmolar dextrose for chronic insertional and midportion Achilles tendinosis. AJR Am J Roentgenol. 2010; 194(4): 1047-1053.

44. Shrier I, Matheson GO, Kohl HW, III. Achilles tendonitis: are corticosteroid injections useful or harmful? Clin J Sport Med. 1996; 6(4): 245-250.

45. Sofka CM, Adler RS, Positano R, Pavlov H, Luchs JS. Haglund's Syndrome: Diagnosis and Treatment Using Sonography. HSS J. 2006; 2(1): 27-29.

46. Speed CA. Injection therapies for soft-tissue lesions. Best Practice and Research Clinical Rheumatology. 2007; 21(2): 333-347.

47. Tatari H, Kosay C, Baran O, Ozcan O, Ozer E, Ulukus. Effect of heparin on tendon degeneration: an experimental study on rats. Knee Surg Sports Traumatol Arthrosc. 2001; 9(4): 247-253.

48. van Sterkenburg MN, de Jonge MC, Sierevelt IN, van Dijk CN. Less Promising Results With Sclerosing Etoxysclerol Injections for Midportion Achilles Tendinopathy: A Retrospective Study. Am J Sports Med. 2010; 38(11)2226-32

49. Willberg L, Sunding K, Ohberg L, Forssblad M, Fahlstrom M, Alfredson H. Sclerosing injections to treat midportion Achilles tendinosis: a randomised controlled study evaluating two different concentrations of Polidocanol. Knee Surg Sports Traumatol Arthrosc. 2008; 16(9): 859-864.

50. Yelland MJ, Sweeting KR, Lyftogt JA, Ng SK, Scuffham PA, Evans KA. Prolotherapy injections and eccentric loading exercises for painful Achilles tendinosis: a randomised trial. Br J Sports Med. 2011; 45(5): 421-428.

"Satisfaction consists in freedom from pain, which is the positive element of life."

Arthur Schopenhauer

Chapter 14

Endoscopic Surgery for Retrocalcaneal Bursitis

Johannes I. Wiegerinck, Ruben Zwiers, C. Niek van Dijk

Take Home Message

• *It is important to remove enough bone to prevent recurrent or persistent conflict between the calcaneus and the Achilles tendon.*

• *Endoscopic surgery is an effective procedure for the treatment of a chronic retrocalcaneal bursitis.*

• *Endoscopic calcaneoplasty provides high patient satisfaction and a low complication rate with rapid sports resumption.*

Introduction

If non-surgical treatment fails, endoscopic calcaneoplasty is a well-established procedure for patients with chronic retrocalcaneal bursitis [11]. Endoscopic procedures offer the advantages of any minimally invasive surgical procedure when compared with open surgical approaches. These advantages include low morbidity, short duration of surgery, improved scar healing, a shorter rehabilitation time and a quicker resumption of sport [1, 2, 8, 9]. This chapter focuses on the indications and surgical technique of endoscopic calcaneoplasty.

Indications

After six months of non-surgical treatment, surgical treatment becomes an option if conventional lateral radiographs show hypertrophy of the postero-superior aspect of the calcaneus and signs of chronic retrocalcaneal bursitis. The latter can be identified by a diminished radiolucency of the retrocalcaneal recess [10] (Figure 1). MRI or ultrasound can be useful to confirm the diagnosis [7].

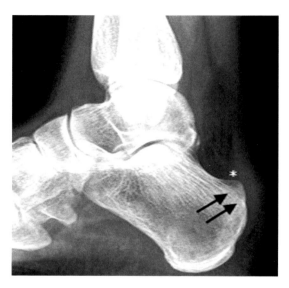

Figure 1. Conventional radiology before endoscopic calcaneoplasty. Pre-operative X-ray with hypertrophy of the postero-superior aspect of the calcaneus (arrows) and infiltration of the retrocalcaneal recess by the fluid-filled retrocalcaneal bursa(*).

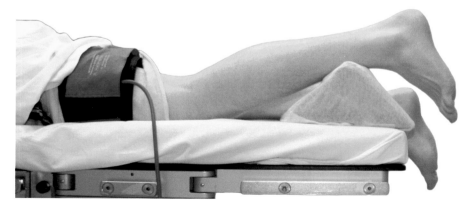

Figure 2. Patient positioning. The patient is placed in a prone position (alternatively the patient can be positioned supine). A tourniquet is placed around the upper leg. The feet are just over the edge, with a bolster under the affected lower leg. The other foot is positioned to ensure the surgeon has sufficient working area.

Surgical Technique

Surgery is performed in an ambulatory setting under general or regional anaesthesia. The patient is placed in the prone position [8, 9]. An alternative, but less used, position is the semi-prone with the hip supported and rotated or a full supine position[1-5, 9]. In the prone position the feet are positioned just over the edge of the operating table with the involved leg elevated (Figure 2). Subsequently, important anatomical structures are marked. These include both the medial and lateral border of the Achilles tendon and the calcaneus (Figure 3). First, the lateral portal is made (Figure 3A) just lateral to the Achilles tendon at the level of the superior aspect of the calcaneus. The skin is incised using a small vertical incision.

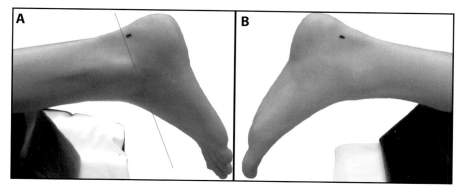

Figure 3. Portal placement. The ankle is placed in plantigrade position. A line is drawn through the tip of the fibula parallel to the foot sole. The incision for the lateral portal in endoscopic calcaneoplasty is placed 1.5-2.0 cm below this line (red).

The retrocalcaneal space is penetrated with a blunt trocar and a 4.5 mm 30° arthroscopic shaft is introduced. To locate the medial portal, a spinal needle is introduced under direct vision (Figure 4).

201

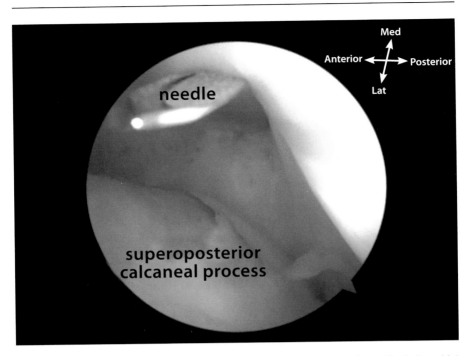

Figure 4. Creating the medial portal. Introduction of the spinal needle (left ankle) under direct vision for placement of the medial portal.

This portal is made medial to the Achilles tendon, again at the superior aspect of the calcaneus. After preparing the medial portal by a vertical stab incision, a 5.5 mm shaver is introduced and visualized by the arthroscope. To provide a better view, the retrocalcaneal space is dissected with a blunt trocar. At this moment the superior surface of the calcaneus is visualized and resected. The full radius resector faces the bone throughout the process to prevent iatrogenic damage to the Achilles tendon. Per-operatively impingement between the Achilles tendon and the calcaneus can be assessed by dorsiflexing the foot. Full dorsiflexion of the foot can elicit impingement between the Achilles tendon and the postero-superior calcaneal edge. Subsequently, the foot is brought into plantar flexion and the postero-superior calcaneal rim is removed. As this bone is fairly soft it can be removed using an aggressive full radius resector. Both portals can be used interchangeably for the arthroscope and the resector (Figure 5).

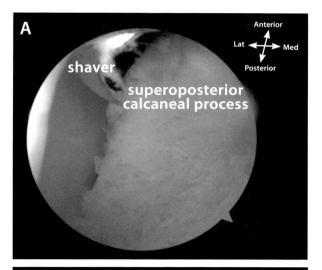

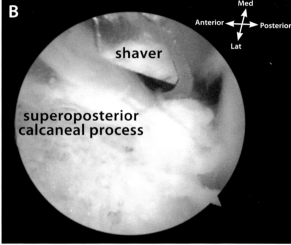

Figure 5. Endoscopic calcaneoplasty. Removal of bone at the postero-medial border of the calcaneus with an arthroscope in the lateral portal (A). Removal of bone at the lateral border of the calcaneus after a change of portals (B).

It is important to remove sufficient bone at the postero-medial and lateral corner by changing portals intermittently. The synovial resector is moved beyond the posterior edge onto the lateral and medial wall of the calcaneus to smoothen the edges. Full plantar flexion of the foot is necessary to visualize the Achilles tendon insertion. This region is smoothened by placing the bonecutter against the calcaneus on the insertion site. The resector is reintroduced to remove loose debris and smoothen other possible rough edges. Fluoroscopic control may be useful to ascertain whether sufficient bone has been resected. Skin sutures are used to close the incisions to prevent sinus formation. A 10 ml 0.5% bupivacaine/morphine solution is injected at the incision site and the surrounding skin. Post-operative treatment is functional and weight-bearing is allowed as tolerated. Active range-of-motion exercises are advised from day one for at least ten minutes, three times a day. The patient may return to regular shoes as tolerated. A conventional lateral radiograph can be made to ascertain whether sufficient bone has been excised (Figure 6).

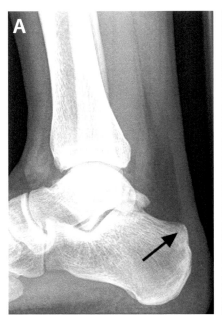
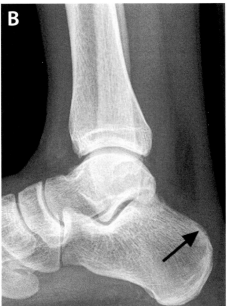

Figure 6. Pre- and post-operative X-ray of the left foot of a 38 year old patient, the postero-superior part of the calcaneus is sufficiently excised (arrow A, B).

Results

Four studies report on the outcome of this two-portal endoscopic technique [3-5, 8]. The first describes the results of patients who were operated on in a prone position. The other three report the results with patients treated in a supine position. Finally one study was found reporting on patients treated with an alternative technique using an additional portal [12].

Scholten and van Dijk [8] published the results of 39 procedures of endoscopic calcaneoplasty in 36 patients. The average age was 35 years. The patients had a painful swelling of the soft tissue of the posterior heel, medial and lateral of the Achilles tendon on physical examination, without pain on palpation of the tendon itself. Non-surgical management for at least six months did not relieve symptoms. The mean follow-up after endoscopic calcaneoplasty was 4.5 years. There were no surgical complications except from one patient who experienced an area of hypoesthesia over the heel pad. Post-operatively there were no infections, tenderness or problematic scars, and all patients were content with their small incisions. Except for two of them, all patients improved. The Ogilvie-Harris score was rated fair by four patients, six rated good and 24 had excellent results. Work and sport resumption was achieved at an average of five weeks and 11 weeks, respectively.

Jerosch and co-workers [3] reported on 164 patients, 81 males and 84 females, with an age range between 16-67 years, operated between 1999 and 2010. A postero-superior calcaneal exostosis was identified in each patient on conventional lateral radiography. None of the included patients had cavus deformities or clinical varus of the hind foot. All patients had failed non-surgical treatment for at least six months. The mean follow-up after surgical intervention was 46.3 months. According to the Ogilvie-Harris score, 155 patients had good or excellent results, while nine patients had fair or poor results. All the post-operative radiographs showed sufficient resection of the calcaneal spur. Only minor post-operative complications were observed.

In 2003, Leitze and co-workers [4] published a series of 30 consecutive patients (33 procedures) treated by endoscopic decompression of the retrocalcaneal space. All patients had unsatisfying non-surgical management of retrocalcaneal bursitis, a symptomatic postero-superior calcaneal exostosis, and/or insertional Achilles tendinopathy. Three patients were excluded. The AOFAS increased from 61.8 points preoperative to 87.5 points postoperative. At an average of 22 months follow-up 19 patients had an excellent outcome and five good. Fair and poor outcomes were reported in three cases. The results of this endoscopically-treated group were compared with a group of 17 heels in 14 patients treated with open surgery. No statistically significant differences in AOFAS, recovery time or complications were found.

Ortmann and McBride [5] reported the results of 30 patients (32 feet) with retrocalcaneal bursitis treated with a similar two-portal endoscopic approach. All patients had persisting complaints after non-surgical measures. During the procedure the inflamed bursa and bony prominence were resected. The postoperative follow-up averaged 35 months. The mean pre-operative AOFAS was 61 versus 97 postoperatively. Twenty-nine heels had excellent or good results. There was one patient with a poor outcome, requiring an open procedure with Achilles tendon augmentation. In one patient an acute Achilles tendon rupture occurred. After primary repair this patient returned to her preoperative activity level.

In a recent study by Wu and co-workers [12], an adjustment to this endoscopic technique was introduced. Compared with the two-portal technique, an additional proximal postero-lateral portal was used just lateral and 5 cm proximal to the insertion of the Achilles tendon. This portal is mainly used as viewing portal. Due to the larger distance to the prominence this portal might provide a better view. Twenty-five patients, diagnosed with a calcaneal prominence and pain in the retrocalcaneal region, were treated with this three-portal technique. The mean follow-up was 41 months. Mean AOFAS improved from 63.3 pre-operatively to 86.8 points at final follow-up. Twenty-one patients had an excellent or good result, and four had fair or poor results. According to the Ogilvie Harris score, there were 22 excellent or good, and three fair or poor results. No complications occurred.

In a number of patients a partial tear of the Achilles tendon was reported [2]. The damage is probably due to repetitive contact between the Achilles tendon and the postero-superior calcaneal prominence. Even though this tear can be quite large, a complete avulsion of the Achilles tendon has never been found during endoscopic calcaneoplasty [1-5, 8, 9]. When performing an endoscopic calcaneoplasty, the medial and lateral insertional areas of the Achilles tendon onto the calcaneus remain intact. In an open resection, however, most of the lateral and medial insertional areas of the Achilles tendon are also detached. This may explain the reports of Achilles tendon avulsions after open resection of a postero-superior calcaneal prominence [2].

Conclusion

To successfully treat patients with an endoscopic resection of the postero-superior calcaneal process it is important that enough bone is removed to prevent recurrent and repetitive trauma of the calcaneus against the Achilles tendon [4-6, 8, 9]. Regardless of the surgeon's preference for a supine or prone position, endoscopic calcaneoplasty has been demonstrated to have a high patient satisfaction and a low complication rate with early return to sports [3-5, 8, 9, 11]. In addition, endoscopic surgery provides several advantages including low morbidity, early functional rehabilitation, day-case treatment and improved scar healing when compared to the results for the open technique [4, 11].

References

1. Jerosch J, Nasef NM. Endoscopic calcaneoplasty--rationale, surgical technique, and early results: a preliminary report. Knee Surg Sports Traumatol Arthrosc 2003;11(3):190-195.

2. Jerosch J, Schunck J, Sokkar SH. Endoscopic calcaneoplasty (ECP) as a surgical treatment of Haglund's syndrome. Knee Surg Sports Traumatol Arthrosc 2007;15(7):927-934.

3. Jerosch J, Sokkar S, Ducker M, Donner A. Die enoskopische Kalkaneoplastik (EKP) beim Haglund-Syndrom. Indikation, OP-Technik, Befunde, Ergebnisse. Z Orthop Unfall 2012.

4. Leitze Z, Sella EJ, Aversa JM. Endoscopic decompression of the retrocalcaneal space. J Bone Joint Surg Am 2003;85-A(8):1488-1496.

5. Ortmann FW, McBryde AM. Endoscopic bony and soft-tissue decompression of the retrocalcaneal space for the treatment of Haglund deformity and retrocalcaneal bursitis. Foot Ankle Int 2007;28(2):149-153.

6. Pauker M, Katz K, Yosipovitch Z. Calcaneal ostectomy for Haglund disease. J Foot Surg 1992;31(6):588-589.

7. Pierre-Jerome C, Moncayo V, Terk MR. MRI of the Achilles tendon: a comprehensive review of the anatomy, biomechanics, and imaging of overuse tendinopathies. Acta Radiol 2010;51(4):438-454.

8. Scholten PE, van Dijk CN. Endoscopic calcaneoplasty. Foot Ankle Clin 2006;11(2):439-46, viii.

9. van Dijk CN, van Dyk GE, Scholten PE, Kort NP. Endoscopic calcaneoplasty. Am J Sports Med 2001;29(2):185-189.

10. van Sterkenburg MN, Muller B, Maas M, Sierevelt IN, van Dijk CN. Appearance of the weight-bearing lateral radiograph in retrocalcaneal bursitis. Acta Orthop 2010;81(3):387-390.

11. Wiegerinck JI, Kok AC, van Dijk CN. Surgical treatment of chronic retrocalcaneal bursitis. Arthroscopy 2012;28(2):283-293.

12. Wu Z, Hua Y, Li Y, Chen S. Endoscopic treatment of Haglund's syndrome with a three portal technique. Int Orthop 2012;36(8):1623-1627.

"Assumptions allow the best in life to pass you by."

John Sales

Chapter 15

Endoscopic Techniques in Mid-portion Achilles Tendinopathies

Hajo Thermann, Ralph M. Fisher, Sven Feil, Ruben Zwiers, C. Niek van Dijk

Take Home Message

- *It is probable that neovascularization, accompanied by nociceptive nerve fibres at the ventral aspect of the Achilles tendon, is responsible for the pain in patients with mid-portion Achilles tendinopathy. It is questionable whether the degeneration of the tendon contributes to the pain, since the tendon itself is aneural. Debridement of the paratenon is often necessary for successful treatment.*

- *Endoscopic debridement yields good results compared with open procedures, with fast rehabilitation and a low complication rate.*

Introduction

Surgery is often considered in patients with chronic Achilles tendinopathy if non-surgical treatment fails. Around 25% of patients may eventually require surgery [9-11]. The technique used for the surgical management of tendinopathy depends on the progress of the disease. Local degeneration and thickening are usually treated by excision and curettage. An Achilles tendon that is inadequate due to extensive degeneration may have to be reconstructed. Isolated paratendinopathy can be treated by the excision of the affected paratenon.

Generally, open surgery is associated with a higher complication rate than endoscopic treatment as well as a longer rehabilitation period, often 4-12 months [1, 6, 13]. Hence, minimally-invasive techniques for the treatment of Achilles tendinopathy have been developed.

In patients with combined tendinopathy and paratendinopathy, the question is whether both pathologies contribute to the complaints. An anatomic cadaver study described degenerative changes of the Achilles tendon in as much as 34% of subjects who had no complaints [7]. Khan and co-workers found abnormal morphology in 65% (37 of 57) of symptomatic tendons and in 32% (9 of 28) of asymptomatic Achilles tendons that were assessed using ultrasound [8]. Therefore, it is questionable whether degeneration of the tendon itself is the main cause of the pain. It is suggested that the ingrowth of neovessels, with accompanying nerves at the anterior aspect of the tendon [5], is one possible cause of pain [2-4, 15]. 'Denervation' of the Achilles tendon by the release of the peritendineum from the Achilles tendon proper may, therefore, be sufficient to resolve such complaints.

Endoscopic debridement as a minimally-invasive procedure allows the surgeon –using two small incisions – complete access to the tendon, especially the anterior part of it. The debridement leads to rapid post-operative pain relief in many cases. In this chapter, three endoscopic approaches to treat Achilles tendinopathy are described.

Surgical technique

I – Treatment of mid-portion Achilles tendinopathy (by addressing the paratenon and plantaris tendon only)

This surgical technique, first described by Steenstra and van Dijk [16], focuses on the management of the paratendinopathy only; the nodular, thickened tendon proper is left untouched even when an intratendinous lesion is present.

Local, epidural, spinal and general anaesthesia can be used for this procedure. The patient is placed in the prone position. A tourniquet is placed around the thigh of the affected leg. Because the surgeon needs to be able to obtain full plantar and dorsiflexion, the foot is placed right over the end of the table.

A 2.7 mm 30° arthroscope for the endoscopy of combined tendinopathy and paratendinopathy is most commonly used. This small-diameter arthroscope yields an excellent picture comparable with the standard 4 mm arthroscope; however, it cannot deliver the same amount of irrigation fluid as the larger arthroscope.

The distal portal is located on the lateral border of the Achilles tendon, 2-3 cm distal to the tendon nodule. The proximal portal is located medial to the border of the Achilles tendon, 2-4 cm above the nodule. When the portals are placed this way, it is usually possible to visualize and work around the complete surface of the tendon, over a span of approximately 10 cm.

The distal portal is made first. After making the skin incision, a mosquito clamp is introduced, followed by a blunt 2.7 mm trocar in the craniomedial direction. With this blunt trocar, the peritendineum is approached, and is blindly released from the tendon (Figure 1A). Subsequently, the 2.7 mm arthroscope is introduced. To minimize the risk of iatrogenic damage, the arthroscope should be kept directly on the tendon. At this point, it should be ascertained whether the surgeon is in the right layer between the deepest layer of the paratenon and the Achilles tendon (Figure 1B). If not, this layer must be identified and a further release can be performed.

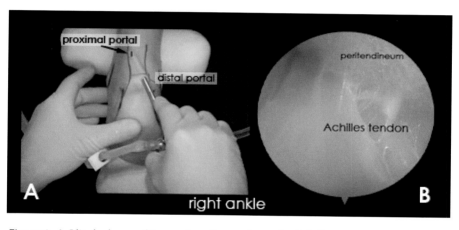

Figure 1. A. Blind release of the peritendineum from the Achilles tendon. B. Endoscopic view: the peritendineum is released from the Achilles tendon.

The proximal portal is made by introducing a spinal needle, followed by a mosquito clamp and probe. The plantaris tendon can be identified at the antero-medial border of the Achilles tendon. In a typical case of paratendinopathy, the plantaris tendon, the Achilles tendon and the peritendineum are tight together in the process. The removal of the local thickened peritendineum on the antero-medial side of the Achilles tendon at the level of the nodule and the release of the plantaris tendon are the goals of this part of the procedure. In patients where the fibrotic peritendineum is firmly attached to the tendon, a release is performed. Neovessels are sometimes found and can be removed with a 2.7 mm full radius shaver. Changing portals can be helpful. At the end of the procedure, it must be possible to move the arthroscope over the complete symptomatic area of the Achilles tendon.

Aftercare consists of a compressive dressing for 2-3 days. Patients are encouraged to actively perform range of motion exercises. Full weight-bearing is allowed as tolerated.

II – Endoscopic treatment of mid-portion tendinopathy with minor and major degenerations

This alternative technique was published in 2009 by Thermann and co-workers [17]. This approach focuses on the varying severity of the pathologies of mid-portion tendinopathy.

Local, spinal and general anaesthesia can be applied for the procedures. During surgery, the patient lies in the prone position with his feet beyond the edge of the table so that the ankle joint is fully movable. A tourniquet is recommended.

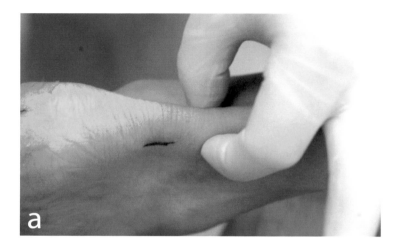

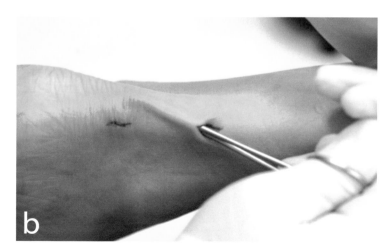

Figure 2. A. The Achilles tendon from the postero-medial side. Palpation of the nodular thickening and location of the distal portal 2-4 cm distally. B. The Achilles tendon from the postero-medial side. Splitting of the subcutaneous layers with a mosquito clamp, to prepare space for the instruments.

A 4.0 mm 30° arthroscope is used. This allows for a good view with sufficient flow. The locations of the portals are approximately 6-8 cm proximally and distally to the medial nodular thickening of the Achilles tendon (Figure 2A). After the stab incisions are performed, a mosquito clamp is used for the separation of the subcutaneous layer (Figure 2B) to create space for the arthroscope and the shaver.

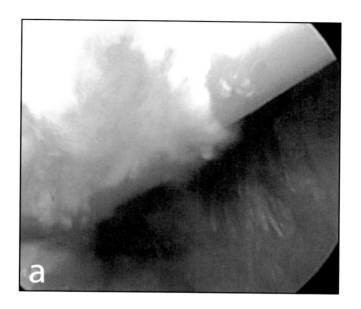

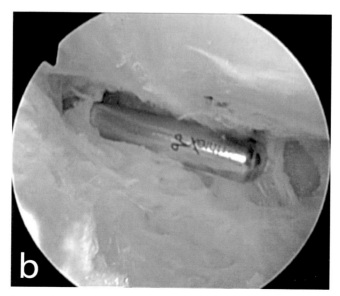

Figure 3. A. Endoscopic view of the surgical procedure. Interior view of the tendon and releasing of the tendon from the ventral soft tissue. B. Endoscopic view of the surgical procedure. Smooth surface of the partially debrided Achilles tendon.

After the insertion of the instruments, the entire anterior part of the tendon can be visualized (Figure 3A). By using the shaver, the anterior soft tissue can be debrided from the tendon (Figure 3B). By changing the positioning of the instruments, the dorsal aspects of the tendon can also be presented and debrided. Furthermore, the peritendineum can be debrided and a ventral tendon release and decompression of the thickened tendon is performed (Figure 4A).

For small tendon degenerations, a longitudinal splitting by a retrograde incision is performed (Figure 4B).

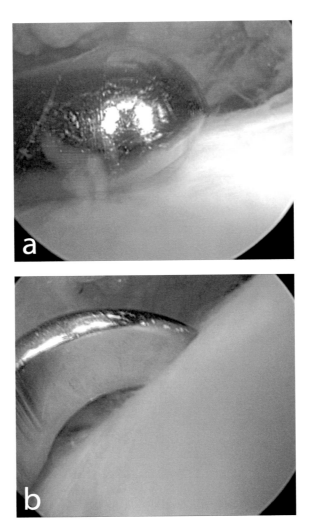

Figure 4. A. Endoscopic view of the surgical procedure. Debridement of the peritendineum around the complete tendon circumference. B. Endoscopic view of the surgical procedure. Longitudinal incisions are performed using a retrograde knife blade.

214

In case of a simple debridement of the Achilles tendon, adapted range of motion exercises are begun on the first post-operative day. Partial weight-bearing is recommended for 14 days. Proprioceptive training, strength training and aqua jogging should be started after wound healing. Particular focus is directed towards the stretching exercises of the entire flexor chain. After 6-12 weeks, light jogging on an even surface is started. Competition-specific training should not be performed before four to six months after surgery.

III Surgical technique – major tendon degeneration

For more significant degeneration (<40% of severe tendon degeneration) that may be defined as 'chronic rupture', a mere tendon splitting is not sufficient. In such a case, the degenerated tissue needs to be excised (Figure 5A). According to the tendon defect after debridement, a PDS "frame' suture (1.3 mm) may be necessary to improve tendon stability (Figure 5B).

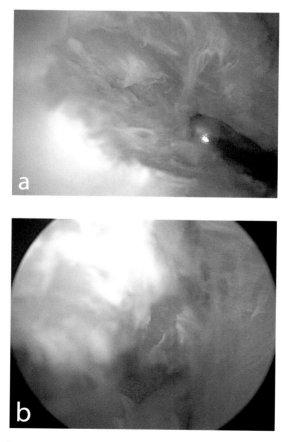

Figure 5. A. Endoscopic view of the surgical procedure. Massive endoscopic debridement of degenerated tendon tissue using a shaver. B. Endoscopic view of the surgical procedure. The PDS cord within the tendon after the construction of the frame suture.

For this 'frame' suture with a 1.3 mm PDS cord, three additional portals are needed. Two of them are located laterally, at the height of the already existing medial incisions. The third incision should be located centrally between the proximal and distal portals to protect the sural nerve (Figure 6A). Using a classic percutaneous suture technique, the suture is pulled in from the proximal medial portal to the lateral portal. From there, the suture is pulled to the distal lateral portal via the central portal, then back to the medial side and up to the proximal medial portal via the central portal (Figure 6B). Finally, both ends are tied together in 5° plantarflexion (Figure 6C).

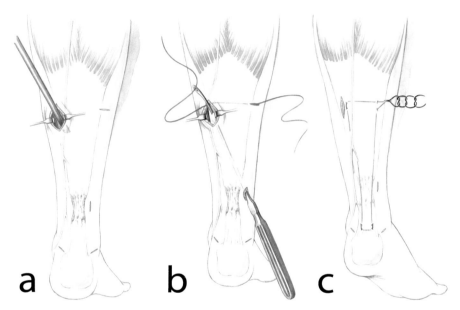

Figure 6. A. Exploration of the tendon ends in the epifascial area to identify the sural nerve. B. The 1.3 mm PDS cord is pulled from medial to lateral with preservation of the nerve. The nerve is retained with a small Hohmann retractor. Thereafter the suture is pulled distally and laterally. Then back to the medial side and finally to the medial and proximal portal. C. The framework is tied using a triple knot. The knot is burried under the subcutaneous tissue.

Discussion

Steenstra and Van Dijk have reported on results in 20 patients treated by means of the release of the paratendinopathy alone [16]. All the patients had a combination of paratendinopathy and tendinopathy, and had had their complaints for more than two years. They had undergone a period of at least six months of physiotherapy before surgery. The results were analysed with a follow-up of six years. There were no complications. Most patients were able to resume their sporting activities after four to eight weeks. All the patients had significant pain relief. The results of the subjective outcome scores used were comparable to a cohort of people without Achilles tendon complaints.

Maquirriain and co-workers reported the outcomes of seven patients who underwent an endoscopic release for chronic Achilles tendinopathy, with similar results. The mean Achilles Tendinopathy Scoring System of this group improved from 39 points pre-operatively to 89 points post-operatively, and there were no complications [12]. Vega and co-workers published a modified endoscopic technique in 2008. Pathological tissue was endoscopically removed, and multiple longitudinal tenotomies were performed using a retrograde knife blade. They reported a series of eight patients with excellent outcomes, return to previous sports activities and no complications [18].

Pearce and co-workers described their results in a consecutive series of 11 patients with mid-portion Achilles tendinopathy [14]. All the patients were treated non-surgically for at least six months before they underwent endoscopic surgery according to the technique described by Streenstra and co-workers [16]. The mean pre-operative AOFAS hindfoot score was 68 points, and it improved significantly to a mean of 92 points at final follow-up. Moreover, the AOS scores for pain (28% pre-op to 8% post-op) and disability (38% pre-op to 10% post-op) improved significantly. The mean SF-36 scores also improved. No complications occurred, and eight of the 11 patients were satisfied with the result.

Thermann and co-workers reported short-term clinical results after endoscopic debridement in patients with Achilles mid-portion tendinopathy [17]. The results showed a significant reduction in pain just six weeks after surgery. Furthermore, in terms of function, satisfaction and the VISA-A the results were good.

Conclusion

Endoscopic surgery for mid-portion Achilles tendinopathies shows promising results. However, further studies with larger cohorts and longer follow-up are required to optimize the techniques.

References

1. Abramowitz Y, Wollstein R, Barzilay Y. Outcome of resection of a symptomatic os trigonum. J Bone Joint Surg Am 2003;85-A(6):1051-1057.
2. Alfredson H, Forsgren S, Thorsen K, Fahlstrom M, Johansson H, Lorentzon R. Glutamate NMDAR1 receptors localised to nerves in human Achilles tendons. Implications for treatment? Knee Surg Sports Traumatol Arthrosc 2001;9(2):123-126.
3. Alfredson H, Ohberg L, Forsgren S. Is vasculo-neural ingrowth the cause of pain in chronic Achilles tendinosis? An investigation using ultrasonography and colour Doppler, immunohistochemistry, and diagnostic injections. Knee Surg Sports Traumatol Arthrosc 2003;11(5):334-338.
4. Andersson G, Danielson P, Alfredson H, Forsgren S. Presence of substance P and the neurokinin-1 receptor in tenocytes of the human Achilles tendon. Regul Pept 2008;150(1-3):81-87.
5. Bjur D, Alfredson H, Forsgren S. The innervation pattern of the human Achilles tendon: studies of the normal and tendinosis tendon with markers for general and sensory innervation. Cell Tissue Res 2005;320(1):201-206.
6. Hamilton WG, Geppert MJ, Thompson FM. Pain in the posterior aspect of the ankle in dancers. Differential diagnosis and operative treatment. J Bone Joint Surg Am 1996;78(10):1491-1500.
7. Kannus P, Jozsa L. Histopathological changes preceding spontaneous rupture of a tendon. A controlled study of 891 patients. J Bone Joint Surg Am 1991;73(10):1507-1525.
8. Khan KM, Forster BB, Robinson J. Are ultrasound and magnetic resonance imaging of value in assessment of Achilles tendon disorders? A two year prospective study. Br J Sports Med 2003;37(2):149-153.
9. Kvist M. Achilles tendon injuries in athletes. Ann Chir Gynaecol 1991;80(2):188-201.
10. Maffulli N, Walley G, Sayana MK, Longo UG, Denaro V. Eccentric calf muscle training in athletic patients with Achilles tendinopathy. Disabil Rehabil 2008;30(20-22): 1677-1684. 3
11. Maffulli N. Augmented repair of acute Achilles tendon ruptures using gastrocnemius-soleus fascia. Int Orthop 2005;29(2):134. 2
12. Maquirriain J, Ayerza M, Costa-Paz M, Muscolo DL. Endoscopic surgery in chronic Achilles tendinopathies: A preliminary report. Arthroscopy 2002;18(3):298-303.
13. Marotta JJ, Micheli LJ. Os trigonum impingement in dancers. Am J Sports Med 1992;20(5):533-536.
14. Pearce CJ, Carmichael J, Calder JD. Achilles tendinoscopy and plantaris tendon release and division in the treatment of non-insertional Achilles tendinopathy. Foot Ankle Surg 2012;18(2):124-127.
15. Peers KH, Brys PP, Lysens RJ. Correlation between power Doppler ultrasonography and clinical severity in Achilles tendinopathy. Int Orthop 2003;27(3):180-183.
16. Steenstra F, van Dijk CN. Achilles tendoscopy. Foot Ankle Clin 2006;11(2):429-38, viii.
17. Thermann H, Benetos IS, Panelli C, Gavriilidis I, Feil S. Endoscopic treatment of chronic mid-portion Achilles tendinopathy: novel technique with short-term results. Knee Surg Sports Traumatol Arthrosc 2009;17(10):1264-1269.
18. Vega J, Cabestany JM, Golano P, Perez-Carro L. Endoscopic treatment for chronic Achilles tendinopathy. Foot Ankle Surg 2008;14(4):204-210.

"The body is an instrument, the mind its function, the witness and reward of its operation."

George Santayana

Chapter 16

Endoscopic Repair of Achilles Tendon Ruptures

Mahmut N. Doral, Gürhan Dönmez, Egemen Turhan, Gazi Huri, Onur Bilge, Murat Bozkurt, Defne Kaya, Feza Korkusuz

Take Home Message

- *Endoscopy-assisted percutaneous Achilles tendon repair allows direct visualization of the synovia and protects the paratenon.*

- *Achilles tendoscopy techniques may reduce the risk of sural nerve injury.*

- *Early functional post-operative rehabilitation following surgery may improve the surgical outcome.*

- *Percutaneous repair of the Achilles tendon under endoscopic control with local infiltration anaesthesia is a safe technique with good outcomes and minimal risk of complications when compared with open surgery or minimally invasive approaches.*

Abstract

Among all injuries, Achilles tendon rupture has a substantial potential to cause significant morbidity. Only 50-60% of elite athletes are able to return to their pre-injury levels following the injury. Recent studies suggest early weight-bearing and strengthening exercises to accelerate a return to sports. Therefore, and regardless of technique, it is important to design a strong suture construct to allow early weight-bearing and strengthening exercises without compromising repair, as well as to avoid wound complications. Recently minimally invasive approaches for the treatment of acute Achilles tendon ruptures have been described to achieve a better outcome and an early return to sport. The purpose of this chapter is to describe less invasive treatment options for Achilles tendon ruptures.

Introduction

Acute Achilles tendon rupture is one of the most common injuries of the foot and ankle. After rotator cuff and quadriceps tendon ruptures, it is reported as the third most frequent major tendon rupture in the body [17, 24]. Despite several non-surgical and surgical treatment options, there is no clear consensus in terms of the most optimal surgical technique for acute ruptures of the Achilles tendon. However, surgical treatment options such as open repair, mini-open and percutaneous repair with or without endoscopic assistance have gained popularity over non-surgical treatment during the last decade [28].

In order to avoid relatively high complication rates due to open procedures, such as delayed wound healing, skin necrosis and adhesions, percutaneous repair techniques have been described. However, a percutaneous approach may lead inadequate repair, with poor contact of the rupture sides and it may increase the risk of sural nerve injuries [29]. Therefore, researchers have recently recommended "endoscopy-assisted repair" procedures as a reasonable solution in order to overcome these problems [11, 36, 37].

The aim of this chapter is to describe the surgical technique and review the literature of endoscopic-assisted Achilles tendon repairs.

Surgical Technique

The selection of the patient for endoscopic-assisted percutaneous Achilles tendon repair is important. A history of previous Achilles tendon surgery and the presence of skin lesions around the surgical side are relative contraindications. The recommended time for the repair is 7-10 days after the injury and the distal part of the tendon should be long enough - more than 2 cm – in order to achieve a firm and reliable grasp of the distal tendon.

The surgery is performed with the patient in the prone position and with the injured foot in approximately 15° plantar flexion in order to achieve the best portal location. The surgery is performed under local anaesthesia and without a tourniquet. Full communication with the patient is ensured as the active motion of the ankle is important. Before starting the procedure, the rupture site and the location of the gap are marked (Figure 1).

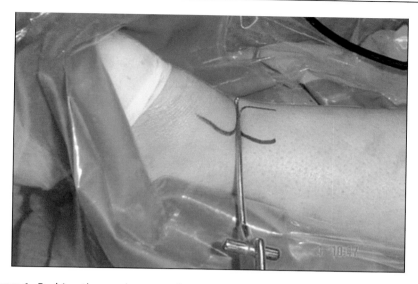

Figure 1. Probing the gap between the ruptured tendon ends.

Subsequently, to minimize local bleeding, proximally (about 5 cm) and distally (about 4 cm) to the tendon gap, the skin, subcutis and paratenon are infiltrated with a 20–50 mL 0.9% saline solution with local anaesthetic (1% Citanest® 5 mL + 0.5% Marcain® 5 mL) around the eight planned stab incisions, four incisions are mid-medial and four mid-lateral to the tendon, distributed evenly proximally and distally to the ruptured area (Figure 2).

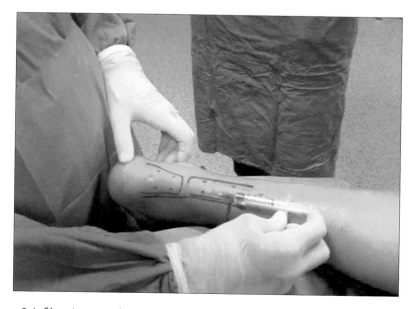

Figure 2. Infiltrative anesthesia.

Special attention is paid to the lateral side, particularly the proximal area, where the sural nerve is located and crosses the Achilles tendon. Using the nick-and-spread technique, the stab incisions are later enlarged and used for needle entry. The patient is asked to report any paraesthesia in the sural nerve area during infiltration. When this is experienced, the puncture site is shifted approximately 0.5–1 cm towards the middle. The tendon and paratenon are examined with a 4.5 mm 30° arthroscope via the distal medial incision, and the injured foot is positioned in approximately 15° plantar flexion (Figure 3). After the level of the rupture is determined, the continuity of the surrounding synovial tissue, its thickness and its vascularization are evaluated.

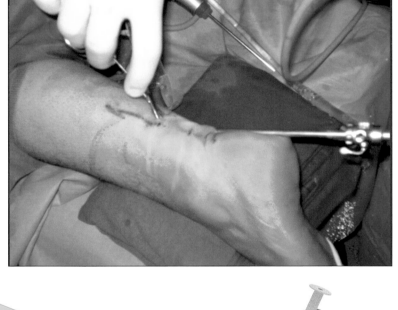

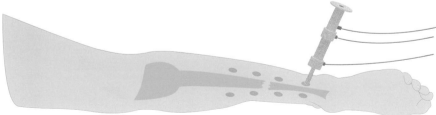

Figure 3. The placement of the arthroscope from distal medial incision.

The torn ends of the Achilles tendon are inspected and, if necessary, manipulated within the paratenon. The passing of the suture through the Achilles tendon is also controlled under endoscopic visualization. A PDS No. 5 double loop (Ethicon Inc, Johnson & Johnson, Somerville, NJ, USA) suture with a modified Bunnell configuration is used. The needle with the PDS or Ethibond suture is first introduced through the upper medial portal. To ensure that the Achilles tendon is fully caught by the needle, the tendon is gently palpated between the thumb and the index finger of the opposite hand. The first stitch is a transverse one, and the needle emerges from the upper lateral portal. The needle is then retrieved, introduced again through it, and passed through the upper lateral portal towards portal 3. The procedure is repeated in a proximal-to-distal direction going from portal 3 to portal 4, from portal 4 to portal 5, from portal 5 to portal 6, from portal 6 to portal 7, and from portal 7 to portal 8, the distal-most lateral portal. At this point, the needle is retrieved from portal 8, and thereafter introduced through it again and passed through the distal-most lateral portal toward portal 5. The procedure described above is thereafter repeated backwards in a distal-to-proximal direction until the needle is finally returned to the upper medial portal. Initially, the suture from the proximal medial incision is passed out from the medial incision just above the ruptured tendon, making sure that the proximal stump of the tendon is squeezed between the thumb and the index fingers of the surgeon. Then, the suture from the same incision is passed out from the lateral stab incision just above the tendon. Finally, as in the first step, the suture is passed through this distal stab incision, passed on to proximal, and then out from the superior medial side again (Figure 4).

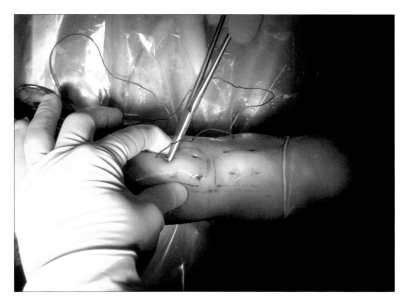

Figure 4. A modified Bunnel suture configuration is used. Initially, the suture passes from the superomedial stab incision (No: 1). The suture is carried distally with zig-zag fashion in the sequence of the number of the stab incisions.

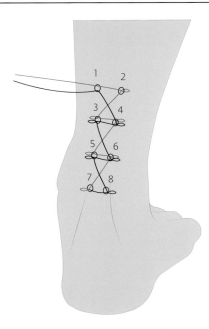

Figure 4. Final step for suturing process is carrying the suture to proximal and then out from the superomedial portal again.

During suture passage, the arthroscope is placed alternatively in the various entry portals, and the Achilles tendon is inspected from the medial and lateral aspects. The proximal and distal stumps are also inspected from the proximal and distal directions to make sure that the tendon stumps are clearly juxtaposed. The sutures are placed in the tendon at different levels in the coronal plane to ensure that the risk of cutting out is minimized during tensioning. Finally, the sutures are tensioned and tied in the proximal medial entry portal with the ankle in neutral position while checking the tendon approximation using the arthroscope (Figure 5).

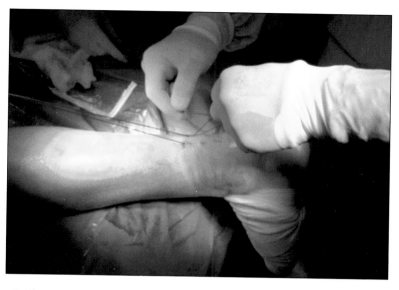

Figure 5. The sutures are tied with the ankle in neutral position.

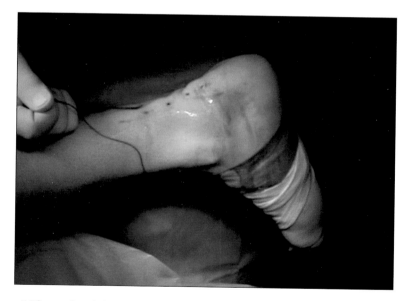

Figure 6. The patient is instructed to actively dorsi- and plantar-flex the ankle in order to make sure that appropriate tension is present.

Following the repair, the active motion of the ankle between 90° to neutral is examined. Subsequently, in order to check whether the appropriate tension at the repair side was obtained, the same examination is repeated while the knee is in 90° flexion (Figure 6). Before securing the sutures, a final endoscopic evaluation is performed (Figure 7).

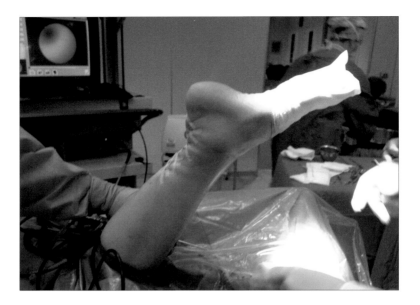

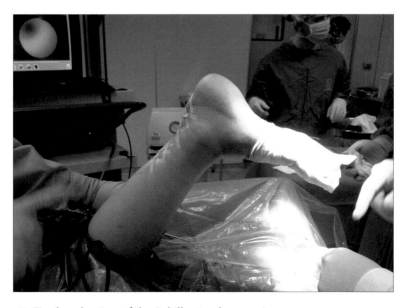

Figure 7. Final evaluation of the Achilles tendon repair.

Meanwhile, to enhance the healing response of the ruptured tendon, platelet-rich plasma (PRP) is injected at the end of the operation (Figure 8). The application of autologous growth factors via PRP is a promising way to improve the biological tissue healing response and has been shown to be safe and effective. However, it is an issue where further investigations and long-term results are required to improve knowledge [2,9,21,26,35].

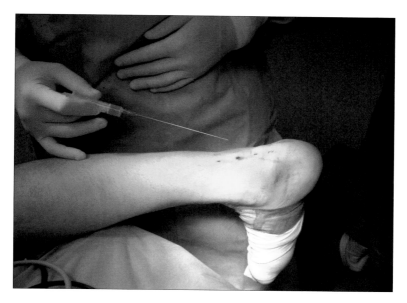

Figure 8. Injection of PRP.

Immediate passive range of motion training is started after surgery and the patient is allowed to engage in full weight-bearing mobilization using a walking brace in the neutral position for at least three weeks.

Discussion

As a result of the increasing incidence of Achilles tendon ruptures, it has become the focus of many studies and meta-analyses during the last decade. Although there are several publications that support non-surgical treatment, recently the number of the studies that promote the surgical treatment has significantly increased, especially for athletes. The management of Achilles tendon ruptures should be based on reducing morbidity, enabling an early return to full function and minimizing complications. It is clearly reported that non-surgical treatment leads to higher re-rupture rates [40, 41]. In a systematic review, the re-rupture rate after non-surgical treatment was approximately 12% [23]. In addition, it is difficult to obtain the original tendon length after non-surgical treatment, which is the primary goal. Numerous open surgical procedures have been proposed to repair Achilles tendon ruptures, ranging from a simple end-to-end suture with Bunnell or Kessler-type techniques, to more complex repairs, sometimes with the use of fascial reinforcement or tendon grafts. However, there is no single, uniformly superior technique for open surgical techniques. Joint stiffness, muscle hypotrophy, adhesions, infection, scarification, algodystrophy, deep venous thrombosis and especially wound break-down, are some of the potential complications of open procedures, which in fact are not rare [3, 4, 25, 33].

The percutaneous repair technique was first described by Ma and Griffith to reduce the complication risk [29]. Although it has the advantage of fewer wound problems, it includes difficulties in achieving proper contact of the tendon stumps and adequate initial fixation [28]. Moreover, the percutaneous technique may lead to tendon lengthening due to a lack of inadequate approximation of the tendon-ends. The technique is also criticized because it provides only approximately 50% of the initial strength afforded by open repair and has a higher re-rupture rate (6.4%) than open repair [18, 39]. Therefore, it is less often recommended for patients with high demands [4, 18, 30]. Wagnon and Akayi reported that this method has a risk of sural nerve entrapment [38]. Cadaveric dissections with computer-assisted modelling in the sagittal and transverse planes revealed that the sural nerve crosses the Achilles tendon at, on average, 11 cm proximal to the calcaneal tubercle and, on average, 3.5 cm distal to the musculo-tendinous junction [8]. Therefore, the nerve is especially vulnerable to iatrogenic injury during surgery in this area, particularly in relation to minimally invasive procedures [1, 8]. Since minimally invasive percutaneous repair techniques do not provide direct visualization of the torn tendon-ends, the percutaneous repair of Achilles tendon ruptures under endoscopic control has been suggested to overcome this limitation [15, 27].

The major advantage of endoscopy-assisted percutaneous repair is in allowing direct visualization of the process, especially the evaluation of the juxtaposition of the torn ends without damaging the paratenon [6, 16, 32, 34]. Furthermore, it also reduces the risk of iatrogenic sural nerve damage by direct visualization. Knowledge of the local anatomy is crucial to place the stab wounds in areas less likely to damage the sural nerve [10]. In an anatomical study, Chan and co-workers reported on the risk of sural nerve entrapment at the proximal medial portal with the endoscopic-assisted technique. They suggested the modification of the technique by grasping the tendon-end with Allis tissue forceps before passing the suture [7]. El Shazly and co-workers described endoscopic-assisted Achilles tendon augmentation with a graft loop technique that was found to be safe for the sural nerve and medial neurovascular structures [14, 16].

Lui has described an endoscopic-assisted repair using a Krackow locking suture [28]. He described a mini-open approach for Achilles tendon repair using the Krackow locking suture, which may improve the strength of repair and maintain the advantage of minimally invasive tendon repair. By means of the release of the medial edge of the crural fascia, the Achilles tendon can be easily mobilized and the Krackow locking suture can be applied through a 1.5 cm medial wound [28]. Carmont and Maffulli recommended a mini-open technique, with a 1.2–1.5 cm transverse incision at the level of the rupture, to directly visualize whether the appropriate juxtaposition of the ruptured tendon-ends was achieved[6]. This method of percutaneous repair permits a less invasive approach to the tendon and accurate opposition of the tendon-ends and minimizes the risk of sural nerve injury.

Fortis and co-workers repaired Achilles tendon ruptures in 20 patients between the ages of 28 and 47 using an endoscopic-assisted percutaneous technique [15]. They evaluated the functional outcomes and complications in a 2.5 years follow-up. All the patients achieved good to excellent outcomes and were able to stand on the tiptoe of the operated leg, and none had limitations in their daily activities. However, they reported less maximum torque and lower work performance for the injured leg as compared with the non-operated leg.

Moreover, complications due to prolonged immobilization, such as arthrofibrosis, joint stiffness, calf hypotrophy, damage of the articular cartilage and deep vein thrombosis, may be prevented since the endoscopic percutaneous technique allows early active range of motion training and weight-bearing after a short period of cast immobilization [13, 20]. In terms of the importance of early active range of motion after Achilles tendon repair, Huri and co-workers described an endobutton-assisted repair technique. They compared an endobutton-assisted modified Bunnell technique and the Krackow suture technique. In the endobutton technique, the button implant was placed under the surface of the calcaneus through a transcalcaneal tunnel. Then a No. 2 Ethibond (Ethicon Inc., Somerville, NJ) suture, which was mounted on the button implant, was pulled proximally through the tunnel. Finally, the Achilles tendon was repaired using a modified Bunnell technique with a No. 2 Ethibond suture. They reported superior biomechanical properties of the endobutton-assisted percutaneous repair over the conventional open repair technique [19]. Buchgraber and Pässler compared the results of immobilization and functional post-operative treatment after using a standardized mini-invasive technique for Achilles tendon rupture repair [5]. They revealed that patients undergoing functional post-operative rehabilitation with early weight-bearing were hospitalized for shorter periods and lost fewer days from work than those treated with immobilization. The re-rupture rate was the same as with cast immobilization but lower than after open surgical repair or non-surgical functional treatment alone [22].

Conclusion

The percutaneous repair of the Achilles tendon under endoscopic control is a safe technique with good functional outcomes and minimal risk of complications when compared with open surgery or other minimally invasive approaches. It might be more cost-effective than open techniques. Furthermore, this procedure protects the paratenon and should thereby enhance biologic healing [12]. The preservation of paratenon also decreases the gliding resistance of the extrasynovial tissue [31, 32]. Direct visualization and manipulation of the tendon-ends also provides stable repair that allows early weight-bearing, and can be recommended in athletes. Despite its promising results, potential problems such as sural neuralgia (transient hypoesthesia) and deficits have been reported [15].

References

1. Apaydin N, Bozkurt M, Loukas M, Vefali H, Tubbs RS, Esmer AF. Relationships of the sural nerve with the calcaneal tendon: an anatomical study with surgical and clinical implications. Surg Radiol Anat. 2009;31(10):775-780.

2. Aspenberg P, Virchenko O. Platelet concentrate injection improves Achilles tendon repair in rats. Acta Orthop Scand. 2004;75(1):93-99.

3. Bhandari M, Guyatt GH, Siddiqui F, Morrow F, Busse J, Leighton RK, Sprague S, Schemitsch EH. Treatment of acute Achilles tendon ruptures a systematic overview and meta-analysis Clin Orthop Relat Res. 2002;400:190-200.

4. Bradley JP, Tibone JE. Percutaneous and open surgical repairs of Achilles tendon ruptures. Am J Sports Med. 1990;18(2):188-195.

5. Buchgraber A, Pässler HH. Percutaneous repair of Achilles tendon rupture. Immobilization versus functional postoperative treatment. Clin Orthop Relat Res. 1997;341:113–122.

6. Carmont MR, Maffulli N. Modified percutaneous repair of ruptured Achilles tendon. Knee Surg Sports Traumatol Arthrosc. 2008;16(2):199–203.

7. Chan KB, Lui TH, Chan LK. Endoscopic-assisted repair of acute Achilles tendon rupture with Krackow suture: an anatomic study. Foot Ankle Surg. 2009;15(4):183-186.

8. Citak M, Knobloch K, Albrecht K, Krettek C, Hufner T. Anatomy of the sural nerve in a computer-assisted model: implications for surgical minimal-invasive Achilles tendon repair. Br J Sports Med. 2007;41(7):456–458.

9. de Mos M, van der Windt AE, Jahr H, van Schie HT, Weinans H, Verhaar JA, van Osch GJ. Can platelet-rich plasma enhance tendon repair? A cell culture study. Am J Sports Med. 2008;36(6):1171–1178.

10. Doral MN, Alam M, Bozkurt M, Turhan E, Atay OA, Dönmez G, Maffulli N. Functional anatomy of the Achilles tendon. Knee Surg Sports Traumatol Arthrosc. 2010;18(5):638-643.

11. Doral MN, Bozkurt M, Turhan E, Ayvaz M, Atay OA, Uzümcügil A, Leblebicioğlu G, Kaya D, Aydoğ T. Percutaneous suturing of the ruptured Achilles tendon with endoscopic control. Arch Orthop Trauma Surg. 2009;129(8):1093-1101.

12. Doral MN, Tetik O, Atay OA, Leblebicioğlu G, Oznur A. Achilles tendon diseases and its management. [Article in Turkish] Acta Orthop Traumatol Turc. 2002;36 Suppl 1:42-46.

13. Doral MN. What is the effect of the early weight-bearing mobilisation without using any support after endoscopy-assisted Achilles tendon repair? Knee Surg Sports Traumatol Arthrosc. 2013;21(6):1378-1384.

14. El Shazly O, Abou Elsoud MM, Desouky A. Endosopic Achilles tendon augmentation with a graft loop anatomic and radiologic study. Foot Ankle Surg. 2011;17(3):173-177.

15. Fortis AP, Dimas A, Lamprakis AA. Repair of Achilles tendon rupture under endoscopic control. Arthroscopy. 2008;24(6):683-688.

16. Halasi T, Tállay A, Berkes I. Percutaneous Achilles tendon repair with and without endoscopic control. Knee Surg Sports Traumatol Arthrosc. 2003;11(6):409-414.

17. Hattrup SJ, Johnson KA. A review of ruptures of the Achilles tendon. Foot Ankle. 1985;6(1):34-38.

18. Hockenbury RT, Johns JC. A biomechanical in vitro comparison of open versus percutaneous repair of tendon Achilles. Foot Ankle. 1990;11(2):67-72.

19. Huri G, Biçer OS, Özgözen L, Uçar Y, Garbis NG, Hyun YS. A novel repair method for the treatment of acute Achilles tendon rupture with minimally invasive approach using button implant: A biomechanical study. Foot and Ankle Surgery, 2013; doi: 10.1016/j.fas.2013.06.12 (In Press).

20. Kangas J, Pajala A, Siira P, Hämäläinen M, Leppilahti J. Early functional treatment versus early immobilization in tension of the musculotendinous unit after Achilles rupture repair: a prospective, randomized, clinical study. J Trauma. 2003;54(6):1171-1180.

21. Kashiwagi K, Mochizuki Y, Yasunaga Y, Ishida O, Deie M, Ochi M. Effects of transforming growth factor-beta 1 on the early stages of healing of the Achilles tendon in a rat model. Scand J Plast Reconstr Surg Hand Surg. 2004;38(4):193–197.

22. Kaya D, Doral MN, Nyland J, Toprak U, Turhan E, Donmez G, Citaker S, Atay OA, Callaghan MJ. Proprioception level after endoscopically guided percutaneous Achilles tendon. Knee Surg Sports Traumatol Arthrosc. 2013;21(6):1238-1244.

23. Kocher MS, Bishop J, Marshall R, Briggs KK, Hawkins RJ. Operative versus nonoperative management of acute Achilles tendon rupture: expected-value decision analysis. Am J Sports Med. 2002;30(6): 783–790.

24. Lipscomb PR, Weiner AD. Rupture of muscles and tendons. Minn Med. 1956;39(11):731–736.

25. Lo IK, Kirkley A, Nonweiler B, Kumbhare DA. Operative versus nonoperative treatment of acute Achilles tendon ruptures. A quantitive review. Clin J Sport Med. 1997;7(3):207-211.

26. Lopez-Vidriero E, Goulding KA, Simon DA, Sanchez M, Johnson DH. The use of platelet-rich plasma in arthroscopy and sports medicine: optimizing the healing environment. Arthroscopy. 2010;26(2):269–278.

27. Lui TH. Endoscopic-assisted Achilles tendon repair with plantaris tendon augmentation. Arthroscopy. 2007;23(5):556.e1–556.e5.

28. Lui TH. Surgical tip: Repair of acute Achilles rupture with Krackow suture through a 1.5 cm medial wound. Foot Ankle Surg. 2010;16(1):28-31.

29. Ma GW, Griffith TG. Percutaneous repair of acute closed ruptured Achilles tendon: a new technique. Clin Orthop Relat Res. 1977;128:247-255.

30. Maffulli N. Current concepts review: rupture of the Achilles tendon. J Bone Joint Surg Am. 1999;81(7):1019-1036.

31. McClelland D, Maffulli N. Percutaneous repair of ruptured Achilles tendon. J R Coll Surg Edinb. 2002;47(4):613–618.

32. Momose T, Amadio PC, Zobitz ME, Zhao C, An KN. Effect of paratenon and repetitive motion on the gliding resistance of tendon of extrasynovial origin. Clin Anat. 2002;15(3):199-205.

33. Mortensen HM, Skov O, Jensen PE. Early motion of the ankle after operative treatment of a rupture of the Achilles tendon: a prospective randomized clinical and radiographic study. J Bone Joint Surg Am. 1999;81(7):983-990.

34. Rebeccato A, Santini S, Salmaso G, Nogarin L. Repair of the Achilles tendon rupture: a functional comparison of three surgical techniques. J Foot Ankle Surg. 2001;40(4):188–194.

35. Sánchez M, Anitua E, Azofra J, Andía I, Padilla S, Mujika I. Comparison of surgically repaired Achilles tendon tears using platelet-rich fibrin matrices. Am J Sports Med. 2007;35(2):245–251.

36. Thermann H, Tibesku CO, Mastrokalos DS, Pässler HH. Endoscopically assisted percutaneous Achilles tendon suture. Foot Ankle Int. 2001;22(2):158-160.

37. Turgut A, Günal I, Maralcan G, Köse N, Göktürk E. Endoscopy, assisted percutaneous repair of the Achilles tendon ruptures: a cadaveric and clinical study. Knee Surg Sports Traumatol Arthrosc. 2002;10(2):130-133.

38. Wagnon R, Akayi M. The Webb-Bannister percutaneous technique for acute Achilles' tendon ruptures: a functional and MRI assessment. J Foot Ankle Surg. 2005;44(6):437–444.

39. Webb JM, Bannister GC. Percutaneous repair of the ruptured tendo Achillis. J Bone Joint Surg (Br). 1999;81(5):877–880.

40. Wills CA, Washburn S, Caiozzo V, Prietto CA. Achilles tendon rupture. A review of the literature comparing surgical versus nonsurgical treatment. Clin Orthop Relat Res. 1986;207:156-163.

41. Wong J, Barrass V, Maffulli N. Quantitative review of operative and nonoperative management of Achilles tendon ruptures. Am J Sports Med. 2002;30(4):565-575.

"Learn the rules before you break them."

Dalai Lama

CHAPTER 17

MINIMALLY INVASIVE SURGERY FOR RETROCALCANEAL BURSITIS

Hajo Thermann, Christoph Becher

Take Home Message

• In insertional Achilles tendon tendinopathy, all pathologies need to be addressed to achieve a satisfactory result.

• The endoscopic-assisted minimally invasive technique combines all the advantages of both open and endoscopic approaches.

Introduction

Patrik Haglund was the first to describe a painful hindfoot condition resulting from a deformity consisting of a superolateral calcaneal prominence in 1928[2]. The initial description of the syndrome represents the complex nature of symptoms with painful healing involving osseous deformity and retrocalcaneal bursitis, with or without insertional Achilles tendon tendinopathy[3,7,8,14,16]. Distinguishing between insertional Achilles tendinopathy and retrocalcaneal bursitis or osseous impingement is difficult, since both may be a continuum of the same disease process and may also coexist[8].

Lateral radiographs show the osseous deformity of the calcaneus and possible calcifications at the insertion of the Achilles tendon. Ultrasonography and magnetic resonance imaging (MRI) can provide additional information about the Achilles tendon and the bursae, and can be useful in pre-operative planning.

If non-surgical treatment fails over a time period of at least three months, surgical treatment might be considered. As a primary goal, bursectomy and the removal of the prominent superior calcaneal tuberosity is necessary to prevent further impingement of the bursae between the calcaneus and the Achilles tendon. In coexisting insertional Achilles tendinopathy, with or without calcifications, the tendon should be debrided of all diseased tissue.

Open surgery is a safe and successful procedure [1, 11, 12, 14, 17] but may be associated with wound and soft tissue problems as well as long rehabilitation periods [4,9,11,13,15]. The endoscopic technique may have the advantage of fewer complications and shorter post-operative recovery times [5, 7, 10, 16], but it can be technically challenging even for experienced surgeons. A fluoroscopic control is imperative to ensure appropriate resection. Still, and especially at the beginning of the learning curve, incomplete resection (dune-type) may occur and fibrotic degenerative changes (which can easily be diagnosed by digital palpation in an open technique) are not easily detected. Remaining fibrotic tissue may have an influence on the kinematics (stone in a rope) and may prevent surgical success. Thus, a "minimally invasive technique" using a small, open approach, and the endoscopic options to combine the advantages of the open and endoscopic techniques, are reported in this chapter.

Surgical Technique

The patient is placed in the prone position and the other leg is lowered to provide enough space for the free handling of the endoscopic instruments when performing from the medial side. A tourniquet is recommended - this is needed to prevent substantial bleeding and blurred vision. A needle is placed over the tip of the calcaneal prominence from lateral and the incision for open surgery is performed approximately 1-1.5 cm distally and 1 cm proximally (Figure 1). The bursa is resected and the complete superior calcaneal prominence is depicted.

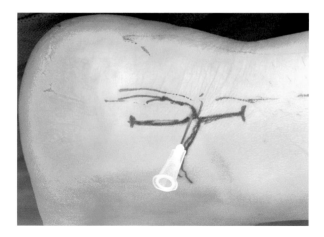

Figure 1. Lateral approach to the insertional area of the Achilles tendon.

234

A small Hohmann retractor is placed at the medial side of the tuber calcanei and the distal insertion of the Achilles tendon is inspected. The lateral part of the Achilles tendon insertion at the (often bulky or prominent) tuber is removed so as to give a clear view of the osseous resection (Figure 2).

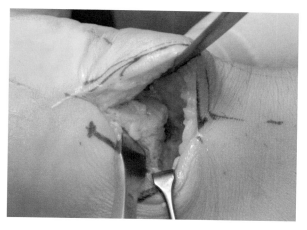

Figure 2. Complete exposure of the (postero-superior) calcaneal exostosis.

The amount of bone should be estimated on the pre-operative lateral radiograph. Usually, the amount of resection includes the bony prominence by measuring a 10°-15° inclination angle from the horizontal line of the posterior part of the calcaneus (Figure 3).

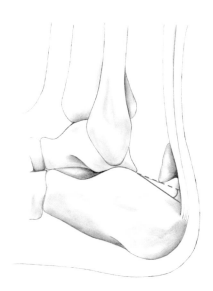

Figure 3. Depiction of the bony resection line.

By using a 10 mm chisel, the bony resection is performed and the fragments are excised. Small bony spurs as found by digital palpation are mostly discovered at the medial or deep distal part, where they are smoothened. The remaining bulky lateral part of the tuber calcanei is thereafter resected using a chisel (Figure 4).

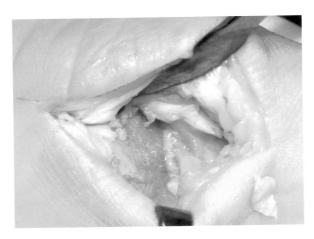

Figure 4. Complete resection of the (postero-superior) calcaneal exostosis.

The lateral approach is provisionally closed by leaving a small endoscopic portal. Typically, a 5.0 mm 30° arthroscope is introduced horizontally to the medial side and a counter-incision is performed. A 4.0 mm full-radius shaver is then introduced from the medial portal and a debridement of the Achilles tendon insertion is performed where necessary (Figure 5).

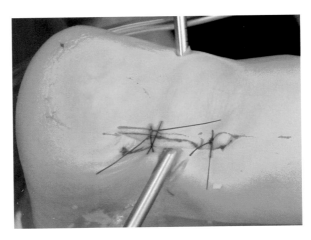

Figure 5. Endoscopic technique: 5.0 mm arthroscope / 4.0 mm shaver.

After the initial debridement, the tendon is palpated percutaneously through the lateral stab wound by a needle and resected using a shaver (Figure 6).

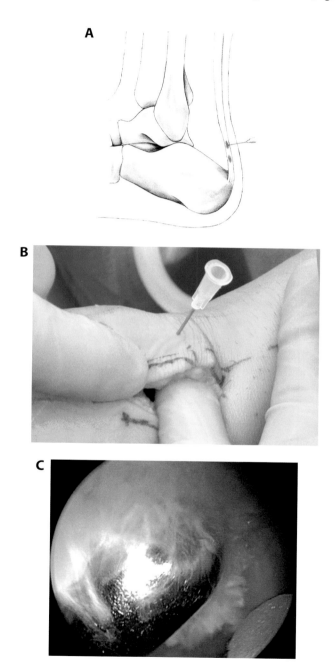

Figure 6. A,B. Depiction of the marking technique. C. Debridement of the Achilles tendon.

Further debridement around the resection area of the tuber calcanei and denervation is accomplished using a shaver, electrocautery or radiofrequency, when available (Figure 7).

A plaster splint in slight plantar flexion may be applied for first post-operative day to reduce post-operative pain.

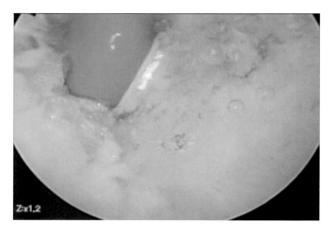

Figure 7. Radiofrequency for debridement, denervation and haemostasis.

Post-operative Rehabilitation

2nd Day:
Removal of the drain and splint. Cryotherapy. NSAID. Elevation. Free ankle movement as tolerated.

2nd – 14th Day:
Partial weight-bearing up to 15 kg. Increasing range of motion of the ankle, and stretching of the gastrocnemius-soleus complex (Figure 8).

2nd – 12th Week:
Stretching of the gastrocnemius-soleus complex and the flexor muscles (Figure 8), biking and aqua jogging. Strength training.

3rd – 6th Month:
Increasing activities. Start of sports specific-training depending on pain with increases up to competitive level.

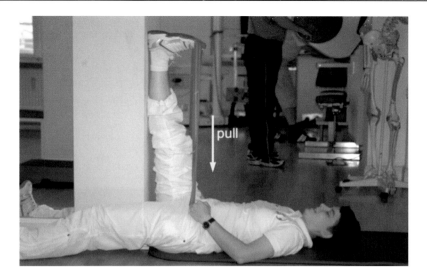

Figure 8. Stretching of the flexor muscle chain as an important part of the post-operative rehabilitation.

Discussion

In many cases, a painful heel at the insertional area of the Achilles tendon represents a complex of pathologies. After the failure of non-surgical management, open surgery is often regarded as the "gold standard". Options to approach the pathology include medial, lateral and posterior Cincinnati-type or tendon-splitting incisions [1, 11, 12, 14, 17]. However, open surgery may have several limitations with wound and soft tissue problems, and wound breakdown, infection, tenderness and altered sensation around the scar, Achilles tendon avulsion, stiffness and long rehabilitation periods have all been reported [4, 9, 11, 13, 15]. These disadvantages may occur when good exposure requires large incisions to remove an adequate amount of bone. The endoscopic technique may have the advantage of fewer complications, decreased post-operative recovery times and better visualization of all parts of the retrocalcaneal space [5, 7, 10, 16]. However, the endoscopic approach can be technically challenging and it may not be possible to remove large spurs with full-thickness intratendinous calcifications [7, 10]. Furthermore, it can be time-consuming, especially in case of deformity.

The evaluation of surgical interventions is predominantly retrospective [6]. The technical approaches and methods for the evaluation of the results present large variations, making them difficult to compare. Many authors have used the AOFAS (American Orthopaedic Foot and Ankle Society) Ankle-Hindfoot Scale, which is not specific to Achilles tendon pathologies. Both open and endoscopic techniques have produced good results, but they have limitations in treating the complex pathology. The study of Leitze and co-workers comparing the open and endoscopic approaches for decompression showed no differences in terms of functional outcomes and recovery times [7]. However, patients treated endoscopically had fewer complications and a better cosmetic result [7]. The endoscopic-assisted minimally invasive technique combines all the advantages of both the open and endoscopic approaches. Sufficient resection of the (postero-superior) calcaneal exostosis can be visualized well. Adequate visualization is imperative to preventing further impingement of the bursa between the calcaneus and Achilles tendon.

Conclusion

In insertional Achilles tendon tendinopathy, all pathologies need to be addressed simultaneously to achieve a satisfactory result. The endoscopic-assisted minimally invasive technique combines all the advantages of both the open and endoscopic approaches. The short-term results are encouraging.

References

1. Carmont MR, Maffulli N. Management of insertional Achilles tendinopathy through a Cincinnati incision. BMC Musculoskelet Disord 2007;8:82.

2. Haglund P. Beitrag zur Klinik der Achillessehne. Zeitschr Orthop Chir 1928;49-58.

3. Heneghan MA, Pavlov H. The Haglund painful heel syndrome. Experimental investigation of cause and therapeutic implications. Clin Orthop Relat Res 1984;(187):228-234.

4. Huber HM, Waldis M. Die Haglund-Exostose: eine Operationsindikation und ein kleiner Eingriff? Z Orthop Ihre Grenzgeb 1989;127(3):286-290.

5. Jerosch J, Schunck J, Sokkar SH. Endoscopic calcaneoplasty (ECP) as a surgical treatment of Haglund's syndrome. Knee Surg Sports Traumatol Arthrosc 2007;15(7):927-934.

6. Kearney R, Costa ML. Insertional achilles tendinopathy management: a systematic review. Foot Ankle Int 2010;31(8):689-694.

7. Leitze Z, Sella EJ, Aversa JM. Endoscopic decompression of the retrocalcaneal space. J Bone Joint Surg Am 2003;85-A(8):1488-1496.

8. Myerson MS, McGarvey W. Disorders of the Achilles tendon insertion and Achilles tendinitis. Instr Course Lect 1999;48:211-218.

9. Nesse E, Finsen V. Poor results after resection for Haglund's heel. Analysis of 35 heels in 23 patients after 3 years. Acta Orthop Scand 1994;65(1):107-109.

10. Ortmann FW, McBryde AM. Endoscopic bony and soft-tissue decompression of the retrocalcaneal space for the treatment of Haglund deformity and retrocalcaneal bursitis. Foot Ankle Int 2007;28(2):149-153.

11. Pauker M, Katz K, Yosipovitch Z. Calcaneal ostectomy for Haglund disease. J Foot Surg 1992;31(6):588-589.

12. Saxena A, Cheung S. Surgery for chronic Achilles tendinopathy. Review of 91 procedures over 10 years. J Am Podiatr Med Assoc 2003;93(4):283-291.

13. Saxena A, Maffulli N, Nguyen A, Li A. Wound complications from surgeries pertaining to the Achilles tendon: an analysis of 219 surgeries. J Am Podiatr Med Assoc 2008;98(2):95-101.

14. Sella EJ, Caminear DS, McLarney EA. Haglund's syndrome. J Foot Ankle Surg 1998;37(2):110-114.

15. Taylor GJ. Prominence of the calcaneus: is operation justified? J Bone Joint Surg Br 1986;68(3):467-470.

16. van Dijk CN, van Dyk GE, Scholten PE, Kort NP. Endoscopic calcaneoplasty. Am J Sports Med 2001;29(2):185-189.

17. Yodlowski ML, Scheller AD, Jr., Minos L. Surgical treatment of Achilles tendinitis by decompression of the retrocalcaneal bursa and the superior calcaneal tuberosity. Am J Sports Med 2002;30(3):318-321.

> *"Do not anticipate trouble, or worry about what may never happen. Keep in the sunlight."*
>
> *Benjamin Franklin*

Chapter 18

Minimally Invasive Surgery for Mid-portion Achilles Tendinopathy

Nicola Maffulli, Umile G. Longo, Vincenzo Denaro

Take Home Message

- *The aim of the surgical management of Achilles tendinopathy is to excise fibrotic adhesions, remove and debride areas of failed healing, possibly stimulating viable cells to initiate protein synthesis and to promote healing.*

- *Multiple longitudinal tenotomies have been proposed to trigger neoangiogenesis in the Achilles tendon, with increased blood flow providing improved nutrition and a more favourable environment for healing.*

- *Pathological nerve ingrowth accompanies pathological neovascularization in the tendinopathic tendon, and it has been considered as a possible cause of the pain. It is possible to disrupt the abnormal neoinnervation in order to interfere with the sensation of pain caused by tendinopathy with minimally invasive approaches.*

Introduction

The aim of the open surgical management of Achilles tendinopathy is to excise fibrotic adhesions and the surrounding thickened soft tissues, restore vascularity, remove or debride areas of failed healing - possibly stimulating viable cells to initiate protein synthesis - and to promote healing [2, 5].

Multiple longitudinal tenotomies have been proposed to remove appreciable macroscopic lesions and to trigger neoangiogenesis in the Achilles tendon, with increased blood flow [6] providing improved nutrition and a more favourable environment for healing.

Ideal candidates for multiple percutaneous longitudinal tenotomies include patients with isolated tendinopathy with no involvement of the paratenon, a well-defined nodular lesion less than 2.5 cm long in whom non-surgical management has failed, and without any signs of paratendinopathy [13]. This procedure may be guided by ultrasound to confirm the precise location of the area of tendinopathy [13, 16, 17]. It is a simple procedure and can be performed in an ambulatory setting under local anaesthesia without using a tourniquet. It requires minimal follow-up care, and it produces no significant complications and no long-term morbidity.

Percutaneous longitudinal ultrasound-guided internal tenotomy of the Achilles tendon can be also performed on an outpatient basis. However, it requires high-resolution ultrasound to properly locate the tendinopathic area and place the initial stab incision [13, 16, 17]. The technique is not as effective in patients with combined tendinopathy and paratendinopathy.

The above-mentioned techniques attempt to address the tendinopathic lesion. However theories on the aetiology of tendinopathy are changing as are its techniques [9, 10]. New theories suggest that pathological nerve ingrowth accompanies pathological neovascularization in the tendinopathic tendon, and it has been considered as a possible cause of the pain. Some authors have attempted to disrupt the abnormal neoinnervation in order to interfere with the sensation of pain caused by tendinopathy. Endoscopy [19], electrocoagulation [1] and minimally invasive stripping [3, 4, 8, 11] have all been described to achieve this aim. Endoscopy allows for the direct visualization of the area of tendinopathy and makes it possible to use a motorized shaver or diathermy to destroy any neovessels.

Multiple percutaneous longitudinal tenotomies

The patient lies prone on the operating table with the feet protruding beyond the edge and the ankles resting on a padded sandbag [13]. The tendon is accurately palpated and the area of maximum swelling and/or tenderness is marked and checked again by ultrasound scanning. The skin and the subcutaneous tissues over the Achilles tendon are infiltrated with 10 to 15 mL of plain 1% lignocaine (Lignocaine Hydrochloride, Evans Medical Ltd, Leatherhead, England).

A surgical scalpel is inserted parallel to the long axis of the tendon fibres in the marked area(s) with the cutting edge pointing cranially. This initial stab incision is made in the central portion of the diseased tendon. Keeping the blade still, a full passive ankle dorsi-flexion movement is performed. Once the position of the blade had been reversed, full passive plantar-flexion is applied. A variable, approximately 3 cm-long area of tenolysis is thus obtained. The procedure is repeated 2 cm medially and proximally, medially and distally, laterally and proximally and laterally and distally to the site of the first stab wound.

Multiple percutaneous longitudinal tenotomies under local anaesthetic were performed on 52 runners with unilateral Achilles tendinopathy and non-responsive to non-surgical management [13]. Forty-eight patients were reviewed at an average of 22.1 months post-operatively. The results were rated as excellent in 25 patients, good in 12, fair in seven and poor in four. Four patients developed subcutaneous hematomas. One patient developed a superficial infection at one of the incision sites, which was managed by oral antibiotics with full recovery. Three patients complained of hyper-sensitivity in response to the incisions; this was resolved by rubbing hand cream over the incisions several times a day. One patient developed painful hypertrophic scars on three of the five incisions, but corticosteroid injections yielded good functional and cosmetic results. The isometric strength and endurance of the gastrocnemius-soleus complex was measured just before the procedure, and at six weeks and six months following. Both were within 10% of the normal contralateral limb by the sixth post-operative month.

Ultrasound-guided percutaneous tenotomy

The patient is positioned as described for the previous technique. The tendon is accurately palpated and the area of maximum swelling and/or tenderness is marked and checked by ultrasound scanning [16]. The skin is prepared with an antiseptic solution and a sterile longitudinal 7.5 MHz US probe is used to confirm the area of tendinopathy. Before infiltration of the skin and subcutaneous tissues over the Achilles tendon with 10 mL of 1% Carbocaine (Pierrel, Milan, Italy), 7 mL of 0.5% Carbocaine is used to infiltrate the space between the tendon and the paratenon. This brisement procedure attempts to free the paratenon from the tendon by disrupting adhesions between the two structures.

Under ultrasound guidance, a Number 11 surgical scalpel blade (SwannYMorton, England) is inserted parallel to the long axis of the tendon fibres in the centre of the area of tendinopathy, as assessed by high-resolution ultrasound imaging. The cutting edge of the blade points caudally and penetrates the whole thickness of the tendon. With the blade held still, a full passive ankle flexion is produced.

All subsequent tenotomies are performed through this same stab incision unless there is an extensive area of tendinosis or an additional area of tendon disease. The scalpel blade is then retracted to the surface of the tendon inclined 45 degrees on the sagittal axis, and the blade is inserted medially through the original tenotomy. With the blade held still, a full passive ankle flexion is performed. The whole procedure is then repeated with the blade inclined 45 degrees laterally to the original tenotomy and inserted laterally through the original tenotomy. Again, with the blade kept still, a full passive ankle flexion is produced. The blade is then partially retracted to the posterior surface of the

Achilles tendon, reversed 180 degrees so that its cutting edge points cranially, and the procedure is repeated, with care taken to dorsiflex the ankle passively. Preliminary cadaveric studies demonstrated that, on average, a 2.8 cm tenotomy is obtained using this technique. A steristrip (3M United Kingdom PLC, Bracknell, Berkshire, England) can be applied to the stab wound or else the stab wound can be left open [7, 12].

Seventy-five athletes with unilateral Achilles tendinopathy underwent ultrasound-guided percutaneous longitudinal tenotomy under local anaesthetic infiltration after a failure of non-surgical management [16]. Sixty-three patients were reviewed at least 36 months after the operation. Thirty-five patients were rated excellent, 12 good, nine fair and seven poor. Nine of the 16 patients with a fair or poor result underwent a formal exploration of the Achilles tendon 7-12 months after the index procedure. The operated tendons remained thickened and the ultrasonographic appearance of operated tendons remained abnormal even eight years after the operation. Isometric maximal muscle strength and isometric endurance gradually returned to values similar to their contralateral un-operated tendon.

Minimally invasive stripping

Local or general anaesthesia is used, according to surgeon or patient preferences. The patient is positioned prone. The skin preparation is performed in the usual fashion.

Four skin incisions are made. The first two incisions are 0.5 cm longitudinal incisions at the proximal origin of the Achilles tendon, just medial and lateral to the origin of the tendon. The other two incisions are also 0.5 cm long and longitudinal, but 1 cm distal to the distal end of the tendon insertion on the calcaneus.

A mosquito is inserted into the proximal incisions and the Achilles tendon is freed of the peritendinous adhesions. A Number 1 un-mounted Ethibond (Ethicon, Somerville, NJ) suture thread is inserted proximally, passing through the two proximal incisions (Figure 1). The Ethibond is retrieved from the distal incisions, over the posterior aspect of the Achilles tendon. Using a gentle see-saw motion, similar to using a Gigli saw (Figure 2), the Ethibond suture thread is made to slide posterior to the tendon, which is stripped and freed from the fat of Kager's triangle.

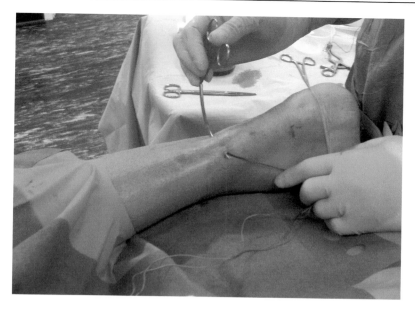

Figure 1. A mosquito is inserted into the proximal incisions and the Achilles tendon is freed of the peritendinous adhesions. A Number 1 unmounted Ethibond (Ethicon, Somerville, NJ) suture thread is inserted proximally, passing through the two proximal incisions.

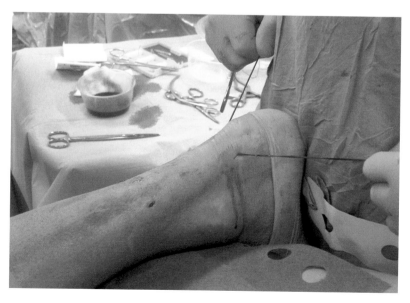

Figure 2. The Ethibond is retrieved from the distal incisions over the posterior aspect of the Achilles tendon. Using a gentle see-saw motion, similar to using a Gigli saw, the Ethibond suture thread is made to slide posterior to the tendon, which is stripped and freed from the fat of Kager's triangle.

247

The procedure is repeated for the posterior aspect of the Achilles tendon. If necessary, longitudinal percutaneous tenotomies parallel to the tendon fibres are made [13, 15, 16].

A removable scotch cast support with Velcro straps can be applied if deemed necessary. In such cases, the cast is used for 10-14 days.

Post-operatively, patients are allowed to mobilize full weight-bearing. After two weeks, the cast - if used - is removed and physiotherapy is begun, focusing on proprioception, the plantar-flexion of the ankle, inversion and eversion.

Naidu and co-workers [14] described a minimally invasive circumferential paratenon release for the management of patients with tendinopathy of the main body of the Achilles tendon.

These techniques [4, 14] are safe and inexpensive, with the potential to offer an alternative option for the management of chronic Achilles tendinopathy before open surgery. Further studies are required to clarify their role in the management of patients with Achilles tendinopathy.

Endoscopy – assisted treatment

Tendoscopy may allow endoscopic access to several tendons, including the Achilles tendon [19]. This operative technique provides access to the posterior aspect of the ankle and sub-talar joints. In addition, extra-articular structures of the hindfoot such as the os trigonum, the flexor hallucis longus (FHL) and the deep portion of the deltoid ligament can be accessed.

Thermann and co-workers [18] described a different technique for the endoscopic debridement of the ventral neovascularized area, the peritenon and the Achilles tendon, with good short-term clinical results in eight patients.

Conclusion

In conclusion, chronic mid-portion Achilles tendinopathy is characterized by impaired performance due to Achilles tendon pain and swelling located typically 2–7 cm from the insertion onto the calcaneus. The source of the pain has not yet been clarified. Several explanations have been suggested and, therefore, a wide range of surgical options are available. Classical approaches address the intratendinous degenerative changes when present. Surgical measures include open excision of the degenerative tendon. The aim of classical surgical management of Achilles tendinopathy is to excise fibrotic adhesions and the surrounding thickened soft tissues, restore vascularity, and remove and debride areas of failed healing. Multiple longitudinal tenotomies have been proposed to trigger neoangiogenesis in the Achilles tendon, with increased blood flow providing improved nutrition and a more favourable environment for healing. Pathological nerve ingrowth accompanies pathological neovascularization in the tendinopathic tendon, and it has been considered as a possible cause of the pain. It is possible to disrupt the abnormal neoinnervation in order to interfere with the sensation of pain caused by tendinopathy with minimally invasive approaches. Pain relief can be obtained by the destruction of the sensory nerves running from the paratenon into the Achilles tendon proper in patients with chronic Achilles tendinopathy: denervation of the Achilles tendon by releasing the paratenon may be the most important part of the majority of such surgical procedures.

References

1. Boesen MI, Torp-Pedersen S, Koenig MJ, et al. Ultrasound guided electrocoagulation in patients with chronic non-insertional Achilles tendinopathy: a pilot study. Br J Sports Med. 2006;40(9):761-766.

2. Kannus P, Jozsa L. Histopathological changes preceding spontaneous rupture of a tendon. A controlled study of 891 patients. J Bone Joint Surg Am. 1991;73-A:1507-1525.

3. Khanna A, Friel M, Gougoulias N, Longo UG, Maffulli N. Prevention of adhesions in surgery of the flexor tendons of the hand: what is the evidence? Br Med Bull. 2009;90:85-109.

4. Longo UG, Ramamurthy C, Denaro V, Maffulli N. Minimally invasive stripping for chronic Achilles tendinopathy. Disabil Rehabil. 2008;30(20-22):1709-1713.

5. Longo UG, Ronga M, Maffulli N. Achilles tendinopathy. Sports Med Arthrosc. 2009;17(2):112-126.

6. Maffulli N. Re: Etiologic factors associated with symptomatic Achilles tendinopathy. Foot Ankle Int. 2007;28(5):660; author reply 660-661.

7. Maffulli N, Dymond NP, Regine R. Surgical repair of ruptured Achilles tendon in sportsmen and sedentary patients: a longitudinal ultrasound assessment. Int J Sports Med. 1990;11(1):78-84.

8. Maffulli N, Longo UG, Denaro V. Letter to the editor: Minimally invasive paratenon release for non-insertional Achilles tendinopathy. Foot Ankle Int. 2009;30(10):1027-1028.

9. Maffulli N, Longo UG, Denaro V. Novel approaches for the management of tendinopathy. J Bone Joint Surg Am. 2010;92(15):2604-2613.

10. Maffulli N, Longo UG, Loppini M, Denaro V. Current treatment options for tendinopathy. Expert Opin Pharmacother. 2010;11(13):2177-2186.

11. Maffulli N, Longo UG, Oliva F, Ronga M, Denaro V. Minimally invasive surgery of the Achilles tendon. Orthop Clin North Am. 2009;40(4):491-498.

12. Maffulli N, Pintore E, Petricciuolo F. Arthroscopy wounds: to suture or not to suture. Acta Orthop Belg. 1991;57(2):154-156.

13. Maffulli N, Testa V, Capasso G, Bifulco G, Binfield PM. Results of percutaneous longitudinal tenotomy for Achilles tendinopathy in middle- and long-distance runners. Am J Sports Med. 1997;25(6):835-840.

14. Naidu V, Abbassian A, Nielsen D, Uppalapati R, Shetty A. Minimally invasive paratenon release for non-insertional Achilles tendinopathy. Foot Ankle Int. 2009;30(7):680-685.

15. Sayana MK, Maffulli N. Eccentric calf muscle training in non-athletic patients with Achilles tendinopathy. J Sci Med Sport. 2007;10(1):52-58.

16. Testa V, Capasso G, Benazzo F, Maffulli N. Management of Achilles tendinopathy by ultrasound-guided percutaneous tenotomy. Med Sci Sports Exerc. 2002;34(4):573-580.

17. Testa V, Maffulli N, Capasso G, Bifulco G. Percutaneous longitudinal tenotomy in chronic Achilles tendonitis. Bull Hosp Jt Dis. 1996;54(4):241-244.

18. Thermann H, Benetos IS, Panelli C, Gavriilidis I, Feil S. Endoscopic treatment of chronic mid-portion Achilles tendinopathy: novel technique with short-term results. Knee Surg Sports Traumatol Arthrosc. 2009;17(10):1264-1269.

19. van Dijk CN. Hindfoot endoscopy. Foot Ankle Clin. 2006;11(2):391-414.

"Small is beautiful."

E. F. Schumacher

CHAPTER 19

MINIMALLY INVASIVE AND PERCUTANEOUS SURGERY FOR ACHILLES TENDON RUPTURES

Robin R. Elliot, W. James White, James D. F. Calder

Take Home Message

• *Modern techniques combine the benefits of visualizing tendon apposition at the rupture site with percutaneous methods.*

• *Knowledge of the anatomy of the sural nerve is essential.*

• *Consider early functional rehabilitation.*

• *A venous thromboembolism risk assessment and discussion regarding prophylaxis should be carried with all patients.*

Introduction

There remains no consensus regarding the gold standard treatment of acute ruptures of the Achilles tendon. If the clinician and patient opt for surgery, there is further debate regarding which of the recognized surgical procedures produces the best outcome. Non-surgical treatment may lead to problems associated with increased risk of re-rupture, lengthening of the tendon and poor function, whereas surgery introduces additional risks of wound breakdown, infection, scar adhesions and sural nerve damage. Percutaneous and mini-open surgical repair techniques were developed in order to minimize the potential risks of surgery and to improve functional outcomes. In general, these techniques have met their stated goals, but this has not always been the case, as will be explained in this overview.

Basic science

The pathology underpinning the mechanism of failure of the Achilles tendon is still not fully understood, but some of the intrinsic characteristics of tendons – namely hypovascularity and hypocellularity – may explain its slow healing. Tendon healing occurs through described phases: inflammation, proliferation, repair and remodelling. During the healing process, tendons respond to stress in a similar manner to bones: they remodel, becoming stronger and stiffer. This is achieved by an increase in collagen synthesis and an alteration in fibre alignment. For this reason, early range of movement training is now widely believed to be an important component of the post-operative rehabilitation regime.

The suture material strongly influences the biomechanical performance of multi-strand tendon repairs and is an important consideration for the surgeon [13].

Treatment Techniques

Although open surgical repair was described as early as the tenth century AD [4], Ma and Griffiths were the first to describe a percutaneous repair technique for acute Achilles rupture [18]. Their construct incorporates a Bunnell suture through the proximal stump and a box suture through the distal stump (Figure 1). The sutures are passed via six stab incisions, three on either side of the tendon.

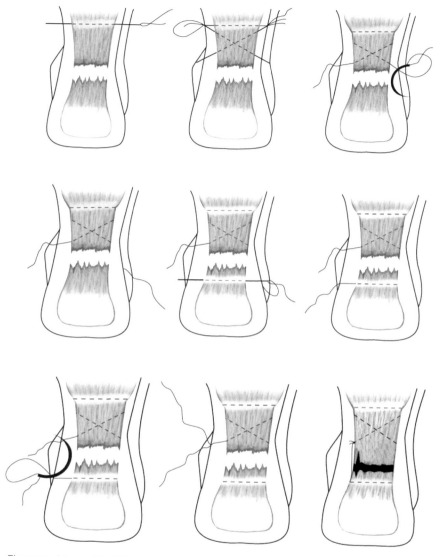

Figure 1. Ma and Griffiths' technique for the percutaneous repair of an acute ruptured Achilles tendon.

This technique has been modified to improve gapping resistance at the repair site by using more passes of the suture material through the distal stump [7,9]. A two-cohort study (237 patients) comparing this modified percutaneous technique to a standard open repair found equivalent functional outcomes in both groups, but less overall complications in the percutaneous group [8].

Webb and Bannister developed their percutaneous technique with the specific aim of reducing the incidence of sural nerve injury, which appeared to be at significant risk when performing percutaneous repairs [27]. Their technique uses only three skin incisions, which are placed away from the lateral side of the tendon in order to protect the sural nerve (Figure 2). A similar technique has been described by McClelland and Maffulli [22].

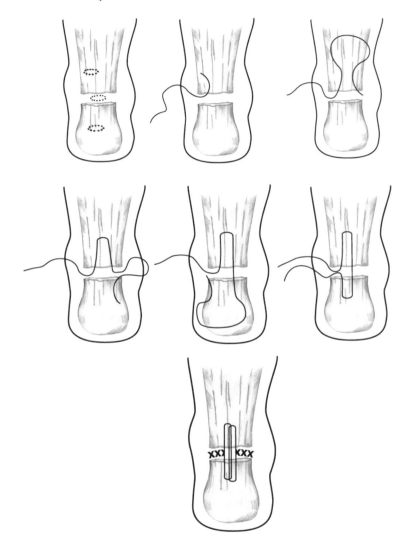

Figure 2. Webb and Bannister's technique.
Diagrams showing: 1a) the position of the three skin incisions, 1b) the suture entering the middle incision, passing through the tendon and out of the proximal incision, 1c) the suture re-entering the proximal incision, back through the tendon and exiting from the middle incision, 1d) again entering the middle incision, passing through the distal tendon and out of the distal incision, 1e) capturing of the distal tendon stump, 1f) completion of the box stitch, and 1g) the placing of a second suture in the tendon before tying both sutures.

The Tenolig® device (Fournitures Hospitalieres Industrie, France) is a percutaneous technique which uses a harpoon device (Figure 3); however, a case series of 124 patients treated using this device reported significant complications, including suture and device failure, and a high rate of re-rupture (10%) and sural nerve damage (5.2%) [19.] A cadaveric study [9] revealed malaligned stumps in four of five tendons repaired with the Ma and Griffiths technique. However, the clinical significance of the malalignment is unclear as, in clinical practice, the functional outcome of the Ma and Griffiths technique is acceptable.

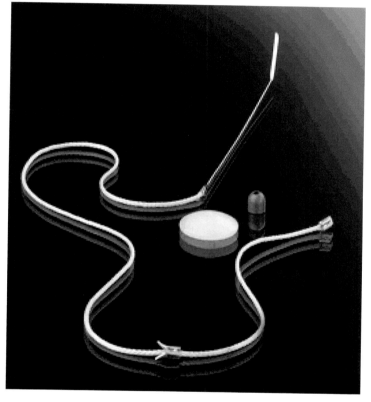

Figure 3. 'Harpoon tenorrhaphy'.
Two stab incisions are made 4-5 cm proximal to the rupture. The harpoon is passed through the proximal stump, the rupture site and the distal stump by palpation, exiting through the skin either side of the calcaneus. The construct is tensioned through barbs proximally and lead crimps distally. The wire is removed after six weeks.

A number of surgeons have made efforts to devise mini-open approaches to Achilles tendon repair. Such techniques have certain advantages, as one can see the rupture site, remove interposed tissue and see whether appropriate tendon stump juxtaposition has been achieved [2, 12, 25].

Kakiuchi reported on a technique that employed a combined percutaneous and limited open repair [13]. The gap in the tendon is palpated and a small incision is made at this level, allowing the tendon stumps to be identified. A repair is then performed percutaneously, assisted by the use of two crude suture-passing devices, fashioned from bent 2 mm Kirschner wires, which are passed beneath the paratenon (Figure 4). This technique ensures good tendon apposition and the sutures are placed well away from the ruptured area of the tendon.

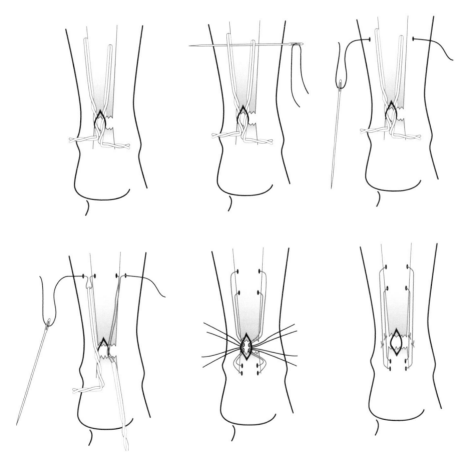

Figure 4. Kakiuchi repair.

The principles of Kakiuchi's technique together with information obtained from a cadaveric study led to the development of a guiding instrument to perform this type of repair [2]. This instrument is now marketed as a single-use, rigid polymer device called Achillon (Integra Lifesciences Corporation, USA), which has a shape (8° V angle) and cross-sectional area (81 mm²) based upon the anatomy of the tendons of the cadaveric specimens (Figure 5).

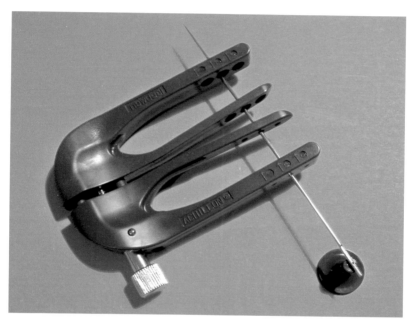

Figure 5. The Achillon device.

The Achillon system combines the percutaneous passage of the sutures with the benefit of visual control at the repair site. The likelihood of sural nerve entrapment is reduced because the sutures are retrieved by the inner arms of the device, which are placed beneath the paratenon layer. A single incision is made at the level of the rupture and the procedure can be performed under local anaesthesia (Figure 6).

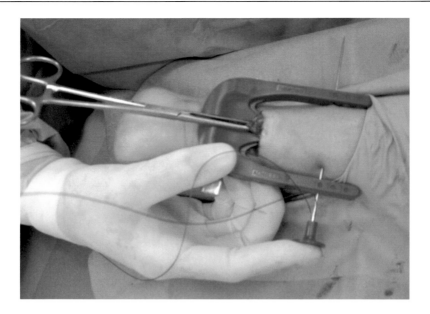

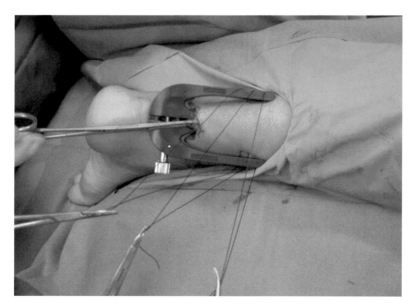

Figure 6. (A) Passing suture (B) Sutures in situ prior to the removal of the introducer.

Technical Considerations

Identification of the correct level for skin incision is important in visualizing the apposition of the tendon-ends as the sutures are tied. Although a longitudinal incision was originally described, a horizontal incision leads to better healing and a more cosmetically acceptable scar. The optimal placement of this incision appears to be approximately 1 cm distal to the palpable proximal stump, allowing the proximal end to be drawn down under tension and the distal stump to be brought up to the wound level by plantar flexion of the ankle.

The Achillon device is made of polycarbonate and care must be taken to ensure that the arms do not twist or bend, as this can lead to the suture needle missing the guide hole. Finally, all the sutures should be tested individually to ensure that they have a good hold in the tendon and are individually capable of drawing the tendon stump to the level of the wound.

Post-operative rehabilitation

Traditionally, acutely repaired Achilles tendon ruptures have been treated post- operatively in a plaster cast, which is serially altered to bring the foot to a plantigrade position over approximately 6-8 weeks. This may lead to calf muscle hypotrophy, joint stiffness, adhesion formation and an increased risk of deep vein thrombosis. In recent times, more functional rehabilitation regimes have gained popularity [6].

Studies have shown that early functional rehabilitation can increase the strength of healed tendons [14] and shorten the rehabilitation time [16]. Percutaneous and mini-open techniques reduce problems with wound healing and, therefore, may be most suited to early mobilization. Patients are given a functional ankle orthotic device, applied in theatre at the time of surgery. The foot is positioned at 20° plantarflexion during wound healing, as this is the optimal position for skin perfusion [26]. Early weight-bearing is encouraged and, from two weeks, free plantarflexion, limiting dorsiflexion past plantigrade. Physiotherapy is commenced at two weeks.

Complications (and how to reduce them)

Infection

Infection is significantly reduced when comparing percutaneous and open surgical techniques (0% vs. 19.6%) [14]. Any surgical procedure should be undertaken with care in patients with diabetes or vascular disease, smokers and those treated with corticosteroids. However, it could be argued that these patients would benefit even more from a minimally invasive approach. The surgeon must handle the soft tissues carefully. A tourniquet is not required for mini-open and percutaneous repair.

Re-rupture

Re-rupture and wound breakdown have been shown to correlate strongly with patient outcome scores and justify re-rupture as a relevant outcome in treatment evaluation [23].

A recent meta-analysis has shown the risk of re-rupture to be reduced threefold with operative techniques with a reduced risk of re-rupture in the percutaneous pooled group (2.1% vs. 4.3%) [14]. Post-operative functional bracing with early weight-bearing and mobilization may lead to a stronger repair and less chance of re-rupture. Five studies have compared re-rupture rates between immobilized and functionally-braced groups post-surgery, none of which found a significant difference. Results were pooled in a recent Cochrane review by Khan and co-workers, which gave a pooled incidence of 7/140 (5.0%) in the cast immobilization group and 3/133 (2.3%) in the functional brace group [13].

Sural nerve damage

A sound knowledge of the anatomy of the sural nerve and care taken when passing sutures should help to prevent damage to the sural nerve. Anatomical studies have shown a significant degree of variability in the location of the sural nerve in relation to the Achilles tendon [1, 27,] which can complicate attempts to avoid entrapment. Exposure of the nerve through extended incisions [21] and the use of the Achillon device [2] have been shown to reduce the incidence of nerve injury.

Adhesion Formation

There is less concern in terms of wound healing when using mini-open and percutaneous methods. For this reason, mobilization can be started early in the post-operative period. This early motion at the repair site combined with a less invasive repair reduces the chance of troublesome adhesions forming. There is no conclusive evidence yet that the use of hyaluronate preparations will reduce adhesions.

Thromboembolism

There is a relatively high risk of deep venous thrombosis (DVT) in patients with Achilles tendon rupture. Lapidus and co-workers showed a rate of >35 % of below-knee DVT in 91 patients placed in immobilization post-surgical repair. There has been ongoing debate regarding the routine use of thromboprophylaxis for these patients. Lapidus and co-workers randomized 105 patients to a placebo-controlled double-blinded randomized study [15]. It also showed levels of 34% and 36% of DVT in both groups. There was a lower rate of above-knee DVT in the treated group, although not clinically significant. They concluded that, although not clinically shown to reduce the rate of DVT (as it is high risk after the surgical treatment of an Achilles tendon rupture and with potentially lethal complications), "effective thromboprophylaxis is desirable." Long-term effects of immobilization, such as the risk of post-thrombotic syndrome, need to be investigated further.

Outcome

The lack of well-conducted studies into the outcomes after Achilles rupture and the efficacy of different treatment modalities is highlighted by two meta-analyses on this subject [14, 29]. Maffulli and co-workers showed that the study methodology has improved over time, however, Khan and co-workers found only 12 studies that were worthy of inclusion in their meta-analysis. They showed a pooled rate of re-rupture of 4.3% (two of 46) in the open group and 2.1% (one of 48) in the percutaneous group. Percutaneous repair was associated with a lower complication rate (excluding re-rupture) compared with open operative repair. Patients who had been managed with a functional brace post-operatively (allowing for early mobilization) had a lower complication rate compared with those who had been managed with a cast.

More recent studies have compared open versus percutaneous techniques. Gigante and co-workers randomized 40 patients to two groups treated with open surgery or percutaneous repair with the implementation of the Tenolig device (Group Fourniture Hospitalier, France). Both groups received the same post-operative regime. Post-operative assessment was performed objectively, subjectively as well as bilateral ultrasound scanning and isokinetic testing. There was no significant difference between the two groups other than increased ankle circumference, which had no functional effect. They recommend the use of percutaneous techniques in non-professional sportsmen and women due to the previously observed reduction in soft tissue and wound complications with comparable function and safety [9].

Assal and co-workers reported on a consecutive series of 87 patients managed using the Achillon device [2]. The results revealed good and excellent AOFAS scores (mean 96 points) at an average 26 month follow up, with no significant difference between the injured and uninjured sides in terms of isokinetic and endurance testing. All the patients returned to their previous levels of sporting activity. In addition, there were no cases of wound infections or sural nerve disturbance. Calder and Saxby replicated these favourable results in a review of 46 patients treated with this technique [3]. Ceccarelli and co-workers compared the modified Ma and Griffith repair with the Achillon system in a prospective two cohort study in which both groups were treated post-operatively with the same semi-functional rehabilitation regime using a walker boot [5]. The two groups were equivalent in terms of complications (no infections, no re-ruptures, no sural nerve injuries), AOFAS scores and return to sports activity.

In vitro studies have examined the strength of the Achillon repair [11]. Ismail and co- workers studied matched groups of sheep Achilles tendons that were repaired, using either the Achillon or a Kessler suture, and tested for mean load to failure. The Achillon was found to be a mechanically sound method of repair, with comparable tensile strength to a Kessler repair (153 N ±60 versus 123 N ±24). It should be noted, however, that the Achillon suture used a total of six strands of suture material versus four strands used in the Kessler repair. Longo and co-workers compared the Achillon suture configuration to a modified percutaneous repair of sheep Achilles tendons and showed no difference between the biomechanical performances in the two groups (mean strength, load, stiffness, mode of failure and failure elongation) [17].

Conclusion

Surgical techniques for treating acute Achilles rupture are changing and there appears to be an increasing role for percutaneous and mini-open techniques. Some studies suggest that these techniques can give results equivalent to or better than those of an open repair, with the added benefit of fewer complications without compromising the strength of repair. Evidence suggests that early functional rehabilitation with early weight-bearing can increase the strength of healed tendons and shorten rehabilitation times; early mobilization may be desirable in patients treated with these methods. Some form of thrombo-prophylaxis should be given in view of the significant risk of DVT. Further well-conducted, prospective, randomized studies are needed to settle the debate over the best treatment for an acute rupture of the Achilles tendon; however, a combined minimally invasive/percutaneous technique with early functional rehabilitation and early weight-bearing appears to be the current gold standard.

References

1. Aktan Ikiz I, Ucerler H, Bilge O. The anatomic features of the sural nerve with an emphasis on its clinical importance. Foot Ankle Int. 2005;26:560-567.
2. Assal M, Jung M, Stern R . Limited open repair of Achilles tendon ruptures: a technique with a new instrument and findings of a prospective multi-center study. J Bone Joint Surg Am. 2002;84:161- 170.
3. Calder JD, Saxby TS. Early, active rehabilitation following mini-open repair of Achilles tendon rupture: a prospective study. Br J Spots Med. 2005;39:857-859.
4. Carlstedt CA. Mechanical and chemical factors in tendon healing. Effects of indomethacin and surgery in the rabbit. Acta Orthop Scand, Suppl. 1987; 224.
5. Ceccarelli F, Berti L, Giuriati L . Percutaneous and minimally invasive techniques of Achilles tendon repair. Clin Orthop Relat Res. 2007 [Epub ahead of print. .
6. Cetti R, Henriksen LO, Jacobsen KS. A new treatment of ruptured Achilles tendons. A prospective randomized study. Clin Orthop Relat Res. 1994;308:155-165.
7. Cretnik A, Zlapjpah L, Smrkolj V . The strength of percutaneous methods of repair of the Achilles tendon: a biomechanical study. Med Sci Sports Exerc. 2000;32:16-20.
8. Cretnik A, Kasanovic M, Smrkolj V. Percutaneous versus open repair of the ruptured Achilles tendon: a comparative study. Am J Sports Med. 2005;33:1369-79.
9. Gigante A, Moschini A, Verdenelli A, Del Torto M, Ulisse S, de Palma L. Open versus percutaneous repair in the treatment of acute Achilles tendon rupture: a randomized prospective study. Knee Surg Sports Traumatol Arthrosc. 2008 16:204-209
10. Hockenbury R, Johns J. A biomechanical in vitro comparison of open versus percutaneous repair of tendon Achilles. Foot Ankle. 1990;11:67-72.
11. Ismail M, Karim A, Calder J. The Achillon Achilles tendon repair - is it strong enough? [Abstract. EFORT Congress 2007.
12. Kakiuchi M. A combined open and percutaneous technique for repair of tendo Achillis: Comparison with open repair. J Bone Joint Surg Br. 1995;77:60-63.
13. Khan RJK, Fick D, Brammar TJ, Crawford J, Parker MJ. Surgical interventions for treating acute Achilles tendon ruptures. Cochrane Database of Systematic Reviews 2004, Issue 3. Art. No.: CD003674. DOI: 10.1002/14651858.CD003674.pub2.
14. Khan R, Fick D, Keogh A . Treatment of Acute Achilles Tendon Ruptures. A Meta-Analysis of Randomized, Controlled Trials. J Bone Joint Surg Am. 2005;87:2202-2210.
15. Lapidus L, Rosfors S . Prolonged Thromboprophylaxis with Dalteparin After Surgical Treatment of Achilles Tendon Rupture: A Randomized, Placebo-Controlled Study. J Orthop Trauma. 2007 21:52-57
16. Lawrence TM, Davis RC. A biomechanical analysis of suture materials and their influence on a four-strand flexor tendon repair. J Hand Surg. 2005;30: 836-841.
17. Longo UG, Forriol F, Campi S, Maffulli N, Denaro V. A biomechanical comparison of the primary stability of two minimally invasive techniques for repair of ruptured Achilles tendon. Knee Surg Sports Traumatol Arthrosc. 2012 20:1392-1397
18. Ma GWC, Griffith TG. Percutaneous repair of acute closed ruptured Achilles tendon: a new technique. Clin Orthop Relat Res. 1977;128:247-255.
19. Maes R, Copin G, Averous C. Is percutaneous repair of the Achilles tendon a safe technique? A study of 124 cases. Acta Orthop Belg. 2006;72:179-183.
20. Maffulli N, Tallon C, Wong J . Early weightbearing and ankle mobilization after open repair of acute midsubstance tears of the Achilles tendon. Am J Sports Med. 2003;31:692-700.
21. Majewski M, Rohrbach M, Czaja S . Avoiding sural nerve injuries during percutaneous Achilles tendon repair. Am J Sports Med. 2006;34:793-798.
22. McClelland D, Maffulli N. Percutaneous repair of ruptured Achilles tendon. Journal of the Royal College of Surgeons of Edinburgh. 2002;41:613–618.
23. Metz R . Effect of Complications after Minimally invasive Surgical Repair of Acute Achilles Tendon Ruptures: Report on 211 Cases 20. Am J Sports Med. 2011 39:820
24. Palmes D, Spiegel H, Schneider T . Achilles tendon healing: long-term biomechanical effects of postoperative mobilization and immobilization in a new mouse model. J Orthop Res. 2002;20:939- 946.
25. Park H, Moon D, Yoon J. Limited open repair of ruptured Achilles tendons with Bunnel-type sutures. Foot Ankle Int. 2001;22:985-987.
26. Poynton A, O'Rourke K. An analysis of skin perfusion over the Achilles tendon in varying degrees of plantarflexion. Foot Ankle Int. 2001;22:572-574.
27. Webb JM, Bannister GC. Percutaneous repair of the ruptured tendo Achillis. J Bone Joint Surg Br. 1999;81:877-880.
28. Webb J, Moorjani N, Radford M. Anatomy of the sural nerve and its relation to the Achilles tendon. Foot Ankle Int. 2000;21:475-477.
29. Wong J, Barrass V, Maffulli N. Quantitative review of operative and nonoperative management of Achilles tendon ruptures. Am J Sports Med. 2002;30:565-575.

*"Energy and persistence
conquer all things."*

Benjamin Franklin

Chapter 20

Open Surgery for Insertional Achilles Tendinopathy

Nicola Maffulli, Umile G. Longo, Angelo Del Buono, Vincenzo Denaro

Take Home Message

- *Traditionally, extensile longitudinal incisions for insertional Achilles tendinopathy have been proposed: the surgical approach is to isolate the medial or lateral - or both - aspects of the tendon to perform posterior central splitting and hockey-stick transverse incisions.*

- *The approach may be made through a medial J-shaped incision, a lateral incision or a combination of medial and lateral incisions.*

- *10% of patients with insertional Achilles tendinopathy require surgery.*

- *The Cincinnati transverse approach allows the removal of the hypertrophic bursa, the paratenon and prominent calcaneal tuberosity.*

- *This procedure is safe and allows a wide exposure and adequate debridement of the Achilles tendon insertion. Most patients are able to return to their original level of physical activity following surgery and adequate rehabilitation.*

Introduction

Insertional Achilles tendinopathy accounts for 24% of all tendinopathies involving the Achilles tendon [9]. Diagnosis is usually clinical, characterized by pain, discomfort and impaired sporting activity [11]. Symptoms typically occur at the insertion of the Achilles tendon into the calcaneus. Using ultrasound scans, patients may present an increased antero-posterior diameter of the distal portion of the involved tendon and the occasional loss of the normal intratendinous texture. Plain lateral radiographs may show a bony prominence of the postero-superior corner of the calcaneal tuberosity or calcific deposits in the tendon. As already reported for other tendinopathies, the definitive diagnosis is histological [15]. With the histology, fibrocartilaginous degeneration close to the area of insertional tendinopathy, hyaline collagen degeneration, myxoid changes and fibrinoid degeneration may be observed [13, 14]. In addition, the intra-tendinous substance is disorganized, collagen fibres are disrupted with no parallel orientation and the diameter of some fibres is decreased, and there are changes in the extracellular matrix [18]. Collagen micro-ruptures have been reported, and erythrocytes surround some fibres. This condition is usually self-limiting but, when symptoms are longstanding, non-surgical measures may be indicated. Specifically, stretching exercises of the Achilles tendon, physical therapy, iontophoresis, steroidal and non-steroidal anti-inflammatory drugs, shoe modifications, night splints and extracorporeal shock wave therapy (ESWT), and activity modification [5, 7, 20] are successful in approximately 90% of patients [24]. On the other hand, when symptoms persist after more than six months (10% of patients), surgery will be recommended. Different surgical procedures have been described, including bursectomy, excision of the diseased tendon, removal of the calcific deposit and excision of the prominent posterolateral corner of the calcaneum [23].

The goal of any operation is to reduce pain and improve symptoms in the long-term. However, few studies in the literature report on the treatment of insertional Achilles tendinopathy. All techniques described in the literature involve debridement of the affected tendon, either by detaching the tendon or leaving it intact and debriding any bony spurs that may be causing tendon impingement. In a systematic review by Kearney and Costa on the surgical management of insertional Achilles tendinopathy, only four studies met the inclusion criteria [8].

Traditionally, extensile longitudinal incisions for insertional Achilles tendin opathy have been proposed: the surgical approach is to isolate the medial or lateral - or both- aspects of the tendon to perform posterior central splitting and hockey-stick transverse incisions [21].

The approach may be through a medial J-shaped incision [22], a lateral incision [28] or a combination of medial and lateral incisions [2]. Since all these approaches are prone to complications of wound healing, wound breakdown and iatrogenic nerve injury [19], the current trend is to prefer minimally invasive procedures. Soft tissue endoscopic techniques may successfully manage this condition [16].

The retrocalcaneal endoscopic decompression reduces the skin-related complications [25] and the use of additional tenodesis with an absorbable screw may reduce the risk of infection and the development of fistulas when using non-absorbable and braided sutures [16].

McGarvey and co-workers retrospectively reviewed 22 heels in 21 patients who were treated surgically for insertional Achilles tendinopathy after non-surgical treatments had failed [17]. A single longitudinal incision was performed above the distal insertion of the Achilles tendon. The calcific or degenerative portion of the tendon was identified and dissected free from the surrounding tissue and then excised. If excessive debridement was required (more than 50% of the tendinous insertion), the remaining tendon was reinforced with either bone-anchored sutures or plantaris tendon transfer. The retrocalcaneal bursa was then completely excised, as were any bony prominences that might have been abrading the tendon. The foot was then immobilized in plaster and full activity was resumed after three months. They reported good to excellent results in the majority of patients, with an 82% satisfaction rate, and over half the patients (13/22) were pain-free at 15 months post-surgery.

Yodlowski and co-workers described a similar approach to decompressing the insertion of the Achilles tendon [28]. Using a single skin incision, positioned laterally to the tendon, they retrospectively reviewed 41 heels in 35 patients who had failed non-surgical treatment measures. The insertion of the tendon on the calcaneus was not disturbed as the tendon was retracted, while the bursa, fat pad, degenerative tissue and any calcaneal prominence were all excised or debrided. At three years follow-up, 14 patients reported that their symptoms had completely resolved. 17 patients reported that their symptoms had significantly improved and four patients were improved.

A similar study by Johnson and co-workers investigated the effect of accessing the Achilles tendon insertion via a central tendon-splitting approach [6]. The tendinous insertion was then reinforced with sutures. Twenty-two patients with a mean follow-up of 34 months reported significant improvements in AOFAS ankle hind scores, pain, function, activity, maximum walking distances and capacity to return to work.

A retrospective study by Wagner and co-workers compared two groups of patients who underwent debridement of the Achilles tendon with no or partial detachment of the tendon or else complete detachment and reattachment with suture anchors at a follow-up of three to four years [26]. The decision not to detach, partially detach or fully detach the tendon was based on the amount of bone and diseased tendon. The endpoints evaluated included pain, activity limitation, gait changes, walking distances, return to sport or work and overall satisfaction with the procedure. No differences were noted in any of the endpoints investigated, but the satisfaction rate for the non-detached group was 92% compared with 74% for the detached group. Of note, there were 31 heels included in the non-detached group and 50 in the detached.

Elias and co-workers retrospectively reviewed 40 patients suffering from chronic insertional Achilles tendinopathy who underwent reconstruction of the tendon using a flexor hallucis longus allograft through a single tendon-splitting approach [4]. Mean follow-up was 27 months. The AOFAS ankle hind foot score increased from 56.3 (20-82) pre-operatively to 96.2 (69-100) post-operatively. The visual analogue pain scores also decreased significantly, from 7.5 to 0.3. Upon questioning, all the patients stated that they would undergo the procedure again.

Surgical procedures are not without their risks and complications. Paavola and co-workers prospectively reported an overall 11% complication rate in 432 consecutive patients who underwent open surgical procedures for chronic tendon overuse injury [19]. Of this cohort, 107 (25%) were diagnosed with either retrocalcaneal bursitis, insertional Achilles tendinopathy or both. They reported an overall complication rate of 5%, including one case of skin necrosis, one case of superficial wound infection, one case of fibrotic scar formation and two cases of haematoma formation.

Endoscopic surgery can also be used to treat patients with retrocalcaneal pain. Leitze and co-workers prospectively followed 30 consecutive patients with 33 heels who were diagnosed with a (postero-superior) calcaneal exostosis and/or insertional Achilles tendinopathy [10]. Patients who had major calcific tendinopathy (defined as more than 50% tendon involvement) were excluded. Despite a small patient cohort and the authors not stating how many patients had insertional Achilles tendinopathy only, they saw comparable results to open surgery with fewer complications. This may suggest that there is a place for the endoscopic debridement of patients suffering with insertional Achilles tendinopathy, but further studies are needed in this area.

Carmont and Maffulli described a Cincinnati (transverse) skin incision for insertional Achilles tendinopathy. The incision is performed close to the insertion of the Achilles tendon[1] to obtain a wide exposure of the insertion and the distal portion of the Achilles tendon. In this way, it is possible to free the tendon from adherences and surrounding fibrotic tissues and, when necessary, both superficial and deep Achilles bursectomy may be performed. The same incision allows access to the postero-superior corner of the calcaneus. Arising from the view that Achilles tendinopathy evolves from repeated micro-traumas due to the impingement of the tendon against the posterior tuberosity of the calcaneus, the same incision to perform an osteotomy of the tuberosity is used.

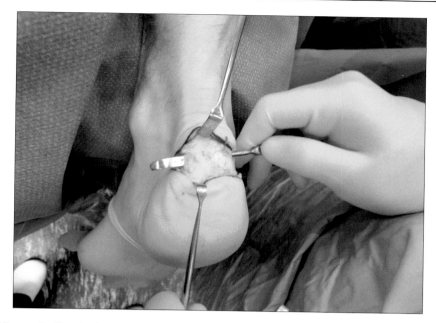

Figure 1. Surgical picture of the semicircular skin incision over the area of tendinopathy.

Surgical technique

The procedure is performed under general anaesthesia, with the patient prone. The Achilles tendon and the calcaneal tuberosity are the pre-operative anatomical markings. A 7-10 cm semicircular skin incision is made over the area of insertional tendinopathy, which is erythematous and swollen with a prominent tuberosity of the calcaneus (Figure 1). The subcutaneous bursa of the Achilles tendon is fully excised, the tendinopathic insertional area is identified (Figure 2), and the degenerated tissue is debrided from the healthy tissue. The space anterior to the tendon is exposed and the bursa anterior to the tendon is carefully excised. Next, the postero-superior corner of the calcaneum is accessed from both the medial and lateral aspects without detaching the tendon from its insertion. An osteotomy of the postero-superior corner of the calcaneus is performed, making sure that no sharp edges of bone are left to impinge on the insertion of the Achilles tendon upon dorsiflexion of the ankle. A below-the-knee weight-bearing cast is applied with the foot plantigrade.

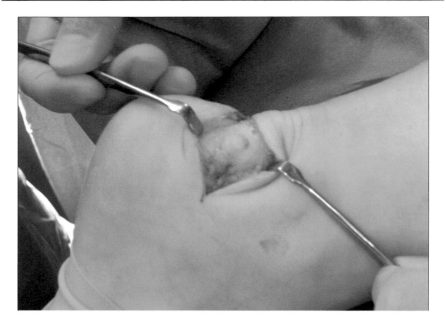

Figure 2. Intraoperative figure depicting the tendinopathic area within the insertional portion of the tendon.

Post-operative management

Patients are discharged on the day of surgery and allowed to bear weight as tolerated on the operated leg. The cast is removed two weeks following the operation. Patients are encouraged to gradually progress to full weight-bearing. Isometric contraction of the gastrosoleus complex and gentle concentric contraction of the calf muscles are begun. Proprioception, active plantar flexion, inversion and eversion exercises are allowed against manual resistance. Stationary cycling and swimming are recommended from the second week after the removal of the cast. At 10 or 12 weeks post-operatively, patients are assessed as to whether they are able to undertake more vigorous physiotherapy. Patients will take almost one year before returning to sport to avoid the possibility that technically well-performed surgery may be compromised by early return.

Clinical results

Maffulli ad co-workers have published a three year follow-up retrospective study on 30 physically-active patients [12]. Two patients reported complications - both cases of delayed wound healing - who healed a few days after oral antibiotic administration. In no instance was a nerve injury noted.

At the final follow-up, all the patients had improved function and fewer symptoms, and achieved an average VISA-A score of 88. Of the 30 patients, 17 reported an excellent result and nine a good result, and all 26 had returned to their pre-injury activity levels after surgery. The remaining four patients did not return to their normal levels of sporting activity, although they modified their sporting activity status without any problem in their daily activities. Since the Cincinnati approach allows for the wide exposure of the area of interest, it is now recommended in patients with calcific insertional tendinopathy - in whom the insertion of the Achilles tendon may have to be partially detached - to remove the calcific deposit(s) in order to properly expose the postero-superior corner of the calcaneum to perform the osteotomy. The Cincinnati approach allows for wide exposure and is less aggressive on soft-tissue.

The hypertrophic bursa, paratenon and prominent calcaneal tuberosity may irritate and compress the tendon. Therefore, through this approach, when removing the retrocalcaneal bursa, the thickened paratenon and the prominent superior calcaneal tuberosity, it is possible to reduce mechanical compression and irritation and relieve pain. The Cincinnati semi-circumferential incision has been used for soft tissue release around the hindfoot in paediatric club foot surgery [3]. The sural nerve may be frequently injured, and numbness around or distal to the incision has been reported [27]. Although this semi-circumferential incision is almost perpendicular to the course of the sural nerve, at the level of the insertion of the Achilles tendon the nerve has split into multiple small branches, and is therefore not at risk. In the hindfoot, once transverse scars have healed, the cosmetic appearance is excellent and they are often difficult to identify, even upon close inspection (Figure 3), and less prone to develop tethering, hypertrophy or contracture, which are commonly related to longitudinal scars.

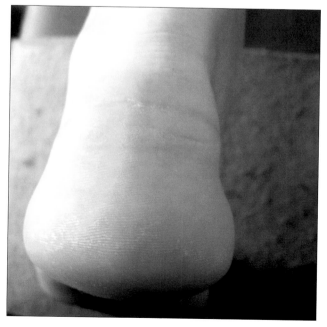

Figure 3. Picture showing the scar's appearance 12 months after surgery.

Conclusion

Insertional Achilles tendinopathy accounts for approximately one-fourth of all tendinopathies involving the Achilles tendon. This condition is usually self-limiting but, when symptoms are unresponsive to non-surgical measures, surgical management may be indicated. Different surgical procedures have been described, including bursectomy, excision of the diseased tendon, and removal of the calcific deposit and the prominent posterolateral corner of the calcaneum. At present, there is insufficient evidence to demonstrate the superiority of any one technique over another.

References

1. Carmont MR, Maffulli N. Management of insertional Achilles tendinopathy through a Cincinnati incision. BMC Musculoskelet Disord. 2007;8:82.

2. Clain MR, Baxter DE. Achilles tendinitis. Foot Ankle. 1992;13(8):482-487.

3. Crawford AH, Marxen JL, Osterfeld DL. The Cincinnati incision: a comprehensive approach for surgical procedures of the foot and ankle in childhood. J Bone Joint Surg Am. 1982;64(9):1355-1358.

4. Elias I, Raikin SM, Besser MP, Nazarian LN. Outcomes of chronic insertional Achilles tendinosis using FHL autograft through single incision. Foot Ankle Int. 2009;30(3):197-204.

5. Fahlstrom M, Jonsson P, Lorentzon R, Alfredson H. Chronic Achilles tendon pain treated with eccentric calf-muscle training. Knee Surg Sports Traumatol Arthrosc. 2003;11(5):327-333.

6. Johnson KW, Zalavras C, Thordarson DB. Surgical management of insertional calcific Achilles tendinosis with a central tendon splitting approach. Foot Ankle Int. 2006;27(4):245-250.

7. Jonsson P, Alfredson H, Sunding K, Fahlstrom M, Cook J. New regimen for eccentric calf-muscle training in patients with chronic insertional Achilles tendinopathy: results of a pilot study. Br J Sports Med. 2008;42(9):746-749.

8. Kearney R, Costa ML. Insertional Achilles tendinopathy management: a systematic review. Foot Ankle Int. 2010;31(8):689-694.

9. Kvist MH, Lehto MU, Jozsa L, al. e. Chronic Achilles paratenonitis. An immunohistologic study of fibronectin and fibrinogen. Am J Sports Med. 1988;16(6):616-623.

10. Leitze Z, Sella EJ, Aversa JM. Endoscopic decompression of the retrocalcaneal space. J Bone Joint Surg Am. 2003;85-A(8):1488-1496.

11. Longo UG, Ronga M, Maffulli N. Achilles tendinopathy. Sports Med Arthrosc. 2009;17(2):112-126.

12. Maffulli N, Del Buono A, Testa V, Capasso G, Oliva F, Denaro V. Safety and outcome of surgical debridement of insertional Achilles tendinopathy using a transverse (Cincinnati) incision. J Bone Joint Surg Br. 93(11):1503-1507.

13. Maffulli N, Longo UG, Denaro V. Novel approaches for the management of tendinopathy. J Bone Joint Surg Am. 2010;92(15):2604-2613.

14. Maffulli N, Longo UG, Loppini M, Denaro V. Current treatment options for tendinopathy. Expert Opin Pharmacother. 2010;11(13):2177-2186.

15. Maffulli N, Longo UG, Maffulli GD, Rabitti C, Khanna A, Denaro V. Marked pathological changes proximal and distal to the site of rupture in acute Achilles tendon ruptures. Knee Surg Sports Traumatol Arthrosc. 2011;19(4):680-687.

16. Maquirriain J. Endoscopic Achilles tenodesis: a surgical alternative for chronic insertional tendinopathy. Knee Surg Sports Traumatol Arthrosc. 2007;15(7):940-943.

17. McGarvey WC, Palumbo RC, Baxter DE, Leibman BD. Insertional Achilles tendinosis: surgical treatment through a central tendon splitting approach. Foot Ankle Int. 2002;23(1):19-25.

18. Movin T, Gad A, Reinholt FP, Rolf C. Tendon pathology in long-standing achillodynia. Biopsy findings in 40 patients. Acta Orthop Scand. 1997;68(2):170-175.

19. Paavola M, Kannus P, Jarvinen TA, Khan K, Jozsa L, Jarvinen M. Achilles tendinopathy. J Bone Joint Surg Am. 2002;84-A(11):2062-2076.

20. Rompe JD, Furia J, Maffulli N. Eccentric loading compared with shock wave treatment for chronic insertional Achilles tendinopathy. A randomized, controlled trial. J Bone Joint Surg Am. 2008;90(1):52-61.

21. Schepsis AA, Jones H, Haas AL. Achilles tendon disorders in athletes. Am J Sports Med. 2002;30(2):287-305.

22. Schepsis AA, Wagner C, Leach RE. Surgical management of Achilles tendon overuse injuries. A long-term follow-up study. Am J Sports Med. 1994;22(5):611-619.

23. Subotnick SI, Sisney P. Treatment of Achilles tendinopathy in the athlete. J Am Podiatr Med Assoc. 1986;76(10):552-557.

24. Sundqvist H, Forsskahl B, Kvist M. A promising novel therapy for Achilles peritendinitis: double-blind comparison of glycosaminoglycan polysulfate and high-dose indomethacin. Int J Sports Med. 1987;8(4):298-303.

25. van Dijk CN, van Dyk GE, Scholten PE, Kort NP. Endoscopic calcaneoplasty. Am J Sports Med. 2001;29(2):185-189.

26. Wagner E, Gould JS, Kneidel M, Fleisig GS, Fowler R. Technique and results of Achilles tendon detachment and reconstruction for insertional Achilles tendinosis. Foot Ankle Int. 2006;27(9):677-684.

27. Webb J, Moorjani N, Radford M. Anatomy of the sural nerve and its relation to the Achilles tendon. Foot Ankle Int. 2000;21(6):475-477.

28. Yodlowski ML, Scheller AD, Minos L. Surgical treatment of Achilles tendinitis by decompression of the retrocalcaneal bursa and the superior calcaneal tuberosity. Am J Sports Med. 2002;30(3):318-321.

"Necessity is the mother of invention."

Plato

Chapter 21

Open Surgical Treatment of Midportion Achilles Tendinopathy

Hajo Thermann, Ralph M. Fischer, Sven Feil, Sean Matuszak, Brian Donley

Take Home Message

- *Open surgical management of tendinopathies of the Achilles tendon should be considered only after failure of non-surgical treatment.*

- *All surgical interventions should include, at a minimum, the surgical debridement of the tendon.*

- *Surgery for severe degenerative and partial ruptures of the Achilles tendon often require an individual approach with individual debridement and reconstruction; adjunctive procedures, such as tendon transfer and gap bridging, may be necessary after extensive tendon debridement.*

- *Wound healing complications are frequent after the surgical treatment of Achilles tendinopathy and should be discussed with, and carefully explained to, the patient and included in the informed consent.*

Introduction

Because both the diagnosis and treatment of Achilles tendinopathy are largely based on empirical data, there is no consensus on treatment. A 2001 Cochrane review determined that, based on the available literature, no conclusions could be drawn about the treatment of Achilles tendinopathy [37]. The reported incidence of painful mid-portion Achilles tendinopathy varies among studies [14, 59]. The incidence is generally higher in the athletic population, with a 7% to 11% incidence reported among runners [54].

Achilles tendinopathy can usually be successfully treated with non-surgical measures; however, non-surgical treatment fails in approximately one third to one quarter of patients [3, 5, 7, 13, 33, 37]. In one long-term study, 29% of patients required surgical intervention [44]. Surgical treatment is successful in approximately 70% of patients in whom non-surgical measures have failed.

While non-surgical treatment is similar for both mid-portion and insertional Achilles tendinopathy, it is important to distinguish between the two when considering surgical intervention. Insertional tendinopathy occurs at the junction of the Achilles and the calcaneal tuberosity and is often associated with a calcaneal exostosis. Mid-portion Achilles tendinopathy occurs approximately 2 to 6 cm above the insertion. This is largely due to the watershed area of vascular supply. Above this area, the tendon receives its blood supply from the musculo-tendinous junction. Below this area, the tendon receives its blood supply from the osseo-tendinous junction [2]. There is a relative avascular area in the central portion of the tendon because of decreased vascular density [62].

Imaging

In patients with mid-portion tendinopathy, radiographs are most often normal. It is important to evaluate a hind foot alignment view because tendinopathy may be associated with pathological varus or valgus deformities [38].

Advanced imaging techniques such as ultrasonography and MRI are important tools for evaluating mid-portion tendinopathy [10, 17]. While the diagnosis is usually made based on history and clinical examination, these imaging studies are useful adjuvants for surgical planning. Ultrasonography is largely user-dependent; however, hypoechoic areas seen on ultrasonography represent areas of pathology. Paavola and co-workers [46] determined that while ultrasonography was useful for identifying areas of pathology, it was unreliable in determining areas of peritendinitis and delineating tendinosis from partial ruptures. Some advantages of ultrasonography are that it can be performed in the office setting, it can be a dynamic study, it is low-cost, and it provides immediate patient feedback in correlation with imaging findings.

MRI is valuable for determining the extent of disease involvement, and in one study it was deemed superior to ultrasonography in identifying areas of pathology. Contrast-enhanced MRI demonstrated areas of pathology that were identified as normoechoic on ultrasound [40]. On axial images, it is possible to estimate the cross-sectional area of tendon involvement. If more than 50% of the tendon is involved, it may be necessary to include an augmentation procedure together with standard debridement. It is important to evaluate signal change within the tendon because tendon volume alone is not as predictive of clinical symptoms [18].

It is important to note that the potential for false positives and false negatives may be high with MRI. Studies have demonstrated that asymptomatic tendons may exhibit abnormal imaging. Khan and co-workers [23] found abnormal morphology in only 65% of symptomatic patients, while only 68% of asymptomatic patients had normal morphology on ultrasound. MRI was better at identifying normal morphology in normal patients (93%); however, only 56% of symptomatic patients demonstrated abnormal morphology. Positive imaging findings must be correlated with clinical symptoms.

Indications for Surgical Treatment

Surgery is generally indicated when non-surgical treatment fails to relieve symptoms. Opinions about the length of time that non-surgical therapies should be tried differ in the literature between three and six months [6, 8, 10, 14, 15, 19, 20, 21, 22]. Our experience has shown that a thickening of the tendon of about 20 mm combined with severe symptoms of tendinopathy should be treated surgically, because further non-surgical treatment will fail and is only time-consuming. Often, the morphological changes in the tendon do not completely correlate with the clinical symptoms of the patient [4, 5]. In chronic tendinopathy with a large intra-tendinous lesion (a partial tear) or the massive thickening of the Achilles tendon, prompt surgical treatment is necessary.

The goal of surgical intervention should be pain relief. It is important to discuss outcomes with patients, including return to sport or activity. Return to activity varies from eight to 15 weeks, while return to competition occurs on average at six months (25 to 27 weeks) [43, 51, 52]. Patients should also have reasonable expectations as to the length of recovery and the process involved. Alfredson and co-workers [5] demonstrated that strength deficits persist up to one year post-operatively, including both concentric and eccentric Achilles strength. A subsequent study by Ohberg, Lorentzon and Alfredson [42] showed that even at maximal recovery, pre-operative strength deficits remain on the surgical side despite pain-free functionality [42]. It is reasonable to counsel patients that return to activity can take up to six months with maximal recovery continuing up to a year after surgery [52]. The length of immobilization and the post-operative physical therapy protocol vary from patient to patient (see section on Post-operative Management).

Surgical Options

Debridement

All surgical interventions should include, at a minimum, the surgical debridement of the tendon. Pre-operative evaluation, including advanced imaging, will help identify the locations of tendinopathy that require excision. Additionally, the intra-operative exploration of the tendon will identify areas of abnormal tendon. A degenerative tendon appears yellow and nodular, as opposed to the glistening smooth white character of a normal tendon. There may also be areas of thickening that may or may not include calcification.

Tendon debridement

With the patient in prone position, a tourniquet is placed around the thigh. Usually, the surgery is done with general anaesthesia, but spinal or local can also be used.

The incision is placed on the antero-medial edge of the palpable thickening of the Achilles tendon (Figure 1a) so as to spare the lateral-lying sural nerve and saphenous vein. The subcutaneous tissue and fascia are incised to expose the paratenon, which is opened slightly medial to the incision to allow inspection of the Achilles tendon, which usually finds xanthochrome, yellowish discolorations and neovascularizations that are easily palpable (Figure 1b). The Achilles tendon is split in a longitudinal direction to expose degenerative areas of the tendon. The localization of the degeneration in the transverse plane should be based on a MR image (medial or lateral). After localization, all degenerative areas are debrided. This is done partly by palpation of the tendon, which is held between the thumb and index finger to feel for any rough resistance that does not macroscopically appear to be clearly pathological. Thorough debridement is essential. If a large portion (>50%) of the tendon is debrided, an augmentation procedure should be added. Individual smaller "knots" that appear macroscopically should be perforated with a Chondropic© or a Mikrofrac© to stimulate tissue regeneration. Anteriorly, all the "neovessels and nerves" are debrided from the tendon. After suturing of the anterior portion of the tendon (Figure 1d), the Krackow technique is used around the dorsal portion with a 3.0 PDS (Figure 1e). Then the paratenon is sutured with a 4.0 PDS continuously, also with a Krackow technique. This is followed by medial closure of the fascia and subcutaneous tissue with a continuous suture.

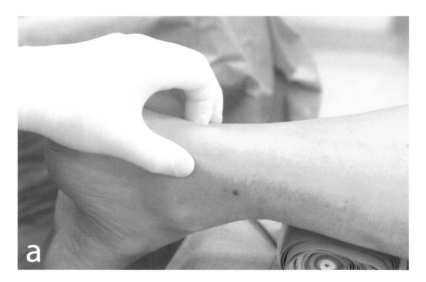

Figure 1A. Palpable thickening of the Achilles tendon.

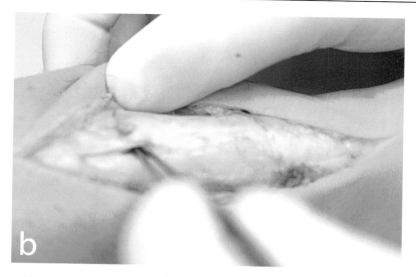

Figure 1B. Inspection and longitudinal splitting of the Achilles tendon.

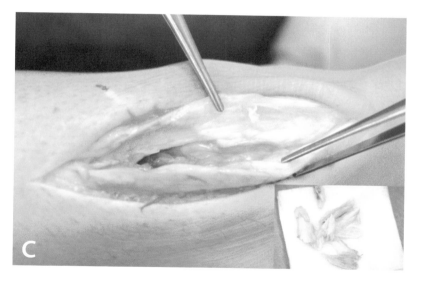

Figure 1C. Radical debridement of the Achilles tendon.

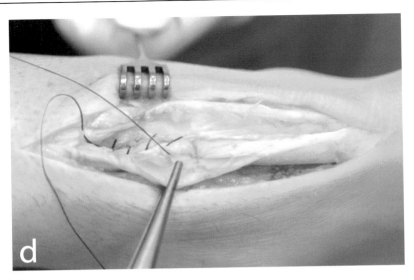

Figure 1D. "Tubulization" of the Achilles tendon with a ventral Krakow suture.

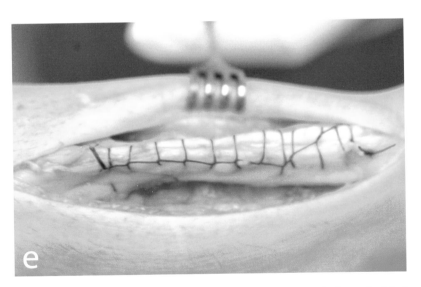

Figure 1E. Closing of the Achilles tendon and finishing of the "tabulation" with dorsal Krakow sutures.

Tendon transfer

Multiple tendon transfers have been described using various tendons and techniques. The flexor digitorum longus, peroneus brevis and flexor hallucis longus (FHL) tendons have been described as possible transfers [35, 47]. The most commonly described transfer involves the flexor hallucis longus, harvested and transferred through a single incision ("short harvest") or through dual incisions ("long harvest").

With single-incision techniques, a postero-medial or central incision provides better access to the FHL than a postero-lateral incision. The FHL is isolated anterior to the Achilles tendon and is released at the most distal point that can be visualized within the incision. The tendon is then brought through posteriorly and attached to the calcaneus with an interference screw. Good-to-excellent results have been obtained in 95% of patients using this technique [11]. Den Hartog [15] described a single-incision technique with satisfactory results in 23 (88%) of 26 patients.

Good results have also been reported with a dual-incision technique. This technique involves a second incision located plantar-medially that allows access to the FHL tendon as it passes deep towards the flexor digitorum tendon at the knot of Henry. This harvest provides a long tendon that can be brought through the posterior incision. Wapner and co-workers [60] described satisfactory results using a dual-incision technique with a bone tunnel and tendon weave in seven patients. Martin and co-workers [36] achieved pain relief in 42 (95%) of 44 patients and satisfactory outcomes in 38 (86%) with complete Achilles tendon excision, as well as transfer of the FHL with a dual-incision technique, while Wilcox and co-workers [61] reported 90% satisfactory results with a dual-incision technique in 20 patients.

Tendon transfer is not without potential morbidity. Loss of the FHL tendon results in up to 30% plantarflexion loss at the ankle, decreased FHL flexion strength, decreased distal phalangeal pressure, and decreased calf circumference [50, 61]. These potential morbidities do not appear to be clinically significant, however [12]. The single incision approach potentially limits the loss of plantarflexion strength because of the inter-tendinous connections at the knot of Henry, which are preserved in the short harvest.

The single-incision approach appears to obtain outcomes similar to those of the dual-incision approach without the potential morbidity of a second incision, increased operative time or potential injury to the medial plantar nerve [12, 20].

Gastrocnemius recession and plantaris excision

Gentchos and co-workers [19] first described gastrocnemius recession for the treatment of chronic Achilles tendinopathy in a case report in 2008. Since that time, other authors have reported success with this procedure in small series of patients. Duthon and co-workers [16] described early results for the treatment of chronic mid-portion Achilles tendinopathy with gastrocnemius recession in 14 patients. They hypothesized that increased force across the Achilles tendon contributed to the "overuse" of the Achilles tendon. By performing a gastrocnemius recession, they theoretically reduced the force across the Achilles tendon. Thirteen of their 14 patients were satisfied with their results, and 11 returned to their pre-injury level of sports. Kiewiet and co-workers [24] reported that all eight of their patients with chronic non-insertional Achilles tendinopathy had excellent pain relief and good functional outcomes after gastrocnemius recession. Gastrocnemius recession may offer a less invasive option for the treatment of refractory Achilles tendinopathy; however, at present long-term outcomes are not available, nor are comparisons to standard treatment options.

The plantaris tendon has also been implicated as a possible cause of pain in patients with Achilles tendinosis [4, 58]. The hypothesis is that medial-sided nodular thickening and pain may be caused by adhesions within or around the plantaris tendon, and that the excision of this tendon may relieve or improve symptoms with a less invasive procedure than a large open debridement of the Achilles tendon. Good results were reported in three patients treated by van Sterkenburg and co-workers [58] after stripping of the plantaris tendon. Alfredson [4] found an enlarged plantaris tendon in close relation to or invaginated in the Achilles tendon in 80% of 73 tendons in 56 patients being treated surgically for chronic Achilles tendinosis; the plantaris tendon was excised in all of these. Lintz and co-workers [28] found, in a biomechanical cadaver study, that the plantaris longus was stiffer and stronger than the Achilles tendon and postulated that it could tether the Achilles tendon and initiate an inflammatory response.

Reconstruction

Extensive debridement may leave a gap within the tendon. Techniques developed for chronic Achilles ruptures can be used in these circumstances to bridge the gap. V-Y tendon advancement has been reported to be successful in bridging gaps of up to 10 cm [1] and turndown fascial flaps have been used to augment V-Y plasty, as well as bridge gaps formed in chronic and acute ruptures [8, 48]. Both of these techniques are reserved for rare circumstances when a large part of the tendon is debrided, leaving insufficient tendon for repair.

Turn-down flap (aponeurosis) for chronic ruptures

In chronic ruptures, the procedure depends on the extent of tendon damage. Purpose of this procedure is the restoration of the tendon instead of a gross resection resulting in a huge defect. The tendon "fragments" are aligned and sutured individually, to regain "natural" tension in slight plantarflexion. This is crucial for tendon healing. A sufficient tendon volume (about 10 to 15 mm in diameter) is needed. For the biomechanical stabilization of the reconstruct, a "stress bypass" by a 1.3 PDS cord in a frame technique (an "internal fixator") has to be applied.

If the tendon reconstruction is small and brittle (less than 10 mm), new tissue will be necessary to guarantee sound tendon healing. This can be accomplished by an augmentation with a 10 mm turn-down flap, placed antero-laterally (to secure skin closure). If this is not sufficient, an additional transfer of the flexor hallucis longus tendon is advisable.

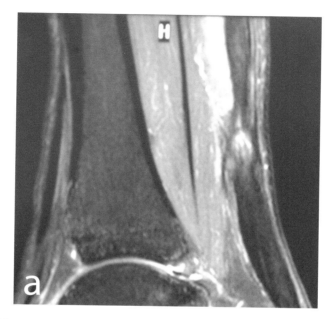

Figure 2A. Magnetic resonance tomography of the Achilles tendon showing a partial rupture and a massive degenerative thickening.

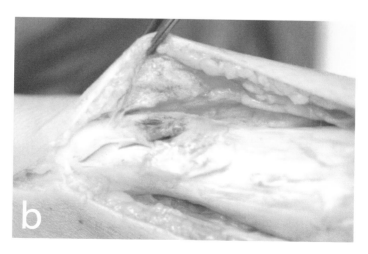

Figure 2B. Visible partial rupture with neovessels and thickening.

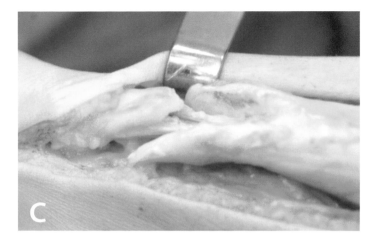

Figure 2C. "Dovetail" reconstruction of the Achilles tendon with intratendinous PDS augmentation.

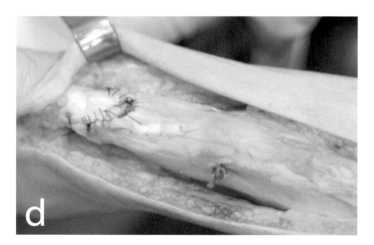

Figure 2D. Repaired Achilles tendon after "superficial" suture finishing.

The approach is made medial to the calcaneal insertion at the musculo-tendinous junction. In most cases, there is a defect with an unstable atrophic scar, which is separated on the distal portion. The Achilles-gastrocnemius-soleus complex is manually mobilized proximally to regain appropriate length and tension in the muscles. Afterwards, only unstable and degenerated tendon tissue are partially or completely ("individually") resected to "streamline" the reconstruction, incorporating the tendon and scar tissue into a solid "neotendon". Reconstruction may include: (1) a "dove tail" technique (Figure 2), (2) a two-flap reconstruction stabilizing the defect (Figure 3), or (3) a lateral turn-down flap for augmentation.

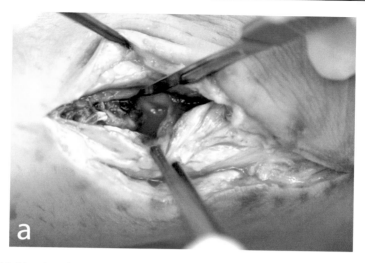

Figure 3A. Massive chronic rupture of the Achilles tendon.

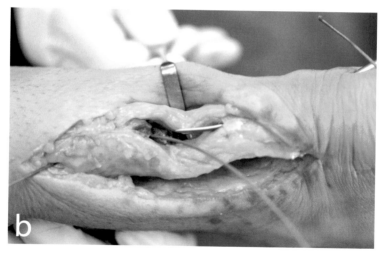

Figure 3B. Intra-tendinous augmentation with the PDS-chord.

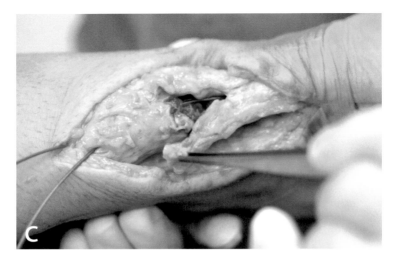

Figure 3C. Intra-tendinous frame suture within the Achilles tendon and tensioning in plantarflexion.

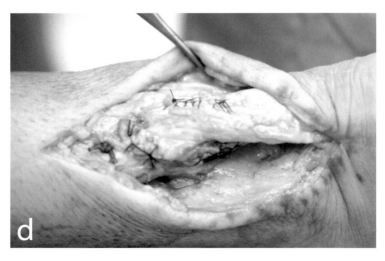

Figure 3D. Individual "sculpturing" and suturing of the Achilles tendon reconstruction.

For the aponeurosis turn-down flap, a lateral, approximately 1 cm-wide and 5 to 7 cm-long flap is prepared. The flap is aligned distally more anterior-laterally using an Ellis clamp.

Then for "stress bypassing" a PDS cord is pulled with an awl intra-tendinously from the proximal-medial to the proximal-lateral side. From the proximal-lateral side to the lateral-distal edge of the tendon, a drill hole (3.5 mm) is performed throughout the tuber calcanei. The PDS cord is inserted laterally through the calcaneus to the medial side and medial-distally pulled through the "neotendon" and medial-proximally back, and knotted medio-proximally (Figure 4) in slight plantarflexion to provide tension for the Achilles-gastrocnemius-soleus complex.

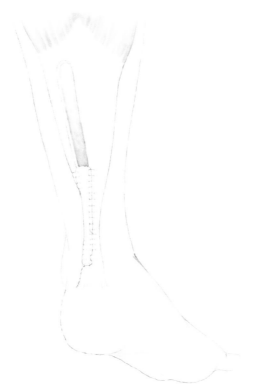

Figure 4. Lateral turn down flap for augmentation.

The "turndown flap" is now sutured with the Krakow technique (Vicryl #2.0) under tension to the antero-lateral "neotendon" to augment and stabilize the entire reconstruct.

287

Grafting

Allografts, as well as synthetic grafts, can be used to bridge tendon gaps, although these techniques are generally used for chronic Achilles ruptures. Allograft Achilles tendon has been used to bridge defects of 10 to 12 cm with good results [9, 27]. Maffulli and co-workers have described multiple free autograft transfers, including a free semitendinosus graft and free gracilis graft [29-31].

Xenografts and synthetic grafts have also been used to augment chronic repairs. In a cadaver model, biomechanical strength testing showed that the augmentation of Achilles tendon repair with an extracellular matrix xenograft reduced gapping and improved load to failure [34]. Synthetic grafts using Dacron, Marlex mesh, carbon fibre and a LARS tendon substitute, have also been studied with favourable results [22]. Acellular human dermal matrix may offer another reconstruction option [26].

Post-operative Management

Post-operative management includes a short period of immobilization in a splint or cast followed by weight-bearing, as tolerated in a walking boot. The initial post-operative splint is placed with the foot in approximately 20 degrees of plantarflexion. The splint is removed at two weeks and is replaced by an Achilles boot with wedges or an Achilles range-of-motion (ROM) boot that allows positioning of the foot in varying degrees of plantarflexion. This allows the patient to bear weight without significant tension on the skin or the repaired tendon. Each week, a wedge is removed or the boot is adjusted until a neutral position is obtained at approximately four weeks. The length of immobilization varies from two to 10 weeks, depending on the procedure performed, and this must be tailored to each individual patient.

Post-operative rehabilitation should focus on ankle ROM and strengthening. Active ROM exercises can be initiated by the patient once the incision is healed at approximately two weeks. Formal physical therapy is also tailored to the individual patient and is dependent on the procedure performed. In general, coordination exercises and isometric exercises can be performed in the boot or walker (self-training by patients after a short briefing). At eight to nine weeks, the rehabilitation programme includes proprioceptive exercises and strength training (plantarflexion), aqua jogging and cycling. Passive mobilization in dorsiflexion is not allowed to prevent the elongation of the new tendon. In a normal healing process within the first two months, emphasis should be placed on the strengthening of the foot flexor muscles and the calf muscle, with only minor limitations in dorsiflexion.

Return-to-work can be as soon as two weeks if the patient is allowed to work with protected weight-bearing in a boot; however, continued swelling and pain are important considerations if the patient is required to be in a standing position for his or her job. Return-to-sport activities can begin at approximately three months with sport-specific training, but return to competitive activity should be delayed until six months after surgery.

Complications

Paavola and co-workers [45] reported a large series of 432 consecutive patients with an 11% complication rate, including wound edge necrosis (3%), superficial infection (2.5%) and sural nerve irritation (1%). Other complications included seroma, haematoma, fibrotic reactions and thrombosis. Other studies confirm a complication rate of approximately 11% with a re-operation rate of approximately 3% [41].

Results of Surgical Treatment

Reported success rates for the surgical management of mid-portion Achilles tendinopathy range from 70% to 100% [13, 25, 32, 38, 57]. Tallon and co-workers [57], in a meta-analysis of 26 articles, found an average success rate of 76%. They also noted that the studies with higher clinical success rates had poorer scientific designs, while the studies with lower success rates were of better scientific quality. The lack of good quality scientific studies and outcome research is a significant reason for the discrepancies and controversy regarding treatment options.

Despite clinically-successful outcomes, it is likely that surgically-treated tendons remain histologically abnormal. Alfredson and co-workers followed 14 patients (16 tendons) for an average of 13 years after open surgical debridement and found thickening of the tendon and persistent structural abnormalities compared with normal tendons [6].

Conclusion

Mid-portion Achilles tendinopathy is usually treated with non-surgical methods. Surgical treatment can be considered if symptoms persist for more than six to 12 months despite an adequate trial of non-surgical treatment. Physical examination is the key component to diagnosis and treatment, with advanced imaging serving as an adjunct for pre-operative planning. Depending on the location and extent of disease, multiple surgical options are available. Simple debridement is effective when less than 50% of the tendon is involved and most of the pathology involves peritendinitis with minimal central involvement. When more than 50% of the tendon is involved and a substantial debridement is required, additional procedures may include FHL transfer, plantaris grafting, turndown fascial flap, lengthening, allografting or synthetic augmentation. Studies vary based on the extent of disease and the procedure, but successful outcomes can be expected in 70% to 100% of patients. Newer techniques have been described, but long-term data are not yet available. Rehabilitation is patient-specific, but return to work and sport can take three to six months. With appropriate patient selection and good surgical technique, surgical intervention is a good option when non-surgical treatment fails to alleviate symptoms.

References

1. Abraham E, Pankovich AM. Neglected rupture of the Achilles tendon. Treatment by V-Y tendinous flap. J Bone Joint Surg Am. 1975;57(2):253-255.
2. Ahmed IM, Lagopoulos M, McConnell P, Soames RW, Sefton GK. Blood supply of the Achilles tendon. J Orthop Res. 1998;16(5):591-596.
3. Alfredson H. Chronic midportion Achilles tendinopathy: an update on research and treatment. Clin Sports Med. 2003;22:727-741.
4. Alfredson H. Midportion Achilles tendinosis and the plantaris tendon. Br J Sports Med. 2011;45: 1023-1025.
5. Alfredson H, Pietilä T, Jonsson P, Lorentzon R. Heavy-load eccentric calf muscle training for the treatment of chronic Achilles tendinosis. Am J Sports Med. 1998;26(3):360-366.
6. Alfredson H, Zeisig E, Fahlström M. No normalization of the tendon structure and thickness after intratendinous surgery for chronic painful midportion Achilles tendinosis. Br J Sports Med. 2009;43:948-949.
7. Anderson DL, Taunton JE, Davidson RG. Surgical management of chronic Achilles tendinitis. Clin J Sports Med. 1992;2:38-42.
8. Christensen I. Rupture of the Achilles tendon: analysis of 57 cases. Acta Chir Scand. 1953;106(1):50-60.
9. Cienfuegos A, Holgado MI, Diaz del Rio JM, Gonzalez Herranz J, Lara Bullón J. Chronic Achilles rupture reconstructed with Achilles tendon allograft: a case report. J Foot Ankle Surg. 2013;52(1):95-98.
10. Comin J, Cook JL, Malliaras P, McCormack M, Calleja M, Clarke A, Connell D. The prevalence and clinical significance of sonographic tendon abnormalities in asymptomatic ballet dancers: a 24-month longitudinal study. Br J Sports Med. 2013;47:89-92.
11. Cottom JM, Hyer CF, Berlet GC, Lee TH. Flexor halluces tendon transfer with an interference screw for chronic Achilles tendinosis: a report of 62 cases. Foot Ankle Spec. 2008;1(5):280-287.
12. Coull R, Flavin R, Stephens MM. Flexor hallucis longus tendon transfer: evaluation of postoperative morbidity. Foot Ankle Int. 2003;24(12):931-934.
13. Courville XF, Coe MP, Hecht PJ. Current concepts review: noninsertional Achilles tendinopathy. Foot Ankle Int. 2009;30(11):1132-1142.
14. de Jonge S, van den Berg C, de Vos RJ, vander Heide HJL, Weir A, Verhgaar JAN, Bierma-Zeinstra SMA, Tol JL. Incidence of midportion Achilles tendinopathy in the general population. Br J Sports Med. 2011;45:1026-1028.
15. Den Hartog BD. Flexor hallucis longus transfer for chronic Achilles tendinosis. Foot Ankle Int. 2003;24(3)233-237.
16. Duthon VB, Lübbeke A, Duc SR, Stern R, Assal M. Noninsertional Achilles tendinopathy treated with gastrocnemius lengthening. Foot Ankle Int. 2011;32(4):375-379.
17. Fredberg U, Bolvig L. Significance of ultrasonographically detected asymptomatic tendinosis in the patellar and Achilles tendons of elite soccer players: a longitudinal study. Am J Sports Med. 2002;30(4):488-491.
18. Gärdin A, Bruno J, Movin T, Kristoffersen-Wiberg M, Shalabi A. Magnetic resonance signal, rather than tendon volume, correlates to pain and functional impairment in chronic Achilles tendinopathy. Acta Radiol. 2006;47(7):718-724.
19. Gentchos CE, Bohay DR, Anderson JG. Gastrocnemius recession as treatment for refractory Achilles tendinopathy: a case report. Foot Ankle Int. 2008;29(6):620-623.
20. Herbst SA, Miller SD. Transection of the medial plantar nerve and hallux cock-up deformity after flexor hallucis longus transfer Achilles tendinitis: case report. Foot Ankle Int. 2006;27(8):639-641.
21. Hess GP, Cappiello WL, Poole RM, Hunter SC. Prevention and treatment of overuse tendon injuries. Sports Med. 1989;8:371-384.
22. Ibrahim SA. Surgical treatment of chronic Achilles tendon rupture. J Foot Ankle Surg. 2009;48(3):340-346.
23. Khan KM, Forster BB, Robinson J, Cheong Y, Louis L, Maclean L, Taunton JE. Are ultrasound and magnetic resonance imaging of value in assessment of Achilles tendon disorders? A two year prospective study. Br J Sports Med. 2003;3e7(2):149-153.
24. Kiewiet NJ, Holthusen SM, Bohay DR, Anderson JG. Gastrocnemius recession for chronic noninsertional Achilles tendinopathy. Foot Ankle Int. 2013;34:481-485.
25. Leach RE, Schepsis AA, Takai H. Long-term results of surgical management of Achilles tendinitis in runners. Clin Orthop Relat Res. 1992;282:208-212.
26. Lee DK. Achilles tendon repair with acellular tissue graft augmentation in neglected ruptures. J Foot Ankle Surg. 2007;46(6)451-455.
27. Lepow GM, Green JB. Reconstruction of a neglected Achilles tendon rupture with an Achilles tendon allograft: a case report. J Foot Ankle Surg. 2006;45(5)351-355.
28. Lintz F, Higgs A, Millett M, Barton T, Raghuvanshi M, Adams MA, Winson IG. The role of the plantaris longus in Achilles tendinopathy: a biomechanical study. Foot Ankle Surg. 2011;17(4):252-255.

29. Maffulli N, Del Buono A, Spiezia F, Maffulli GD, Longo UG, Denaro V. Less-invasive semitendinosus tendon graft augmentation for the reconstruction of chronic tears of the Achilles tendon. Am J Sports Med. 2013;41:865-871.

30. Maffulli N, Longo UG, Gougoulias N, Denaro V. Ipsilateral free semitendinosus tendon graft transfer for reconstruction of chronic tears of the Achilles tendon. BMC Musculoskelet Disord. 2008;9:100.

31. Maffulli N, Spiezia F, Testa V, Capasso G, Longo UG, Denaro V. Free gracilis tendon graft for reconstruction of chronic tears of the Achilles tendon. J Bone Joint Surg Am. 2012;94(10):906-910.

32. Maffulli N, Testa V, Capasso G, Oliva F, Sullo A, Benazzo F, Regine R, King JB. Surgery for chronic Achilles tendinopathy yields worse results in nonathletic patients. Clin J Sport Med. 2006;16(2):123-128.

33. Magnussen RA, Dunn WR, Thomson AB. Nonoperative treatment of midportion Achilles tendinopathy: a systematic review. Clin J Sport Med. 2009;19(1):54-64.

34. Magnussen RA, Glisson RR, Moorman CT III. Augmentation of Achilles tendon repair with extracellular matrix xenograft: a biomechanical analysis. Am J Sports Med. 2011;39(7):1522-1527.

35. Mann RA, Holmes GB Jr, Seale KS, Collins DN. Chronic rupture of the Achilles tendon: a new technique of repair. J Bone Joint Surg Am. 1991;73(2)214-219.

36. Martin RL, Manning CM, Carcia CR, Conti SF. An outcome study of chronic Achilles tendinosis after excision of the Achilles tendon and flexor hallucis longus tendon transfer. Foot Ankle Int. 2005;26(9):691-697.

37. McLauchlan GJ, Handoll HH. Interventions for treatment acute and chronic Achilles tendinitis. Cochrane Database Syst Rev. 2001;(2):CD000232.

38. McShane JM, Ostick B, McCabe F. Noninsertional Achilles tendinopathy: pathology and management. Curr Sports Med Rep. 2007;6(5):288-292.

39. Monto RR. Platelet rich plasma treatment for chronic Achilles tendinosis. Foot Ankle Int. 2012;33(5):379-385.

40. Movin T, Kristoffersen-Wiberg M, Shalabi A, Gad A, Aspelin R, Rolf C. Intraintendinous alterations as imaged by ultrasound and contrast medium-enhanced magnetic resonance in chronic achillodynia. Foot Ankle Int. 1998;19(5):311-317.

41. Nunley JA, Ruskin G, Horst F. Long-term clinical outcomes following the central incision technique for insertional Achilles tendinopathy. Foot Ankle Int. 2011;32(9):850-855.

42. Ohberg L, Lorentzon R, Alfredson H. Good clinical results but persisting side-to-side differences in calf muscle strength after surgical treatment of chronic Achilles tendinosis: a 5-year follow-up. Scand J Med Sci Sports. 2001;11(4):207-212.

43. Paavola M, Kannus P, Orava S, Pasanen M, Järvinen M. Surgical treatment for chronic Achilles tendinopathy: a prospective seven-month follow-up study. Br J Sports Med. 2002;36:178-182.

44. Paavola M, Kannus P, Paakkala T, Pasanen M, Järvine M. Long-term prognosis of patients with Achilles tendinopathy. An observational 8-year follow-up study. Am J Sports Med. 2000;28(5):634-642.

45. Paavola M, Orava S, Leppilahti J, Kannus P, Järvinen M. Chronic Achilles tendon overuse injury: complications after surgical treatment. An analysis of 432 consecutive patients. Am J Sports Med. 2000;28(1):77-82.

46. Paavola M, Paakkala T, Kannus P, Järvinen M. Ultrasonography in the differential diagnosis of Achilles tendon injuries and related disorders. A comparison between pre-operative ultrasonography and surgical findings. Acta Radiol 1998;39(6):612-619.

47. Pérez Teuffer A. Traumatic rupture of the Achilles tendon. Reconstruction by transplant and graft using the lateral peroneus brevis. Orthop Clin North Am. 1974;5(1):89-93.

48. Ponnapula P, Aaranson RR. Reconstruction of Achilles tendon rupture with combined V-Y plasty and gastrocnemius-soleus fascia turndown graft. J Foot Ankle Surg. 2010;49(3):310-315.

49. Rasmussen S, Christensen M, Mathiesen I, Simonson O. Shockwave therapy for chronic Achilles tendinopathy: a double-blind, randomized clinical trial of efficacy. Acta Orthop. 2008;79(2):249-256.

50. Richardson DR, Willers J, Cohen BE, Davis WH, Jones CP, Anderson RB. Evluation of the hallux morbidity of single-incision flexor hallucis longus tendon transfer. Foot Ankle Int. 2009;30(7):627-630.

51. Saxena A. Results of chronic Achilles tendinopathy surgery on elite and nonelite track athletes. Foot Ankle Int. 2003;24(9):712-720.

52. Schepsis AA, Jones H, Haas AL. Achilles tendon disorders in athletes. Am J Sports Med. 2002;30(2):287-305.

53. Schepsis AA, Leach RE. Surgical management of Achilles tendinitis. Am J Sports Med. 1987;15(4):308-315.

54. Schepsis AA, Wagner C, Leach RE. Surgical management of Achilles tendon overuse injuries. A long-term follow-up study. Am J Sports Med. 1994;22(5):611-619.

55. Scott AT, Le IL, Easley ME. Surgical strategies: noninsertional Achilles tendinopathy. Foot Ankle Int. 2008;29(7):759-771.

56. Silbernagel KG, Gustavsson A, Thomeé R, Karlsson J. Evaluation of lower leg function in patients with Achilles tendinopathy. Knee Surg Sports Traumatol Arthrosc. 2006;14:1207-1217.

57. Tallon C, Coleman BD, Khan KM, Maffulli N. Outcome of surgery for chronic Achilles tendinopathy: a critical review. Am J Sports Med. 2001;29(3):315-320.

58. van Sterkenburg MN, Kerkhoffs GM, van Dijk CN. Good outcome after stripping the plantaris tendon in patients with chronic mid-portion Achilles tendinopathy. Knee Surg Sports Traumatol Arthrosc. 2011;19(8):1362-1366.

59. Waldecker U, Hofmann G, Drewitz S. Epidemiologic investigation of 1394 feet: coincidence of hindfoot malalignment and Achilles tendon disorders. Foot Ankle Surg. 2012;18(2):119-123.

60. Wapner KL, Pavlock GS, Hecht PJ, Naselli F, Walther R. Repair of chronic Achilles tendon rupture with flexor hallucis longus tendon transfer. Foot Ankle. 1993;14(8):443-449.

61. Wilcox DK, Bohay DR, Anderson JG. Treatment of chronic Achilles tendon disorders with flexor hallucis longus tendon transfer/augmentation. Foot Ankle Int. 2000;21(12):1004-1010.

62. Zantop T, Tillmann B, Petersen W. Quantitative assessment of blood vessels of the human Achilles tendon: an immunohistochemical cadaver study. Arch Orthop Trauma Surg. 2003;123:501-504.

Chapter 22

Open Surgery for Achilles Tendon Rupture

Jón Karlsson, Nicklas Olsson, Katarina Nilsson Helander,
Gino M.M.J. Kerkhoffs, C. Niek van Dijk

Take Home Message

- *Open surgery is considered the gold standard procedure when operative management is contemplated in patients with acute Achilles tendon ruptures. All other approaches (minimally-invasive and percutaneous) should be compared with open end-to-end repair.*

- *The risk of re-rupture after open end-to-end repair is low; however, the risk of other complications, such as adhesions and wound infections is higher.*

- *Re-rupture risk can be reduced using strict adherence to treatment protocols and patients compliance.*

- *Patients can start exercising range of motion at approximately 10 days post-operatively, or possibly earlier (e.g., immediately after the repair). After 14 days weight-bearing with restricted dorsiflexion could be commenced.*

- *Recent technical advances show as low re-rupture rate as 0%, using stable surgical technique.*

- *A stable surgical technique allows early range of motion training and early weight bearing.*

Introduction

Treatment of Achilles tendon ruptures has long been at the centre of debate. The discussion is, however, mostly concerned with surgical or non-surgical treatment. Both techniques have their strong supporters. Even though the Achilles tendon is considered to be the strongest in the body, it is one of the most commonly ruptured tendons. The rupture occurs in majority of patients during sporting activities in middle-aged males [5]. Total rupture of the Achilles tendon is uncommon in top-level athletes.

The rupture is usually situated approximately 2-6 cm proximal to the insertion to the calcaneus, and the rupture ends are typically severely frayed (Figure 1). Whether the rupture happens in an area of tendinopathy or not is still a matter of debate [8, 15, 22]. However, most patients suffer an Achilles tendon rupture without any prodromal symptoms, like chronic pain, or signs of inflammation. Partial Achilles ruptures are uncommon in cases with a very distinct patient history and in most cases 'partial Achilles tendon rupture' is probably an incorrect diagnosis.

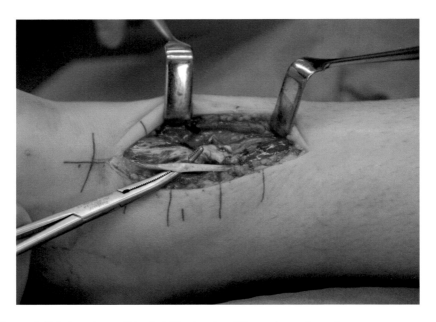

Figure 1. Total rupture of the Achilles tendon. The ends are frayed.

The injury happens suddenly (sometimes dramatically), in patients who have not suffered from pain prior to the rupture. Most researchers suggest that typical "painful" tendinopathy (tendinosis) does not precede an acute Achilles tendon rupture.

Once the correct diagnosis is established; the treatment should be decided, being either surgical or non-surgical. Ultrasound and/or MRI for correct diagnosis is, in fact, one of the main reasons for incorrect diagnosis and delay. The diagnosis is clinical, with positive Thompson's (calf squeeze test) or/and Matle's test [13], inability to walk on the toe, reduced (or even absence of) plantar flexion strength and a palpable gap in the tendon.

Controversy exists in terms of the best treatment, and not even the existing randomized studies - which have been published over the last decade - are able to produce clear and definitive treatment algorithms. Those who prefer surgical treatment refer as a rule to a lower risk of re-rupture after open surgery. Young active athletes are, in the majority of cases, treated with surgery [14, 16, 23]. Even though surgical treatment carries the risk of complications - such as wound break-down, infection, sural nerve injuries and adhesions/stiffness - many patients are in favour of surgical treatment, due to the lower risk of re-rupture [7, 10]. In a recent meta-analysis by Khan and co-workers [10], it was shown that the risk of re-rupture after surgical treatment is approximately 5% and after non-surgical treatment approximately 12%. This difference might be counter-acted by the increase risk of wound infections, up to 10% in some studies after surgical treatment. Wound infections are nowadays - probably due to less invasive surgical approach - mostly superficial and are easily treated with antibiotics and superficial wound care. Wound break-down and necrosis of the Achilles tendon – both feared complications – are very infrequent today.

The issue of immobilization is also of concern. The trend is without doubt towards shorter immobilization period. Early range of motion training, using movable brace and early weight-bearing has been advocated recently. In fact, it has been shown that early, well-protected range of motion training and at least moderately aggressive rehabilitation will result in better outcomes after surgical treatment. In general, the tendency has been for immobilisation to be shortened and motion of the ankle to be started earlier [3, 9, 21].

Selection of surgical treatment

When surgical treatment has been selected the important issue is to make a choice regarding technique and approach. Classically, an end-to-end repair is performed. Open repair can probably be performed up to approximately three weeks following the injury. The exact limit as to when the rupture becomes chronic is arbitrary and debated. Most authors agree in performing a primary end-to-end repair without an augmented repair up to 2-3 weeks.

Surgery can be done using an open, miniopen or percutaneous approach. Even a closed approach using the arthroscope to visualize the tendon ends has been reported . In this chapter, only the open approach will be discussed. The patient should always be placed in a prone position, with the feet over a pillow or beyond the operating table in order to avoid excessive plantar flexion, as over-tightening of the repair will risk tendon shortening of the tendon and loss of motion. On the other hand, lengthening of the tendon (as this will most probably cause reduced plantar flexion strength) should be avoided at any cost. A soft roll may be placed under the tibia. The procedure can be carried out under local, regional or general anesthesia. A bloodless field is not needed. When considering the position of the foot, in order to avoid shortening or lengthening of the tendon, it is prudent to compare the position to the other foot in neutral position and dorsiflexion. It is important to judge the tension of the repair and the balance between the dorsiflexors and the plantarflexors.

Surgical approach

A postero-medial skin incision is preferred in order to minimize any risk of injury to the branches of the sural nerve. Also, this makes access to the plantaris tendon if needed. In some cases, a longitudinal posterior skin incision is used; however, this may create a painful scar. Therefore a postero-medial incision is advocated. The postero-medial incision is usually between 5 and 8 cm long, although the tendency in recent years has been for a shorter incision. After the paratendon is opened, there is easy access to the frayed tendon ends. The healthy tendon should always be exposed at the proximal and distal ends. It is very uncommon for the tendon to be ruptured from bone. In such cases, the treatment is different, often using suture anchors in the calcaneus to secure the tendon to the bone. The skin and subcutaneous tissues should be handled very carefully due to the limited and vulnerable blood supply, in order to reduce the risk of tissue breakdown. After the tendon has been exposed, the gap is cleaned of blood clots and the ends are freed in both directions. Dissection should be minimized, to reduce the risk of additional vascular injury. Usually, the ends of the tendon are debrided and thereafter carefully approached. This can usually be done without major tension. There is much debate concerning suture selection and the surgeon's preference plays a role. In most studies, either non-absorbable or absorbable strong core sutures are used. Generally, two parallel strands are used - e.g. side-to-side absorbable sutures - with the knots hidden inside the tendon gap. However, up to six strands have also been used in order to increase the mechanical strength of the repair. Recent studies have used strong non-absorbable sutures (Orthocord®/ FibreWire®/Ethibond®) in order to maximize the strength of the repair as much as possible (7). The most commonly used suture techniques are Bunnell-, Kessler-modified Kessler- and Krackow-types (Figure 2)[19]. There are no convincing controlled comparisons between these different suture types [6, 18, 19]. In general terms, some kind of a locking-type suture is preferred, such as a Kessler-type of suture. This has been shown to increase the mechanical strength and thereby reduce the risk of re-rupture. Other configurations, like wire pull-out are probably rarely used anymore. The locking mechanism will make it easier to handle the tendon during surgery as well as ensure that the repair does not over-tighten. Whether necessary or not, several smaller non-absorbable sutures are placed at the tendon margins in order to improve the repair and make the overlap between the ruptured ends smoother. On the other hand specific epitenon sutures (i.e. peripheral criss-cross stich) with multiple strands have shown increased load to failure that greatly increases the strength of the core repair [4, 12]. This is not the same as augmentation, which was traditionally used 20-30 years ago, but has today been shown to increase the risk of surgical complications, especially due to the much longer surgical wound and the risk of healing problems [17].

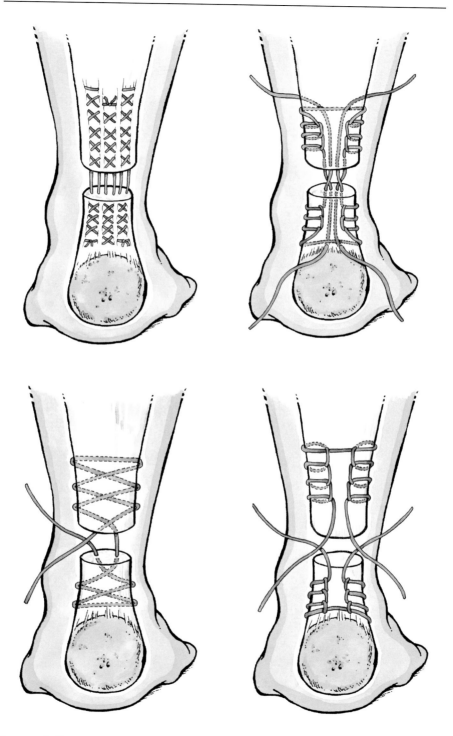

Figure 2. Different types of suture configurations

Augmentation may be considered in case of extreme tissue fraying, very distal rupture, and poor holding strength of the sutures. Some surgeons have used artificial ligaments, such as braided polyester and polypropylene, while others have used the plantaris tendon or a proximal section of the Achilles tendon, either as a free flap, or turn-down flap [1]. There are other more complex and – accordingly - less frequently used possibilities, like allografts and the peroneus tendons. Augmentation will always require a larger incision and the risk of wound complications is thereby increased.

After the repair is completed, the paratendon should always be carefully closed - before the skin is closed with interrupted sutures - without any tension. Post-operatively, the leg is immobilized either using a short leg plaster cast or a brace. Provided the suture strength is judged as satisfactory, range of motion exercises are generally started after approximately 10-14 days. Weight-bearing should be started as early as possible.

Discussion

Comparisons of different open techniques, like the study of Aktas and co-workers [1], who compared end-to-end suture to augmented repair and demonstrated better surgical outcome concerning local tenderness, skin adhesion scar and tendon thickness in the end-to-end suture group. This technique provided a safer and more reliable treatment with a low risk of complications compared with the plantaris tendon augmentation. On the other hand, Ateschrang and co-workers [2] studied open augmentation repair using the Silfverskiöld technique, with a turn-down flap. In 104 patients, the re-rupture rate was 2% and the infection rate 3%. They concluded that the Silfverskiöld augmentation technique was a good alternative, even in athletes. The infection rate was surprisingly low.

Uchiyama and co-workers [23] studied a new technique for surgical Achilles tendon repair designed to allow for more stability and earlier rehabilitation. They operated on 100 patients using the Tsugue suture, where each of five bundles were gathered in the longitudinal direction and fixed with a Bunnell-type suture. They concluded that this surgical technique produced strong repair stability and enabled earlier (two weeks) weight-bearing and range of motion exercises.

Olsson and co-workers [16] studied a similar technique in a randomized controlled study of 100 patients. They compared their surgical outcomes with non-surgical protocols, using a weight-bearing brace for six and eight weeks, respectively. The open surgical technique utilized two strong semi-absorbable core sutures and a running circumferential criss-cross technique to increase the strength of the repair as much as possible in order to reduce the risk of re-rupture (Figure 3). The surgical group underwent an accelerated rehabilitation program. The results were very promising, with 0% re-rupture in the surgical group, compared with 10% re-rupture rate in the non-surgical group. Accordingly, the authors recommended this type of surgical treatment. The complication rate was low, with a few superficial wound infections; all were effectively treated with antibiotics. One patient sustained a partial re-rupture – that was successfully treated without revision surgery.

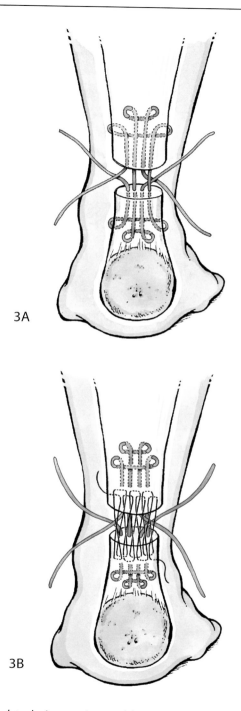

3A

3B

Figure 3. Surgical technique using stable sutures with Fibre-wire and additional sutures at the rupture level. (Figure 3B is reproduced with permission from American Journal of Sports Medicine).

Strauss and co-workers [20] studied the post-operative complications after open end-to-end repair of acute Achilles tendon ruptures. They found that open repair provided consistent good and excellent long-term results. In this study high clinical success rate was associated with a relatively high incidence of post-operative complications. However, with careful attention to the surgical wound, and careful repair of the paratenon and patient adherence to post-operative rehabilitation protocols, open surgical repair using end-to-end suture is a reliable treatment for active patients.

Khan and co-workers [10, 11] stated that there is a lack of consensus in terms of the best option for the treatment of acute Achilles tendon ruptures. They performed a meta-analysis of total [12] randomised controlled trials, involving approximately 800 patients and concerned with the effectiveness of different interventions for the treatment of acute ruptures. They showed that open treatment of acute Achilles tendon ruptures significantly reduced the risk of re-rupture compared with non-surgical treatment; however, surgical treatment was associated with a significantly higher risk of other complications, like infections and wound break-down. They also mentioned that risks may be reduced by performing percutaneous surgery. Also, post-operative splinting, i.e. the use of functional brace reduced the overall complication rate. Despite this well-conducted meta-analysis there is no overall consensus on the optimal treatment of acute Achilles tendon ruptures.

Conclusions

On the basis of the randomized studies, there is evidence that open surgical management of acute Achilles tendon ruptures significantly reduces the risk of re-rupture compared with non-surgical treatment, but it has the drawback of a significantly higher risk of other complications, including wound infection.

These complications may be reduced by performing surgery in a mini-open fashion. Post-operative splinting in a functional brace rather than a cast appears to reduce hospital stay, time off work and sports, and most probably lowers the overall complication rate.

There is inadequate evidence to comment on different suture techniques, different non-surgical management regimes and the different aspects of post-operative cast immobilization. Recent study has shown a very low risk of re-rupture (as low as 0%) using a strong suture technique.

References

1. Aktas S, Kocaoglu B, Nalbantoglu U, Seyhan M, Guven O. End-to-end versus augmented repair in the treatment of acute Achilles tendon ruptures. J Foot Ankle Surg. 2007;46(5):336-340.

2. Ateschrang A, Gratzer C, Ochs U, Ochs BG, Weise K. [Open augmented repair according to Silfverskjold for Achilles tendon rupture: an alternative for athletes?]. Z Orthop Unfall. 2007;145(2):207-211.

3. Costa ML, MacMillan K, Halliday D, et al. Randomised controlled trials of immediate weight-bearing mobilisation for rupture of the tendo Achillis. J Bone Joint Surg Br. 2006;88(1):69-77.

4. Hirpara KM, Sullivan PJ, Raheem O, O'Sullivan ME. A biomechanical analysis of multistrand repairs with the Silfverskiold peripheral cross-stitch. J Bone Joint Surg Br. 2007;89(10):1396-1401.

5. Houshian S, Tscherning T, Riegels-Nielsen P. The epidemiology of Achilles tendon rupture in a Danish county. Injury. 1998;29(9):651-654.

6. Jaakkola JI, Hutton WC, Beskin JL, Lee GP. Achilles tendon rupture repair: biomechanical comparison of the triple bundle technique versus the Krakow locking loop technique. Foot Ankle Int. 2000;21(1):14-17.

7. Jones MP, Khan RJ, Carey Smith RL. Surgical interventions for treating acute achilles tendon rupture: key findings from a recent cochrane review. J Bone Joint Surg Am. 2012;94(12):e88.

8. Jozsa L, Kannus P. Histopathological findings in spontaneous tendon ruptures. Scand J Med Sci Sports. 1997;7(2):113-118.

9. Kerkhoffs GM, Struijs PA, Raaymakers EL, Marti RK. Functional treatment after surgical repair of acute Achilles tendon rupture: wrap vs walking cast. Arch Orthop Trauma Surg. 2002;122(2):102-105.

10. Khan RJ, Carey Smith RL. Surgical interventions for treating acute Achilles tendon ruptures. Cochrane Database Syst Rev. 2010(9):CD003674.

11. Khan RJ, Fick D, Keogh A, Crawford J, Brammar T, Parker M. Treatment of acute achilles tendon ruptures. A meta-analysis of randomized, controlled trials. J Bone Joint Surg Am. 2005;87(10):2202-2210.

12. Kim PT, Aoki M, Tokita F, Ishii S. Tensile strength of cross-stitch epitenon suture. J Hand Surg Br. 1996;21(6):821-823.

13. Maffulli N. The clinical diagnosis of subcutaneous tear of the Achilles tendon. A prospective study in 174 patients. Am J Sports Med. 1998;26(2):266-270.

14. Maffulli N, Longo UG, Maffulli GD, Khanna A, Denaro V. Achilles tendon ruptures in elite athletes. Foot Ankle Int. 2011;32(1):9-15.

15. Maffulli N, Longo UG, Maffulli GD, Rabitti C, Khanna A, Denaro V. Marked pathological changes proximal and distal to the site of rupture in acute Achilles tendon ruptures. Knee Surg Sports Traumatol Arthrosc. 2010.

16. Olsson N, Silbernagel KG, Eriksson BI, et al. Stable surgical repair with accelerated rehabilitation versus nonsurgical treatment for acute achilles tendon ruptures: a randomized controlled study. Am J Sports Med. 2013;41(12):2867-2876.

17. Pajala A, Kangas J, Siira P, Ohtonen P, Leppilahti J. Augmented compared with nonaugmented surgical repair of a fresh total Achilles tendon rupture. A prospective randomized study. J Bone Joint Surg Am. 2009;91(5):1092-1100.

18. Park HG, Moon DH, Yoon JM. Limited open repair of ruptured Achilles tendons with Bunnel-type sutures. Foot Ankle Int. 2001;22(12):985-987.

19. Sadoghi P, Rosso C, Valderrabano V, Leithner A, Vavken P. Initial Achilles tendon repair strength--synthesized biomechanical data from 196 cadaver repairs. Int Orthop. 2012;36(9):1947-1951.

20. Strauss EJ, Ishak C, Jazrawi L, Sherman O, Rosen J. Operative treatment of acute Achilles tendon ruptures: an institutional review of clinical outcomes. Injury. 2007;38(7):832-838.

21. Suchak AA, Bostick GP, Beaupre LA, Durand DC, Jomha NM. The influence of early weight-bearing compared with non-weight-bearing after surgical repair of the Achilles tendon. J Bone Joint Surg Am. 2008;90(9):1876-1883.

22. Tallon C, Maffulli N, Ewen SW. Ruptured Achilles tendons are significantly more degenerated than tendinopathic tendons. Med Sci Sports Exerc. 2001;33(12):1983-1990.

23. Uchiyama E, Nomura A, Takeda Y, Hiranuma K, Iwaso H. A modified operation for Achilles tendon ruptures. Am J Sports Med. 2007;35(10):1739-1743.

"The outcome of any serious research can only be to make two questions grow where only one grew before."

Thorstein Veblen

CHAPTER 23

CURRENT CONCEPTS:

TREATMENT FOR INSERTIONAL ACHILLES TENDINOPATHY AND CHRONIC RETROCALCANEAL BURSITIS

Johannes I. Wiegerinck, Ruben Zwiers, Umile G. Longo, C. Niek van Dijk

Take Home Message

- There is limited evidence for the treatment of insertional Achilles tendinopathy.

- Shockwave therapy is a promising treatment for insertional Achilles tendinopathy.

- Surgical intervention for insertional Achilles tendinopathy has a high patient satisfaction rate.

- Open surgery for retrocalcaneal bursitis has a relatively high complication rate.

- Chronic retrocalcaneal bursitis can be treated well by minimally invasive procedures.

Introduction

Insertional Achilles tendon pathology can be divided into insertional Achilles tendinopathy and chronic retrocalcaneal bursitis. Although symptoms may be similar and these pathologies may coexist, their management differs significantly [29]. An overview of available systematic reviews on the treatment of these pathologies is provided below (Table 1).

Study	Number of Studies Included	Investigated Treatment Modalities	Methodological Quality (AMSTAR)
Insertional Achilles tendinopathy			
Kearney and Costa [14]	11	Non-surgical and surgical treatment	2/11
Wiegerinck and co-workers [32]	14	Non-surgical and surgical treatment	4/11
Retrocalcaneal bursitis			
Wiegerinck and co-workers [33]	15	Surgical treatment	4/11

Table 1. Available systematic reviews.

Insertional Achilles tendinopathy

Two systematic reviews on the management of insertional Achilles tendinopathy are outlined [14, 32].

Kearney and Costa 2010 [14]

Kearney and Costa included 11 studies evaluating the treatment of. Of these, six evaluated surgical techniques following failed non-surgical management and five studies reported on non-surgical treatments. The aim of this review was to evaluate the effect of treatment modalities for insertional Achilles tendinopathy, based on functional outcome scores and pain scales.

The authors reported that, based on the included studies, technical advice about specific procedures could be provided. However, it was not possible to provide

Any evidence in terms of which surgical technique provides better outcomes in terms of function and reducing pain. The level of evidence of studies evaluating non-surgical treatment was higher. One randomized controlled trial (RCT) was included in addition to four prospective studies. As outlined by the authors, the methodological quality of these studies was low. Eccentric training, shockwave treatment and sclerosing injections were evaluated. Eccentric training had a reported 67% patient satisfaction. These results were poorer than those obtained by eccentric exercises for the management of non-insertional Achilles tendinopathy. Shockwave treatment showed to be effective, although the outcome could be affected by certain methodological inconsistencies. The power of the study on sclerosing injections did not allow any conclusions to be drawn. In conclusion, the authors stated that there is a consensus on the best non-surgical methods for the management of patients with insertional Achilles tendinopathy. Eccentric training and shockwave therapy showed some degree of effectiveness [14].

Major Complications	Minor Complications
Achilles tendon rupture	Discomfort
Any re-operation	Superficial infections
Deep venous thrombosis	Minor wound problems
Reflex dystrophy	Scar tenderness/hypertrophy
Persisting neuralgia	Mild form of paraesthesia
Deep infections/major wound problems	Prolonged hospitalization

Table 2. Classification of complications.

Wiegerinck and co-workers 2012 [32]

The study by Wiegerinck and co-workers added an analysis of the quality of therapeutic studies on insertional Achilles tendinopathy as well as an evaluation on which treatment for insertional Achilles tendinopathy is the most effective. The primary outcome measures were a change in numeric pain score (e.g., the Visual Analogue Scale) and reported patient satisfaction. The Coleman Methodology Score (CMS) was used to assess the quality of the included articles. Fourteen trials were included, evaluating 452 procedures in 433 patients. Overall, the quality of the included studies was low – mean CMS: 58 (range 36-78); for surgical studies: CMS: 52 (range 36-67); and non surgical studies: CMS: 62 (range 44-78). Eight studies evaluated non-surgical interventions. Two studies analysed injections (hyperosmolar dextrose and sclerosing polidocanol), both showing a significant decrease in VAS. Four studies evaluated eccentric exercises, each showing a significant decrease in VAS. However, a large group of patients was unsatisfied with the treatment. Furthermore, two studies evaluated extracorporeal shockwave therapy (ESWT). ESWT was shown to be superior to both wait-and-see and an eccentric training regime. Finally, one small study evaluated Laser CO2, TECAR and Cryoultrasound; all showed a significant decrease in VAS. Five surgical techniques evaluated 200 patients, including 211 tendons (procedures) (Table 3) [8, 12, 18, 19, 30, 34]. Five studies reported on patient satisfaction, all showing a relative good outcome regarding patient satisfaction: 163 of 183 patients (89%) reported excellent or good satisfaction [8, 18, 19, 30, 34]. Complications were documented in 52 (23%) cases; including seven major complications (3.1%), the number of complications differed substantially between techniques (Table 2, 3). Furthermore, the authors outlined the importance of proper documentation of tendon calcifications and the diagnostic method in the included studies; in other words, treatment results may differ in patients with a bony pathology compared to a group without bony pathology. Thus, it was stated that imaging is essential in the diagnosis and treatment of insertional Achilles tendinopathy. Nine of 14 studies reported on the presence of a bony disorder in every case [8, 10, 12, 13, 16, 18, 21, 24, 34]. Four of six studies evaluating surgery for insertional Achilles tendinopathy reported on bony disorders [8, 12, 18, 34]. The diagnostic method was based on imaging in 12 studies and was unclear in two studies. It was concluded that there are numerous treatment modalities - surgical and non-surgical – for insertional Achilles tendinopathy. Some differences in outcome between surgical techniques were found, mainly regarding complication rates (Table 3). Despite these differences, patient satisfaction is relatively high in all studies. Wiegerinck and co-workers stated that it was not possible to draw any conclusion regarding the best surgical technique for insertional Achilles tendinopathy. Based on the outcomes of the non-surgical studies, there appears to be no evidence for advising full range eccentric exercises for insertional Achilles tendinopathy, as patient satisfaction is insufficient compared with other treatment modalities. The results of floor level eccentric exercises are promising, as is ESWT; however, more high-level evidence studies are necessary in terms of the best available treatment [32].

Discussion on insertional Achilles tendinopathy

Kearney and Costa [14] concluded that non-surgical treatment is preferred prior to surgical treatment. In addition, they concluded that non-surgical treatment favoured eccentric training and ESWT [14]. The results of the review by Wiegerinck and co-workers showed a large group of unsatisfied patients after eccentric training compared with other non-surgical treatments [8, 9, 13, 24]. The reason for this difference in interpretation of largely equal data is uncertain. Eccentric exercises can be divided between full range of motion and limited (floor-level) exercises. Kearney and Costa did not specify for these different training regimes. In addition, there may be a difference in primary outcomes between the two reviews, leading to a different interpretation of the results. As eccentric training has a substantial effect on decreasing pain, this may be interpreted as effective; Kearney and Costa may have based their conclusion on this, regardless of the level of patient satisfaction.

Both studies conclude that there is a substantial lack of evidence on any currently performed treatment (non-surgical or surgical). A recent review stated to evaluate ESWT for both insertional and mid-portion Achilles tendinopathy [1]. Indeed, studies on both pathologies were included; however, the results did not describe the effects individually and, hence, no conclusion could be drawn regarding the separate pathologies.

Retrocalcaneal bursitis

The initial treatment of chronic retrocalcaneal bursitis is non-surgical and at first consists of activity cessation, a heel raise inlay and non-steroidal anti-inflammatory drugs (NSAIDs). Surgical intervention is an option in case non-surgical treatment fails. No systematic reviews on the non-surgical treatment of retrocalcaneal bursitis were available at the time of publication; in addition, only one systematic review on the surgical treatment of retrocalcaneal bursitis was found [33].

Wiegerinck and co-workers 2012 [33]

In this systematic review, the authors aimed to systematically analyse the results of surgical treatments for retrocalcaneal bursitis. The primary goal was to evaluate the efficiency of the provided treatment based on patient satisfaction and complication rates (divided into major and minor complications, Table 2). The quality of the studies included was assessed using the "GRADE" quality assessment scale. Fifteen trials were included, evaluating altogether 547 procedures in 461 patients. Twelve trials reported on open surgical techniques; three studies evaluated endoscopic techniques. In all open surgical techniques, the postero-superior calcaneal process was resected; all but one also excised the retrocalcaneal bursa. One study performed a calcaneal wedge osteotomy (Zadek or Keck & Kelly) + Substantial differences were found in terms of complications satisfaction (30-42% with no change in complaints) +. Six studies reported opposing results, with good or excellent satisfaction in 81-95% of patients [6, 7, 17, 20, 25, 27]. Likewise, the number of complications differed greatly (Table 4). According to the authors of the included studies, a possible explanation for persisting symptoms after open surgery is inferior visualization compared with arthroscopic intervention.

The postero-superior calcaneal process and retrocalcaneal bursa were resected in all patients when endoscopically treated, and 90% of the patients reported excellent or good satisfaction. The complication ratio was low (Table 4). The quality of the included studies revealed a poor level of methodological quality in most studies. As no RCTs were included, caution should be taken with the interpretation of the findings of this study [4]. There are evident differences in outcomes between techniques. Endoscopic interventions show consistently low complication rates with consistently high patient satisfaction levels compared with open surgical techniques. All authors publishing on endoscopic intervention stated that the procedure requires significant experience on the part of the surgeons involved. The review concluded that there are many different surgical techniques to treat retrocalcaneal bursitis. Regardless of technique, the resection of sufficient bone is essential for a good outcome. Despite the relatively low level of evidence of the included studies, it can be concluded that endoscopic surgery is superior to open intervention for the treatment of [33].

Discussion on retrocalcaneal bursitis

As mentioned, only one systematic review on the surgical treatment of retrocalcaneal bursitis was found. No systematic reviews on the non-surgical treatment of retrocalcaneal bursitis were found. Despite the limitation of a low level of evidence in terms of the treatment of retrocalcaneal bursitis, based on the current evidence it can be concluded that endoscopic surgical treatment for retrocalcaneal bursitis (Chapter 14) is superior to open techniques. An important limitation of studies on retrocalcaneal bursitis is the confusing terminology – this is further discussed in the general discussion of this chapter.

Discussion and Conclusion

An important limitation of studies on insertional Achilles tendinopathy and retrocalcaneal bursitis is the lack of consistent terminology (Chapter 1). As many find the terminology confusing, these pathologies are susceptible to subjective interpretation and different denominations of a combination of clinical symptoms. This can result in a mixture of pathologies in a single study.

We found 29 therapeutic studies that met the inclusion criteria of these systematic reviews [14, 32, 33]. Only one of them was a RCT; three were prospective in design while the remaining were retrospective. The number of high-level studies and the total number of studies for these two different pathologies is low.

Author	No. of Proce-dures	Complications		Surgical Technique		
		Major	Minor	Positioning	Approach	Description of Procedure
Elias[8]	40	0	2	Prone	Longit. mid-line incision over Achilles tendon.	Diseased part of Achilles tendon resected. Post-sup. calcaneal ostectomy+spur resection. If 50-100% of Achilles tendon detached, reattachment and FHL autograft.
McGarvey[19]	22	0	9	Prone	Longit. mid-line inc. through Achilles tendon and insertion.	Calcification debridement if excessive (>50%); plantaris augm. or bone anchors if necessary; retrocalcaneal bursectomy, Achilles tendon defect approximated with absor. sutures.
Johnson[12*]	22	1†	2			Same technique as McGarvey.
Maffulli[18]	21	0	6	Prone	Medial longit. inc. up to 1/3 of Achilles tendon.	Bursectomy, abnormal Achilles tendon appearance were explored by tenotomise (not repaired) and excised, if 1/3 or > of Achilles tendon was detached reattached with bone anchors.
Wagner[30**]	47	2±	2	Prone	Medial J. incision	Achilles tendon and paratenon debridement, no/partial (<50%) Achilles tendon detachment; sup. calcaneal tuberosity resection. Reattachment with four bone anchors.
Yodlowski[34]	41	1†	17	Prone	Lateral longit. Inc. between Achilles tendon and supero-lateral crest of calcaneus	Pre-operative AB iv. Fat pad; bursa; sup. calc. tuberosity resection. Excision of scar tissue; adhesions between Achilles tendon and paratenon. Check for intratendinous calcifications; excised if present. Reattachment of Achilles tendon with bone anchors if necessary.
Totals	226	7 (3.1 %)	45 (20%)			

* = Same surgical technique as McGarvey.
AT = Achilles tendon.
** = Same study comparing complete detachment of the Achilles tendon with partial or no detachment.
AB = Antibiotics.
±= One substantial wound infection; one surgical revision (complete detachment).
†= One deep venous thrombosis.
§ = One Achilles tendon rupture; two major wound problems.

Table 3. Studies describing surgical techniques. Outlined are a number of procedures, major and minor complications, and surgical techniques.

Open Surgical Techniques	Number of Evaluated Procedures	Procedure	Intervention		
			Position	Approach	Procedure & Achilles tendon Involvement
Anderson[2]	35	Open	Prone	Lateral	Anchor reattachment if >50% of Achilles tendon was detached. Resection of posterior-superior process and retrocalcaneal bursa
	31	Open	Prone	Central (Tendon-Split)	Anchor reattachment if >50% of Achilles tendon was detached. Resection of posterior-superior process and retrocalcaneal bursa
Angermann[3]	40	Open	NR	Lateral	Resection of posterior-superior process by means of osteotomy
Chen[6]	30	Open	Supine	Medial	Pre-operative antibiotics. Resection of posterior-superior process
DeVries[7]	22	Open	Prone	Medial J	Complete Achilles tendon detachment. Resection of posterior-superior
Biyani[5]	37	Open	Prone	Lateral	Resection of posterior-superior process with power saw
Lehto[17]	28	Open	NR	Bilateral	No Achilles tendon involvement. Resection of posterior-superior process and retrocalcaneal bursa
Nesse[20]	35	Open	NR	34 Medial 1 Lateral	NR
Pauker[23]	19	Open	NR	18 Lateral 10 Medial	No Achilles tendon involvement. Retrocalcaneal bursa was not removed
Schepsis[25]	21	Open	Prone	Medial J	No Achilles tendon involvement. Resection of posterior-superior process and retrocalcaneal bursa
Taylor[28]	61	Open	Prone	Lateral	Keck & Kelly Osteotomy
	8	Open	Prone	Lateral	Zadek Osteotomy
Sella[27]	16	Open	Supine	Lateral	Resection of posterior-superior process and retrocalcaneal bursa
Watson[31]	14	Open	Prone	Postero-Lateral	Achilles tendon detached and reattached with non-absorbable sutures. Resection of posterior-superior process and retrocalcaneal bursa
Totals Open Techniques	397				
Endoscopic Techniques					
Jerosch[11]	81	Endoscopic	Supine (1st 10 prone)	Two Portal ECP	Two Portal ECP (van Dijk technique)
Ortmann[22]	30	Endoscopic	Supine	Two Portal ECP	Two Portal ECP (van Dijk technique)
Scholten[26]	39*	Endoscopic	Prone	Two Portal ECP	Two Portal ECP (van Dijk technique)
Total Endoscopic	150	Open			

NR = Not reported.   * = Authors were contacted to provide these data.   AT = Achilles tendon.
• = Data acquired through author.   • ECP = Endoscopic Calcaneoplasty.

Table 4. Overview of surgical techniques, complication rates, clinical results, patient satisfaction and quality assessment per study (categorized for open and endoscopic techniques). Totals and weighed means are provided for the open surgical sub-group and the endoscopic sub-group.

Complications		Decrease in pain score / Change in subjective questionnaire (range)	Satisfaction / Other Outcome Data				GRADE
Major	Minor		Excellent	Good	Unchanged	Poor	
0	2	AOFAS pre-operative: 54 (10-72) AOFAS post-operative: 86 (10-100)	Satisfaction NR* Similar groups in age; duration of symptoms				Low
1	3	AOFAS pre-operative: 43 (10-67) AOFAS post-operative: 81 (10-100)					
0	4	Patient Satisfaction	20	8	9	3	Very Low
NR	NR	Patient Satisfaction	27	0	0	3	Very Low
1	3	VAS pre-operative: 7.9 (2-10) VAS post-operative: 1.6 (1-4.5)	10	6	1	0	Low
3	11	Patient Satisfaction	0	21	12	3	Very Low
4	0	Patient Satisfaction	13	10	2	3	Low
3	19	VAS pre-operative: 55 (15-90) VAS post-operative: 15 (0-88)		20	10	5	Very Low
NR	NR	Patient Satisfaction		15	2	2	Very Low
1	0	Patient Satisfaction	13	5	6	0	Very Low
1	109	Patient Satisfaction	25	14	15	7	Very Low
0	9	Patient Satisfaction	5	3	0	0	
3	0	AOFAS post-operative good: 87 AOFAS post-operative poor: 25	0	13	0	3	Low
0	0	AOFAS post-operative: 98.6	0	13	1	0	Low
17 (4.3%)	X 160 (40%)		113 (34%)	128 (39%)	58 (18%)	29 (9%)	Very Low
Endoscopic Techniques							
0	1	Ogilvie Harris	41	34	3	3	Low
1	0	AOFAS pre-operative: 62 (SD: 12.7) AOFAS post-operative: 97 (SD: 6.1)	26	3	0	1	Low
0	1	Ogilvie Harris	24	6	4	2	Low
1 (0.7%)	2 (1.3%)		91 (62%)	43 (29%)	7 (5%)	6 (4%)	Low

NR = Not reported.   * = Authors were contacted to provide these data.   AT = Achilles tendon.
• = Data acquired through author.   • ECP = Endoscopic Calcaneoplasty.

Table 4 – CONTINUED – Overview of surgical techniques, complication rates, clinical results, patient satisfaction and quality assessment per study (categorized for open and endoscopic techniques). Totals and weighed means are provided for the open surgical sub-group and the endoscopic sub-group.

Conclusion

No definitive recommendations can be made in terms of the best treatment for insertional Achilles tendinopathy or retrocalcaneal bursitis. There is a consensus (but no evidence) that non-surgical treatment should be advised prior to surgical intervention.

Regarding insertional Achilles tendinopathy, the effect of eccentric training is doubtful and ESWT is promising. Additional research is necessary to reach stronger conclusions. Surgery for (calcified) insertional Achilles tendinopathy appears to be effective; however - and again - this is based on marginal evidence.

Concerning retrocalcaneal bursitis, subjective outcome scores indicate a degree of effectiveness regardless of the surgical technique. It should be noted that the number of complications was substantially lower and patient satisfaction was substantially higher after endoscopic procedures. The results are, therefore, in favour of the endoscopic approach. This, however, is based on a limited level of evidence and should be interpreted with caution. Future studies should focus on methodological quality in addition to a clear description of the treated pathology.

References

1. Al-Abbad H, Simon JV. The effectiveness of extracorporeal shock wave therapy on chronic Achilles tendinopathy: a systematic review. Foot Ankle Int 2013;34(1):33-41.

2. Anderson JA, Suero E, O'Loughlin PF, Kennedy JG. Surgery for retrocalcaneal bursitis: a tendon-splitting versus a lateral approach. Clin Orthop Relat Res 2008;466(7):1678-1682.

3. Angermann P. Chronic retrocalcaneal bursitis treated by resection of the calcaneus. Foot Ankle 1990;10(5):285-287.

4. Audige L, Bhandari M, Griffin D, Middleton P, Reeves BC. Systematic reviews of nonrandomized clinical studies in the orthopaedic literature. Clin Orthop Relat Res 2004;(427):249-257.

5. Biyani A, Jones DA. Results of excision of calcaneal prominence. Acta Orthop Belg 1993;59(1):45-49.

6. Chen CH, Huang PJ, Chen TB et al. Surgical treatment for (postero-superior) calcaneal exostosis. Kaohsiung J Med Sci 2001;17(8):419-422.

7. DeVries JG, Summerhays B, Guehlstorf DW. Surgical correction of Haglund's triad using complete detachment and reattachment of the Achilles tendon. J Foot Ankle Surg 2009;48(4):447-451.

8. Elias I, Raikin SM, Besser MP, Nazarian LN. Outcomes of chronic insertional Achilles tendinosis using FHL autograft through single incision. Foot Ankle Int 2009;30(3):197-204.

9. Fahlstrom M, Jonsson P, Lorentzon R, Alfredson H. Chronic Achilles tendon pain treated with eccentric calf-muscle training. Knee Surg Sports Traumatol Arthrosc 2003;11(5):327-333.

10. Furia JP. High-energy extracorporeal shockwave therapy as a treatment for insertional Achilles tendinopathy. Am J Sports Med 2006;34(5):733-740.

11. Jerosch J, Schunck J, Sokkar SH. Endoscopic calcaneoplasty (ECP) as a surgical treatment of Haglund's syndrome. Knee Surg Sports Traumatol Arthrosc 2007;15(7):927-934.

12. Johnson KW, Zalavras C, Thordarson DB. Surgical management of insertional calcific Achilles tendinosis with a central tendon splitting approach. Foot Ankle Int 2006;27(4):245-250.

13. Jonsson P, Alfredson H, Sunding K, Fahlstrom M, Cook J. New regimen for eccentric calf-muscle training in patients with chronic insertional Achilles tendinopathy: results of a pilot study. Br J Sports Med 2008;42(9):746-749.

14. Kearney R, Costa ML. Insertional Achilles tendinopathy management: a systematic review. Foot Ankle Int 2010;31(8):689-694.

15. Keck SW, Kelly PJ. Evaluation of surgical treatment of eighteen patients. J Bone Joint Surg Am 1965;47-A:267-273.

16. Knobloch K. Eccentric training in Achilles tendinopathy: is it harmful to tendon microcirculation? Br J Sports Med 2007;41(6):e2.

17. Lehto MUK, Jarvinen M, Suominen P. Chronic Achilles peritendinitis and retrocalcaneal bursitis. Knee Surg Sports Traumatol Arthrosc 1994;2:182-185.

18. Maffulli N, Testa V, Capasso G, Sullo A. Calcific insertional Achilles tendinopathy: reattachment with bone anchors. Am J Sports Med 2004;32(1):174-182.

19. McGarvey WC, Palumbo RC, Baxter DE, Leibman BD. Insertional Achilles tendinosis: surgical treatment through a central tendon splitting approach. Foot Ankle Int 2002;23(1):19-25.

20. Nesse E, Finsen V. Poor results after resection for Haglund's heel. Analysis of 35 heels in 23 patients after 3 years. Acta Orthop Scand 1994;65(1):107-109.

21. Ohberg L, Alfredson H. Sclerosing therapy in chronic Achilles tendon insertional pain-results of a pilot study. Knee Surg Sports Traumatol Arthrosc 2003;11(5):339-343.

22. Ortmann FW, McBryde AM. Endoscopic bony and soft-tissue decompression of the retrocalcaneal space for the treatment of Haglund deformity and retrocalcaneal bursitis. Foot Ankle Int 2007;28(2):149-153.

23. Pauker M, Katz K, Yosipovitch Z. Calcaneal ostectomy for Haglund disease. J Foot Surg 1992;31(6):588-589.

24. Rompe JD, Furia J, Maffulli N. Eccentric loading compared with shock wave treatment for chronic insertional Achilles tendinopathy. A randomized, controlled trial. J Bone Joint Surg Am 2008;90(1):52-61.

25. Schepsis AA, Wagner C, Leach RE. Surgical management of Achilles tendon overuse injuries. A long-term follow-up study. Am J Sports Med 1994;22(5):611-619.

26. Scholten PE, van Dijk CN. Endoscopic calcaneoplasty. Foot Ankle Clin 2006;11(2):439-46, viii.

27. Sella EJ, Caminear DS, McLarney EA. Haglund's syndrome. J Foot Ankle Surg 1998;37(2):110-114.

28. Taylor GJ. Prominence of the calcaneus: is operation justified? J Bone Joint Surg Br 1986;68(3):467-470.

29. van Dijk CN, van Sterkenburg MN, Wiegerinck JI, Karlsson J, Maffulli N. Terminology for Achilles tendon related disorders. Knee Surg Sports Traumatol Arthrosc 2011;19(5):835-841.

30. Wagner E, Gould JS, Kneidel M, Fleisig GS, Fowler R. Technique and results of Achilles tendon detachment and reconstruction for insertional Achilles tendinosis. Foot Ankle Int 2006;27(9):677-684.

31. Watson AD, Anderson RB, Davis WH. Comparison of results of retrocalcaneal decompression for retrocalcaneal bursitis and insertional Achilles tendinosis with calcific spur. Foot Ankle Int 2000;21(8):638-642.

313

32. Wiegerinck JI, Kerkhoffs GM, van Sterkenburg MN, Sierevelt IN, van Dijk CN. Treatment for insertional Achilles tendinopathy: a systematic review. Knee Surg Sports Traumatol Arthrosc 2012.

33. Wiegerinck JI, Kok AC, van Dijk CN. Surgical Treatment of Chronic Retrocalcaneal Bursitis: A Systematic Review. Arthroscopy 2012.

34. Yodlowski ML, Scheller AD, Jr., Minos L. Surgical treatment of Achilles tendinitis by decompression of the retrocalcaneal bursa and the superior calcaneal tuberosity. Am J Sports Med 2002;30(3):318-321.

35. Zadek I. An operation for the cure of achillobursitis. American Journal of Surgery 1939;43:542-546.

"Surgery is always second best. If you can do something else, it's better."

Dr. John Kirklin

Chapter 24

Current Concepts:

Treatment of Mid-portion Achilles Tendinopathy

Ruben Zwiers, Johannes I. Wiegerinck, C. Niek van Dijk

Take Home Message

• *Eccentric exercise is supported by most evidence and is, therefore, the treatment of first choice for mid-portion Achilles tendinopathy.*

• *Other non-surgical treatment modalities have shown promising results; however, further research is required.*

• *There is a lack of evidence regarding the surgical treatment of mid-portion Achilles tendinopathy.*

Introduction

In the treatment of mid-portion Achilles tendinopathy, both non-surgical and surgical options play a role. The initial treatment usually consists of non-surgical management, but in approximately 25% of the patients a surgical intervention is still needed [33, 36, 37]. In this chapter, an overview of the current evidence is provided.

Mid-portion Achilles tendinopathy

Several systematic reviews evaluating the treatment of mid-portion Achilles tendinopathy were identified. However, only six reviews solely report on the treatment of mid-portion Achilles tendinopathy[21, 32, 40, 41, 46, 62]. Since no systematic literature reviews have been conducted in terms of surgical treatment, the main focus here is on non-surgical treatment.

Magnussen and co-workers[40] (2009)

Magnussen and co-workers[40] performed a systematic literature search to provide a clear overview of the available evidence for the non-surgical treatment of mid-portion Achilles tendinopathy. Only prospective randomized controlled trials that focused solely on the treatment of mid-portion Achilles tendinopathy were included. If the localization of the tendinopathy was not adequately described, the study was excluded, resulting in 16 trials eligible for evaluation. Numeric pain scores were used as primary outcome measures, and additionally other common outcome measures, like range of motion, return to activity, peak torque measurements, pain with a variety of provocative tests, and change in tendon diameter, were reported.

Eccentric exercise

Four studies compared eccentric exercise with a control group. In two of these studies, the control group underwent concentric exercises[39, 48, 72], whereas two studies used wait-and-see or normal activity in the control group[44, 59]. One study compared two different treatment protocols consisting of a combination of eccentric and concentric exercises[72]. The four studies comparing eccentric exercise with a control group showed a statistically significant difference in pain score in favour of eccentric exercise.

One study found no differences in pain scores between a group undergoing eccentric exercise without restrictions and eccentric exercise with restrictions on running and jumping[72]. Another trial showed eccentric exercises to be more effective in decreasing pain scores in comparison to night splints alone. However, no differences were detected when the combination of eccentric exercise and night splints were compared with either eccentric exercise or night splints alone[61]. Additionally, one study showed a decrease in pain scores in a group wearing individualized insoles compared with the control group, whereas no difference was reported when comparing those insoles with eccentric training.

Other non-surgical treatment

Two studies that investigated the effectiveness of extracorporeal shockwave therapy in mid-portion Achilles tendinopathy were identified[9, 59]. One compared ESWT with a placebo and did not find any effect after three months[9]. The other study showed a significant improvement compared with a wait-and-see policy, but no benefit over eccentric exercises was reported[59].

316

Two randomized controlled trials compared local steroid injections with a placebo. The first study did not demonstrate any benefit in terms of pain scores 12 weeks after injection [12], while the other reported decreased pain scores four weeks after ultrasound-guided injections [18]. Furthermore three studies were identified that compared other injections with a placebo. Polidocanol [3] and haemodialysate [55] were found to be effective, whereas aprotinin [5] did not appear to improve pain scores. A significant decrease in pain was also reported after iontophoresis with corticosteroids [47] and topical glycerol nitrate [51].

The authors concluded that there is some evidence for beneficial effects of eccentric exercise. Together with its low cost and low risk, this option should be utilized for the initial management. Other treatment options have shown promising results, although further studies are needed.

Meyer and co-workers [46] (2009)

The effectiveness of eccentric exercise was investigated in a systematic review of randomized controlled trials by Meyer and co-workers [46]. Five studies met the inclusion criteria; however, two studies were excluded due to insufficient methodological quality according to the PEDro scale. The three studies included all used the protocol described by Alfredson and co-workers [4]. One study added different speeds of the exercises as reported by Stanish and co-workers [74]. The eccentric exercises were compared with deep friction massage, ultrasound and stretching in the study by Herrington and McCulloch [22], shockwave treatment or a wait-and-see policy in the study by Rompe and co-workers [59] and night splints in the study by Roos and co-workers [61]. In all studies, the outcomes of those subjects who completed eccentric exercises were significantly improved. In two studies, the results in the VISA-A score were significantly better in the eccentric exercise groups compared with the control groups. In the third study, no statistically significant differences were found; however, the authors found the results to be in favour of eccentric exercise. The authors of this systematic review concluded that similar positive outcome results could be achieved with eccentric exercises. However, due to the lack of compliance data, it was not possible to analyse the associations between compliance and outcomes.

Krämer and co-workers [32] (2010)

In 2010 Krämer and co-workers [32] published a systematic review of eccentric training in chronic mid-portion Achilles tendinopathy. Eight randomized controlled trials were included, and all but one reported on mid-portion Achilles tendinopathy alone. Each study evaluated eccentric training for 12 weeks; all reported a decrease of pain in both the intervention and control groups. As pooling of the data was not possible due to heterogeneity, percentages were used to compare the control and intervention groups. All differences in outcomes were expressed as percentages. The mean improvement in the eccentric training group was 50.2% (SD 19.5) and 36.4% (SD 21.8) in the control group. In all but one study, the outcomes were better in the intervention group. The authors of this systematic review concluded that eccentric exercise as a non-surgical treatment modality is promising. However, due to the heterogeneity in outcome measures and methodological limitations, no definite recommendations could be made.

Rowe and co-workers [62] (2012)

Rowe and co-workers [62] systematically searched the literature for studies that evaluated the effectiveness of any non-surgical intervention for mid-portion Achilles tendinopathy. Ultimately, 47 studies were included. Among these studies, five were of excellent quality, 17 of good quality and 25 of poor quality, according to the PEDro scale. The authors rated the strength of evidence supporting each treatment modality according to the number and quality of the articles reporting on that modality. Strong evidence was defined as: "consistent findings among multiple high-quality RCTs"; moderate evidence implied: "consistent findings among multiple low-quality RCTs and/or CCTs and/or one high-quality RCT". "One low-quality RCT and/or CCT" defined limited evidence, and when "inconsistent findings among multiple trials" were found, it was described as conflicting evidence. It was found that the evidence for eccentric loading and extra-corporeal shockwave therapy was strong, whereas for splinting or bracing, active rest, low-level laser therapy and concentric exercises the evidence was moderate. Limited evidence was found for foot orthotics and therapeutic ultrasound, and evidence was conflicting for topical glycerine trinitrate (Table 1).

Strength of Evidence	Criteria	Treatment Modalities
Strong	Consistent findings among multiple high-quality RCTs	– Eccentric exercise – ESWT
Moderate	Consistent findings among multiple low-quality RCTs and/or CCTs and/or one high-quality RCT	– Splinting or bracing – Active rest – LLLT – Concentric exercise
Limited	One low-quality RCT and/or CCT	– In-shoe foot orthoses – Therapeutic ultrasound
Conflicting	Inconsistent findings among multiple trials	– Topcal glycerine trinitrate
No Evidence	No RCTs or CCTs	– Taping – Soft-tissue mobilizations

Table 1. Strength of evidence supporting each treatment modality according to Rowe and co-workers [62]. RCT: Randomized controlled trial; CCT: Case controlled trial.

Malliaras and co-workers [41] (2013)

A recent review by Malliaras and co-workers [41] evaluated the evidence in studies that compared two or more loading programmes in Achilles and patellar tendinopathy. In addition, they reviewed the association between non-clinical outcomes or potential mechanisms and clinical outcomes. Four randomized trials were identified, of which three were of low quality while one was a high quality study. The first study showed that a greater proportion of the patients were satisfied with the results and that a higher proportion returned to a pre-injury level of activity after eccentric exercises in comparison with concentric exercises [39]. The second trial demonstrated the Silbernagel combined-loading programme as leading to lower VAS pain scores and higher patient satisfaction compared with calf raises and stretching [72]. Another study showed that the Stanish and Curwin programme [74] was superior to isotonic loading in terms of pain scores and return to sports [48]. The only high-quality study showed no differences in VISA-A scores between two groups treated with Silbernagel combined-loading, with and without activity restriction [71]. The authors of this systematic review concluded that there was only limited evidence concerning the effectiveness of the different loading programmes.

Gross and co-workers [21] (2013)

Gross and co-workers [21] performed a systematic review evaluating the efficacy of injection therapies for mid-portion Achilles tendinopathy. Only randomized controlled trials and cohort studies with a comparative control group reporting on clinical outcomes following injections in patients with mid-portion Achilles tendinopathy were eligible. This resulted in the inclusion of nine randomized controlled trials. Only one study [13] was of high methodological quality, following the Detsky methodological quality scale. One study reported on PRP [13], one on autologous blood injection [53], two on sclerosing agents [3, 86], one on protease inhibitors [5], one on haemodialysate [55, 55,] two on corticosteroids [18, 12], and one on prolotherapy [88].

In the study by de Jonge and co-workers [13], no difference was found in clinical and sonographic outcomes in the PRP group in comparison with the saline injection group. Both groups showed significant improvement in VISA-A scores and patient satisfaction. Moreover, in the one year follow-up of this population, the outcomes were similar.

Treatment with peritendinous autologous blood injections showed a similar improvement of VISA-A score in comparison with placebo injections in a study by Pearson and co-workers [53]. Alfredson and Ohberg [3] compared sclerosing agent injections with placebo injections, and reported a significant decrease in the VAS score in the group of patients treated with sclerosing injections. Wilberg and co-workers [86] reported no difference in outcome after investigating two concentrations of a sclerosing agent.

Brown and co-workers [5] reported no difference in outcomes after treatment with proteinase inhibitors in comparison with placebo injections. Pförringer and co-workers [55] investigated the injection of deproteinized haemodialysate, and reported a significant reduction of the diameter of the Achilles tendon. In addition, a reduction in pain was reported; however, the follow-up was short. The two studies reporting on outcomes after corticosteroid injections used different outcome measures. Fredberg and co-workers [18] reported that patients who underwent corticosteroid injections had a significantly higher pressure-pain threshold compared with the placebo group. DaCruz and co-workers [12] did not detect any difference in the complete recovery rate.

Gross and co-workers [21] concluded that, based on the current evidence, no definite recommendations could be made for injection treatment. No study has exhibited superiority in terms of any of the injection therapies or long-term efficacy.

Discussion

There is only limited evidence in terms of the treatment of mid-portion Achilles tendinopathy. Six systematic reviews were identified [21, 32, 40, 41, 46, 62,] including five reviews of randomized controlled trials. All reported on non-surgical treatment, three studies solely reviewed eccentric exercise as a treatment modality, and one study reported on injection treatment. 35 randomized controlled trials met the inclusion criteria (Table 2). In addition, Rowe and co-workers [62] also included 19 non-randomized studies, 13 were prospective case studies, and the remaining articles included four case control and two single case studies.

RCT \ Systematic Review	Magnussen [40] (2009)	Meyer [46] (2009)	Krämer [32] (2010)	Rowe [62] (2012)	Malliaras [41] (2013)	Gross [21] (2013)
DaCruz [12] (1988)	o	–	–	–	–	o
Niesen-Vertommen [48] (1992)	o	o	o	o	o	–
Pförringer [55] (1994)	o	–	–	–	–	o
Silbernagel [72] (2001)	o	–	o	o	o	–
Mafi [39] (2001)	o	o	o	o	o	–
Alfredson [2] (2003)	–	–	–	o	–	–
Neeter [47] (2003)	o	–	–	–	–	–
Roos [60] (2004)	o	o	o	o	–	–
Paoloni [51] (2004)	o	–	–	o	–	–
Fredberg [18] (2004)	o	–	–	–	–	o
Alfredson [3] (2005)	o	–	–	–	–	o
Costa [9] (2005)	o	–	–	o	–	–
Knobloch [30] (2006) (1)	–	–	–	o	–	–
De Vos [14] (2006)	o	–	o	o	–	–
Brown [5] (2006)	o	–	–	–	–	o
Mayer [44] (2007)	o	–	–	o	–	–
Petersen [54] (2007)	–	–	o	o	–	–
Knobloch [28] (2007)	–	–	o	o	–	–
Paoloni [52] (2007)	–	–	–	o	–	–
Rompe [58] (2007)	o	o	–	o	–	–
Herrington [22] (2007)	–	o	–	o	–	–
Silbernagel [71] (2007)	o	–	–	o	o	–
Norregaard [49] (2007)	–	–	–	o	–	–
Kane [24] (2008)	–	–	–	o	–	–
Knobloch [29] (2008)	–	–	o	o	–	–
Chester [6] (2008)	–	–	–	o	–	–
Stergioulas [76] (2008)	–	–	–	o	–	–
Tumity [81] (2008)	–	–	–	o	–	–
Rasmussen [56] (2008)	–	–	–	o	–	–
Willberg [86] (2008)	–	–	–	–	–	o
Rompe [57] (2009)			–	o	–	–
De Jonge [15] (2010)				o	–	o
Yelland [88] (2011)				o	–	o
Silbernagel [70] (2011)				o	–	–
Van der Plas [82] (2012)				o	–	–
Pearson [53] (2012)				–	–	o
TOTAL	16	5	8	28	4	9

RCT \ Systematic Review	Magnussen[40] (2009)	Meyer[46] (2009)	Krämer[32] (2010)	Rowe[62] (2012)	Malliaras[41] (2013)	Gross[21] (2013)
Non-RCT						
Niesen-VertAlfredson[4] (1998)				O		
Coisier[11] (2001)				O		
Fahlström[16] (2003)				O		
Ohberg[50] (2004)				O		
Lakshmanan[34] (2004)				O		
Smith[73] (2004)				O		
Shalabi[67] (2004)				O		
Langberg[35] (2007)				O		
Sayana[65] (2007)				O		
Christenson[7] (2007)				O		
Knobloch[27] (2007)				O		
Furia[19] (2008)				O		
Maffulli[37] (2008)				O		
Knobloch[31] (2009)				O		
Vulpiani[85] (2009)				O		
Firth[17] (2010)				O		
Gardin[20] (2010)				O		
Verrall[84] (2011)				O		
Saxena[64] (2011)				O		
TOTAL				19		

Table 2. Overview of the included studies. (1) This article has been withdrawn because it is a redundant publication of an article that was published in the Br J Sports Med.

Due to the large heterogeneity among the studies and the low methodological quality of the randomized controlled trials, none of the authors were able to pool the data, resulting in descriptive systematic reviews. The methodological quality of the six systematic reviews included is assessed using the AMSTAR checklist[68]. This is an 11-item questionnaire for measuring the methodological quality of systematic reviews. The scores of the six included reviews ranged from 2/11 to 6/11 points, indicating limited methodological quality (Table 3).

Study	Number of Studies Included	Selection Criteria	Methodological Quality (AMSTAR)
Magnussen and co-workers [40]	16	– Mid-portion tendinopathy – RCT – English	3 / 11
Meyer and co-workers [46]	5	– At least one group eccentric exercise; control group other treatment modality – Unilateral mid-portion Achilles tendinopathy – RCT – PEDro score > 5	4 / 11
Krämer and co-workers [32]	8	– Chronic Achilles tendinopathy – Eccentric exercise – Comparing ≥2 groups – Prospective RCT – Full text available – German or English	2 / 11
Rowe and co-workers [62]	47	– Mid-portion Achilles tendinopathy – Conservative exercise – Age > 18 – Full text available	5 / 11
Malliaras and co-workers [41]	4	– Achilles tendinopathy – Clinical outcomes of loading programmes, only as a primary intervention – Minimal follow-up 4 wks – Comparing ≥2 groups – RCT or non-randomized controlled clinical trials – English	6 / 11
Gross and co-workers [21]	9	– Mid-portion Achilles tendinopathy – Injection therapy – RCT or non-randomized controlled clinical trials – Age > 18	6 / 11

Table 3. Characteristics of the included systematic reviews.

Magnussen and co-workers [40] provided an overview of the evidence for non-surgical treatment, and concluded that only some evidence is available for eccentric training. Other treatment options show promising results; however, in order to make any recommendation, more research is required. Although both Krämer and co-workers [32] and Meyer and co-workers [46] were not able to draw definite conclusions, they reported that eccentric exercise was an effective treatment option in most studies. Rowe and co-workers [62] demonstrated strong evidence supporting eccentric training and shock-wave therapy. Gross and co-workers [21] concluded that, based on the current evidence, no definite recommendations could be made for injection treatment.

Shrier and co-workers [69] published the first systematic review on Achilles tendinopathy. They found insufficient data to determine the comparative risks and benefits of corticosteroid injections in Achilles tendinopathy. In 2001, McLauchlan and Handoll [45] performed a Cochrane review to assess the effectiveness of various treatment interventions for acute and chronic Achilles tendinitis. In conclusion, there was insufficient evidence from randomized controlled trials to determine which method of treatment would be most appropriate for the treatment of acute or chronic Achilles tendinopathy.

More recently, the role of PRP in the treatment of Achilles tendon injuries was investigated in a systematic review by Sadoghi and co-workers [63]. Only two randomized controlled trials concerning PRP in Achilles tendinopathy were identified. These studies will be discussed in the PRP chapter of this book. Al-Abbad and Simon [1] performed a systematic review to assess the effectiveness of extracorporeal shockwave therapy. Six studies were included, of which four were randomized controlled trials. Only two of the studies reported purely on mid-portion Achilles tendinopathy [34, 59]. However, regarding the results, no distinction was made between insertional and mid-portion tendinopathy. A systematic literature review by Joseph and co-workers [23] sought to assess the effect of deep friction massage in the management of tendinopathies. Due to large heterogeneity exhibited, different types of tendinopathies, study designs and outcome measures, no conclusion could be drawn. Coombes and co-workers [8] performed a systematic review of the efficacy and safety of injections in the treatment of tendinopathies. They found that polidocanol, aprotinin, and PRP injections were no more efficacious than placebos for Achilles tendinopathy. Prolotherapy showed no benefit over eccentric exercise. The clinical effectiveness of low level laser therapy (LLLT) is assessed in a systematic review by Tumility and co-workers [80]. Of the four studies reporting on Achilles tendinopathy, two showed benefits from LLLT, whereas two were inconclusive. No distinction was made between the types of Achilles tendinopathy. A systematic review was performed by Woodley and co-workers [87] to evaluate the evidence for the effectiveness of eccentric exercise treatment in patients with chronic tendinopathies. Of the 20 studies included, only four described patients with Achilles tendinopathies. The authors of this review did not separately report the results of insertional and mid-portion tendinopathies. Kingma and co-workers [26] evaluated the effectiveness of eccentric overload training in patients with chronic Achilles tendinopathy.

Although the authors found an improvement in pain after eccentric training in all studies included, it was not possible to draw any conclusion due to the methodological shortcomings of the studies. Sussmilch-Leitch and co-workers [77] performed a systematic review and meta-analysis of the evidence for physical therapies for Achilles tendinopathies. 23 randomized controlled trials comparing at least one non-surgical, non-pharmacological intervention on pain or altered function were included. Again, different Achilles tendinopathies were combined, although the majority of the studies described mid-portion tendinopathies. The individual RCTs supported the use of eccentric exercises as a treatment modality in patients with Achilles tendinopathy. Additional benefits were shown when laser therapy was used as an adjunct intervention. Similar outcomes were found when shockwave therapy was used as an alternative for eccentric exercise. Only inconclusive evidence for night splints and heel braces as a treatment option was found.

At present, no systematic review on the surgical treatment of mid-portion Achilles tendinopathy has been published. The best available evidence comes from level IV studies. With regards to mid-portion pathology, both open and endoscopic approaches are used. Good results are reported after open surgical treatment [10, 25, 38, 43, 66]. However, these studies have to be interpreted with caution, since an inverse relation between study quality and outcome has been shown [78]. Different techniques for endoscopic approach have shown promising results, with less complications and - possibly - shorter recovery [42, 75, 79, 83]. However, the cohorts remain limited in size and the follow-up is short.

Conclusion

Concerning the non-surgical management, most studies showed eccentric exercise to be an effective treatment modality. Promising results are demonstrated for extracorporeal shockwave therapy in several studies. For all other non-surgical treatment options, the evidence was too limited to make a reliable recommendation. In terms of the surgical treatment of mid-portion Achilles tendinopathy, no definite recommendations can be made.

References

1. Al-Abbad H, Simon JV. The effectiveness of extracorporeal shock wave therapy on chronic Achilles tendinopathy: a systematic review. Foot Ankle Int. 2013; 34(1): 33-41.
2. Alfredson H, Lorentzon R. Intratendinous glutamate levels and eccentric training in chronic Achilles tendinosis: a prospective study using microdialysis technique. Knee Surg Sports Traumatol Arthrosc. 2003; 11(3): 196-199.
3. Alfredson H, Ohberg L. Sclerosing injections to areas of neo-vascularisation reduce pain in chronic Achilles tendinopathy: a double-blind randomised controlled trial. Knee Surg Sports Traumatol Arthrosc. 2005; 13(4): 338-344.
4. Alfredson H, Pietila T, Jonsson P, Lorentzon R. Heavy-load eccentric calf muscle training for the treatment of chronic Achilles tendinosis. Am J Sports Med. 1998; 26(3): 360-366.
5. Brown R, Orchard J, Kinchington M, Hooper A, Nalder G. Aprotinin in the management of Achilles tendinopathy: a randomised controlled trial. Br J Sports Med. 2006; 40(3): 275-279.
6. Chester R, Costa ML, Shepstone L, Cooper A, Donell ST. Eccentric calf muscle training compared with therapeutic ultrasound for chronic Achilles tendon pain - a pilot study. Man Ther. 2008; 13(6): 484-491.
7. Christenson RE. Effectiveness of specific soft tissue mobilizations for the management of Achilles tendinosis: single case study – experimental design. Man Ther. 2007; 12(1): 63-71.
8. Coombes BK, Bisset L, Vicenzino B. Efficacy and safety of corticosteroid injections and other injections for management of tendinopathy: a systematic review of randomised controlled trials. Lancet. 2010; 376(9754): 1751-1767.
9. Costa ML, Shepstone L, Donell ST, Thomas TL. Shock wave therapy for chronic Achilles tendon pain: a randomized placebo-controlled trial. Clin Orthop Relat Res. 2005; 440: 199-204.
10. Coull R, Flavin R, Stephens MM. Flexor hallucis longus tendon transfer: evaluation of postoperative morbidity. Foot Ankle Int. 2003; 24(12): 931-934.
11. Croisier JL, Forthomme B, Foidart-Dessalle M, Godon B, Crielaard JM. Treatment of recurrent tendinitis by isokinetic eccentric exercises. Isokinetics and Exercise Science. 2001; 9(2): 133-141.
12. DaCruz DJ, Geeson M, Allen MJ, Phair I. Achilles paratendonitis: an evaluation of steroid injection. Br J Sports Med. 1988; 22(2): 64-65.
13. de Jonge S, de Vos RJ, Weir A. One-year follow-up of platelet-rich plasma treatment in chronic Achilles tendinopathy: a double-blind randomized placebo-controlled trial. Am J Sports Med. 2011; 39(8): 1623-1629.
14. de Vos RJ, Weir A, Cobben LP, Tol JL. The value of power Doppler ultrasonography in Achilles tendinopathy: a prospective study. Am J Sports Med. 2007; 35(10): 1696-1701.
15. de Jonge S, de Vos RJ, van Schie HT, Verhaar JA, Weir A, Tol JL. One-year follow-up of a randomised controlled trial on added splinting to eccentric exercises in chronic midportion Achilles tendinopathy. Br J Sports Med. 2010; 44(9): 673-677.
16. Fahlstrom M, Jonsson P, Lorentzon R, Alfredson H. Chronic Achilles tendon pain treated with eccentric calf-muscle training. Knee Surg Sports Traumatol Arthrosc. 2003; 11(5): 327-333.
17. Firth BL, Dingley P, Davies ER, Lewis JS, Alexander CM. The effect of kinesiotape on function, pain, and motoneuronal excitability in healthy people and people with Achilles tendinopathy. Clin J Sport Med. 2010; 20(6): 416-421.
18. Fredberg U, Bolvig L, Pfeiffer-Jensen M, Clemmensen D, Jakobsen BW, Stengaard-Pedersen K. Ultrasonography as a tool for diagnosis, guidance of local steroid injection and, together with pressure algometry, monitoring of the treatment of athletes with chronic jumper's knee and Achilles tendinitis: a randomized, double-blind, placebo-controlled study. Scand J Rheumatol. 2004; 33(2): 94-101.
19. Furia JP. High-energy extracorporeal shock wave therapy as a treatment for chronic noninsertional Achilles tendinopathy. Am J Sports Med. 2008; 36(3): 502-508.
20. Gardin A, Movin T, Svensson L, Shalabi A. The long-term clinical and MRI results following eccentric calf muscle training in chronic Achilles tendinosis. Skeletal Radiol. 2010; 39(5): 435-442.
21. Gross CE, Hsu AR, Chahal J, Holmes GB. Injectable Treatments for Noninsertional Achilles Tendinosis A Systematic Review. Foot Ankle Int. 2013.
22. Herrington L, McCulloch R. The role of eccentric training in the management of Achilles tendinopathy: A pilot study. Phys Ther Sport. 2007; 8(4): 191-196.
23. Joseph MF, Taft K, Moskwa M, Denegar CR. Deep friction massage to treat tendinopathy: a systematic review of a classic treatment in the face of a new paradigm of understanding. J Sport Rehabil. 2012; 21(4): 343-353.
24. Kane TP, Ismail M, Calder JD. Topical glyceryl trinitrate and noninsertional Achilles tendinopathy: a clinical and cellular investigation. Am J Sports Med. 2008; 36(6): 1160-1163.
25. Khan KM, Forster BB, Robinson J et al. Are ultrasound and magnetic resonance imaging of value in assessment of Achilles tendon disorders? A two year prospective study. Br J Sports Med. 2003; 37(2): 149-153.

26. Kingma JJ, de KR, Wittink HM, Takken T. Eccentric overload training in patients with chronic Achilles tendinopathy: a systematic review. Br J Sports Med. 2007; 41(6): e3.

27. Knobloch K. Eccentric training in Achilles tendinopathy: is it harmful to tendon microcirculation? Br J Sports Med. 2007; 41(6): e2.

28. Knobloch K, Kraemer R, Jagodzinski M, Zeichen J, Meller R, Vogt PM. Eccentric training decreases paratendon capillary blood flow and preserves paratendon oxygen saturation in chronic Achilles tendinopathy. J Orthop Sports Phys Ther. 2007; 37(5): 269-276.

29. Knobloch K, Schreibmueller L, Longo UG, Vogt PM. Eccentric exercises for the management of tendinopathy of the main body of the Achilles tendon with or without the AirHeel Brace. A randomized controlled trial. A: effects on pain and microcirculation. Disabil Rehabil. 2008; 30(20-22): 1685-1691.

30. Knobloch K, Schreibmueller L, Kraemer R et al. Eccentric training and an Achilles wrap reduce Achilles tendon capillary blood flow and capillary venous filling pressures and increase tendon oxygen saturation in insertional and midportion tendinopathy: a randomized trial. Am J Sports Med. 2006.

31. Knobloch K, Schreibmueller L, Kraemer R, Jagodzinski M, Vogt PM, Redeker J. Gender and eccentric training in Achilles mid-portion tendinopathy. Knee Surg Sports Traumatol Arthrosc. 2010; 18(5): 648-655.

32. Krämer R, Lorenzen J, Vogt PM, Knobloch K. Systematische Literaturanalyse über exzentrisches Training bei chronischer Mid-portion-Achillestendinopathie: Gibt es einen Standard? Sportverletz Sportschaden. 2010; 24(04): 204-211.

33. Kvist M. Achilles tendon injuries in athletes. Ann Chir Gynaecol. 1991; 80(2): 188-201.

34. Lakshmanan P, O'Doherty DP. Chronic Achilles tendinopathy: treatment with extracorporeal shock waves. Foot Ankle Surg. 2004; 10(3): 125-130.

35. Langberg H, Ellingsgaard H, Madsen T et al. Eccentric rehabilitation exercise increases peritendinous type I collagen synthesis in humans with Achilles tendinosis. Scand J Med Sci Sports. 2007; 17(1): 61-66.

36. Maffulli N. Augmented repair of acute Achilles tendon ruptures using gastrocnemius-soleus fascia. Int Orthop. 2005; 29(2): 134.

37. Maffulli N, Walley G, Sayana MK, Longo UG, Denaro V. Eccentric calf muscle training in athletic patients with Achilles tendinopathy. Disabil Rehabil. 2008; 30(20-22): 1677-1684.

38. Maffulli N, Longo UG, Gougoulias N, Denaro V. Ipsilateral free semitendinosus tendon graft transfer for reconstruction of chronic tears of the Achilles tendon. BMC Musculoskelet Disord. 2008; 9(1): 100.

39. Mafi N, Lorentzon R, Alfredson H. Superior short-term results with eccentric calf muscle training compared to concentric training in a randomized prospective multicenter study on patients with chronic Achilles tendinosis. Knee Surg Sports Traumatol Arthrosc. 2001; 9(1): 42-47.

40. Magnussen RA, Dunn WR, Thomson AB. Nonoperative treatment of midportion Achilles tendinopathy: a systematic review. Clin J Sport Med. 2009; 19(1): 54-64.

41. Malliaras P, Barton CJ, Reeves ND, Langberg H. Achilles and patellar tendinopathy loading programmes: a systematic review comparing clinical outcomes and identifying potential mechanisms for effectiveness. Sports Med. 2013; 43(4): 267-286.

42. Maquirriain J, Ayerza M, Costa-Paz M, Muscolo DL. Endoscopic surgery in chronic Achilles tendinopathies: A preliminary report. Arthroscopy. 2002; 18(3): 298-303.

43. Martin RL, Manning CM, Carcia CR, Conti SF. An outcome study of chronic Achilles tendinosis after excision of the Achilles tendon and flexor hallucis longus tendon transfer. Foot Ankle Int. 2005; 26(9): 691-697.

44. Mayer F, Hirschmuller A, Muller S, Schuberth M, Baur H. Effects of short-term treatment strategies over 4 weeks in Achilles tendinopathy. Br J Sports Med. 2007; 41(7): e6.

45. McLauchlan GJ, Handoll HH. Interventions for treating acute and chronic Achilles tendinitis. Cochrane Database Syst Rev. 2001; 2: CD000232.

46. Meyer A, Tumilty S, Baxter GD. Eccentric exercise protocols for chronic non-insertional Achilles tendinopathy: how much is enough? Scand J Med Sci Sports. 2009; 19(5): 609-615.

47. Neeter C, Thomee R, Silbernagel KG, Thomee P, Karlsson J. Iontophoresis with or without dexamethazone in the treatment of acute Achilles tendon pain. Scand J Med Sci Sports. 2003; 13(6): 376-382.

48. Niesen-Vertommen SL, Taunton JE, Clement DB, Mosher RE. The effect of eccentric versus concentric exercise in the management of Achilles tendonitis. Clin J Sport Med. 1992; 2(2): 109-113.

49. Norregaard J, Larsen CC, Bieler T, Langberg H. Eccentric exercise in treatment of Achilles tendinopathy. Scand J Med Sci Sports. 2007; 17(2): 133-138.

50. Ohberg L, Lorentzon R, Alfredson H. Eccentric training in patients with chronic Achilles tendinosis: normalised tendon structure and decreased thickness at follow up. Br J Sports Med. 2004; 38(1): 8-11.

51. Paoloni JA, Appleyard RC, Nelson J, Murrell GA. Topical glyceryl trinitrate treatment of chronic noninsertional Achilles tendinopathy. A randomized, double-blind, placebo-controlled trial. J Bone Joint Surg Am. 2004; 86-A(5): 916-922.

52. Paoloni JA, Murrell GA. Three-year followup study of topical glyceryl trinitrate treatment of chronic noninsertional Achilles tendinopathy. Foot Ankle Int. 2007; 28(10): 1064-1068.

53. Pearson J, Rowlands D, Highet R. Autologous Blood Injection for Treatment of Achilles Tendinopathy? A Randomised Controlled Trial. J Sport Rehabil. 2011; 21(3):218-24.

54. Petersen W, Welp R, Rosenbaum D. Chronic Achilles tendinopathy: a prospective randomized study comparing the therapeutic effect of eccentric training, the AirHeel brace, and a combination of both. Am J Sports Med. 2007; 35(10): 1659-1667.

55. Pförringer W, Pfister A, Kuntz GÃ. The treatment of Achilles paratendinitis: Results of a double-blind, placebo-controlled study with a deproteinized hemodialysate. Clin J Sport Med. 1994; 4(2): 92-99.

56. Rasmussen S, Christensen M, Mathiesen I, Simonson O. Shockwave therapy for chronic Achilles tendinopathy: a double-blind, randomized clinical trial of efficacy. Acta Orthop. 2008; 79(2): 249-256.

57. Rompe JD, Furia J, Maffulli N. Eccentric loading versus eccentric loading plus shock-wave treatment for midportion Achilles tendinopathy: a randomized controlled trial. Am J Sports Med. 2009; 37(3): 463-470.

58. Rompe JD, Nafe B, Furia JP, Maffulli N. Eccentric loading, shock-wave treatment, or a wait-and-see policy for tendinopathy of the main body of tendo Achilles: a randomized controlled trial. Am J Sports Med. 2007; 35(3): 374-383.

59. Rompe JD, Nafe B, Furia JP, Maffulli N. Eccentric loading, shock-wave treatment, or a wait-and-see policy for tendinopathy of the main body of tendo Achilles: a randomized controlled trial. Am J Sports Med. 2007; 35(3): 374-383.

60. Roos EM, Engstrom M, Lagerquist A, Soderberg B. Clinical improvement after 6 weeks of eccentric exercise in patients with mid-portion Achilles tendinopathy - a randomized trial with 1-year follow-up. Scand J Med Sci Sports. 2004; 14(5): 286-295.

61. Roos EM, Engström M, Lagerquist A, Söderberg B. Clinical improvement after 6 weeks of eccentric exercise in patients with mid-portion Achilles tendinopathy: a randomized trial with 1-year follow-up. Scand J Med Sci Sports. 2004; 14(5): 286-295.

62. Rowe V, Hemmings S, Barton C, Malliaras P, Maffulli N, Morrissey D. Conservative management of midportion Achilles tendinopathy: a mixed methods study, integrating systematic review and clinical reasoning. Sports Med. 2012; 42(11): 941-967.

63. Sadoghi P, Rosso C, Valderrabano V, Leithner A, Vavken P. The role of platelets in the treatment of Achilles tendon injuries. J Orthop Res. 2013; 31(1): 111-118.

64. Saxena A, Ramdath Jr S, O'Halloran P, Gerdesmeyer L, Gollwitzer H. Extra-corporeal pulsed-activated Therapy ("EPAT" Sound Wave) for Achilles tendinopathy: a prospective study. Foot Ankle Surg. 2011; 50(3): 315-319.

65. Sayana MK, Maffulli N. Eccentric calf muscle training in non-athletic patients with Achilles tendinopathy. J Sci Med Sport. 2007; 10(1): 52-58.

66. Schepsis AA, Wagner C, Leach RE. Surgical management of Achilles tendon overuse injuries. A long-term follow-up study. Am J Sports Med. 1994; 22(5): 611-619.

67. Shalabi A, Kristoffersen-Wilberg M, Svensson L, Aspelin P, Movin T. Eccentric training of the gastrocnemius-soleus complex in chronic Achilles tendinopathy results in decreased tendon volume and intratendinous signal as evaluated by MRI. Am J Sports Med. 2004; 32(5): 1286-1296.

68. Shea BJ, Grimshaw JM, Wells GA et al. Development of AMSTAR: a measurement tool to assess the methodological quality of systematic reviews. BMC Med Res Methodol. 2007; 7(1): 10.

69. Shrier I, Matheson GO, Kohl HW, III. Achilles tendonitis: are corticosteroid injections useful or harmful? Clin J Sport Med. 1996; 6(4): 245-250.

70. Silbernagel KG, Brorsson A, Lundberg M. The majority of patients with Achilles tendinopathy recover fully when treated with exercise alone: a 5-year follow-up. Am J Sports Med. 2011; 39(3): 607-613.

71. Silbernagel KG, Thomee R, Eriksson BI, Karlsson J. Continued sports activity, using a pain-monitoring model, during rehabilitation in patients with Achilles tendinopathy: a randomized controlled study. Am J Sports Med. 2007; 35(6): 897-906.

72. Silbernagel KG, Thomee R, Thomee P, Karlsson J. Eccentric overload training for patients with chronic Achilles tendon pain--a randomised controlled study with reliability testing of the evaluation methods. Scand J Med Sci Sports. 2001; 11(4): 197-206.

73. Smith M, Brooker S, Vicenzino B, McPoil T. Use of anti-pronation taping to assess suitability of orthotic prescription: Case report. Australian Journal of Physiotherapy. 2004; 50(2): 111-113.

74. Stanish WD, Rubinovich RM, Curwin S. Eccentric exercise in chronic tendinitis. Clin Orthop Relat Res. 1986; 208: 65-68.

75. Steenstra F, van Dijk CN. Achilles tendoscopy. Foot Ankle Clin. 2006; 11(2): 429-38, viii.

76. Stergioulas A, Stergioula M, Aarskog R, Lopes-Martins RA, Bjordal JM. Effects of low-level laser therapy and eccentric exercises in the treatment of recreational athletes with chronic Achilles tendinopathy. Am J Sports Med. 2008; 36(5): 881-887.

77. Sussmilch-Leitch SP, Collins NJ, Bialocerkowski AE, Warden SJ, Crossley KM. Physical therapies for Achilles tendinopathy: systematic review and meta-analysis. J Foot Ankle Res. 2012; 5(1): 15.

78. Tallon C, Coleman BD, Khan KM, Maffulli N. Outcome of surgery for chronic Achilles tendinopathy. A critical review. Am J Sports Med. 2001; 29(3): 315-320.

79. Thermann H, Benetos IS, Panelli C, Gavriilidis I, Feil S. Endoscopic treatment of chronic mid-portion Achilles tendinopathy: novel technique with short-term results. Knee Surg Sports Traumatol Arthrosc. 2009; 17(10): 1264-1269.

80. Tumilty S, McDonough S, Hurley DA, Baxter GD. Clinical effectiveness of low-level laser therapy as an adjunct to eccentric exercise for the treatment of Achilles' tendinopathy: a randomized controlled trial. Arch Phys Med Rehabil. 2012; 93(5): 733-739.

81. Tumilty S, Munn J, Abbott JH, McDonough S, Hurley DA, Baxter GD. Laser therapy in the treatment of Achilles tendinopathy: a pilot study. Photomed Laser Surg. 2008; 26(1): 25-30.

82. van der Plas A, de JS, de Vos RJ. A 5-year follow-up study of Alfredson's heel-drop exercise programme in chronic midportion Achilles tendinopathy. Br J Sports Med. 2012; 46(3): 214-218.

83. Vega J, Cabestany JM, Golano P, Perez-Carro L. Endoscopic treatment for chronic Achilles tendinopathy. Foot Ankle Surg. 2008; 14(4): 204-210.

84. Verrall G, Schofield S, Brustad T, Physio D. Chronic Achilles tendinopathy treated with eccentric stretching program. Foot Ankle Int. 2011; 32(9): 843-849.

85. Vulpiani MC, Trischitta D, Trovato P, Vetrano M, Ferretti A. Extracorporeal shockwave therapy (ESWT) in Achilles tendinopathy. A long-term follow-up observational study. J Sports Med Phys Fitness. 2009; 49(2): 171.

86. Willberg L, Sunding K, Ohberg L, Forssblad M, Fahlstrom M, Alfredson H. Sclerosing injections to treat midportion Achilles tendinosis: a randomised controlled study evaluating two different concentrations of Polidocanol. Knee Surg Sports Traumatol Arthrosc. 2008; 16(9): 859-864.

87. Woodley BL, Newsham-West RJ, Baxter GD. Chronic tendinopathy: effectiveness of eccentric exercise. Br J Sports Med. 2007; 41(4): 188-198.

88. Yelland MJ, Sweeting KR, Lyftogt JA, Ng SK, Scuffham PA, Evans KA. Prolotherapy injections and eccentric loading exercises for painful Achilles tendinosis: a randomised trial. Br J Sports Med. 2011; 45(5): 421-428.

"Faith and knowledge lean largely upon each other in the practice of medicine."

Peter Mere Latham

CHAPTER 25

CURRENT CONCEPTS:
TREATMENT OF ACUTE
ACHILLES TENDON RUPTURES

Ruben Zwiers, Johannes I. Wiegerinck, C. Niek van Dijk

Take Home Message

• *The management of acute Achilles tendon rupture should be adjusted to the patient's lifestyle. Non-surgical management leads to higher re-rupture rates, and surgical treatment leads to higher complication rates other than re-ruptures.*

• *Surgery reduces re-rupture rates, while the risk of other complications is increased.*

• *Subjective outcome scores are recommended to be used as a primary outcome measure.*

• *Post-operative functional bracing leads to a shorter rehabilitation period when compared with immobilization in a cast.*

Introduction

Although several reviews have been published, there remains a lack of consensus in terms of the best management of acute Achilles tendon rupture. Generally, treatment can be divided in surgical and non-surgical treatments. Surgical management is typically reserved for high-demand patients, while the sedentary are treated non-surgically by means of immobilization. This chapter provides an overview of systematic reviews of randomized controlled trials on this topic.

Overview of systematic reviews

Lo and co-workers[19] (1997)

Lo and co-workers[19] performed a quantitative review of surgical versus non-surgical treatments. They identified two prospective randomized trials and 17 case series, and concluded that no clear recommendations could be made. The re-rupture rate for surgical management was found to be substantially lower compared with non-surgical management at the expense of minor and moderate complications after surgical management, the latter being 20-times larger. They concluded that patients with poor healing potential should be treated non-surgically, and that active patients should be offered either surgical or non-surgical management.

Wong and co-workers[43] (2002)

Wong and co-workers[43] identified 125 studies. 83 of them were retrospective, and there were 20 prospective studies, 18 retrospective comparative studies and only four randomized controlled trials. All the studies compared surgical intervention in casts or functional after-treatment with non-surgical management in casts or functional braces. The complications described in each study were divided into three main categories: wound complications (major/minor), general complications (major/minor) and re-rupture.

The patients that were managed non-surgically generally underwent a period of immobilization in a below-the-knee cast in an equinus position for four weeks, and with the ankle placed in a more neutral position for an additional four weeks. Three studies described management only by functional bracing. All reported good functional outcomes and low re-rupture rates. The average duration of immobilization in these studies was only two weeks. Of the 645 patients who underwent non-surgical management, there were 55 (8.5%) who sustained minor general complications, four (0.6%) with major complications, and 63 (9.8%) who had re-ruptures.

247 patients underwent percutaneous repair (different techniques) and immobilization, while 122 patients underwent percutaneous repair and early mobilization. In the percutaneous techniques, the entrapment of the sural nerve was relatively common.

Of the 247 patients in the immobilized group, the number of minor wound complications was 12 (4.9%), the general rate of minor complications was 21 (8.5%), and two patients (0.8%) had major complications. There were nine (3.6%) re-ruptures. The 122 patients in the early-mobilized group sustained eight (6.6%) minor and four (3.3%) major wound complications, and 18 (14.8%) minor and one (0.8%) major general complication. There were eight (6.6%) re-ruptures.

Many different open methods of repair have been described. There were 3,718 Achilles tendon ruptures managed with open repair and immobilization, and 283 Achilles tendon ruptures managed with open repair and early mobilization (Table 1). Of the 3,718 patients managed with open repair and immobilization, there were 457 (12.3%) minor and 86 (2.3%) major wound complications, 301 (8.1%) minor and 29 (0.8%) major general complications, and 82 (2.2%) re-ruptures. Of the 283 patients managed with open repair and early mobilization, there were 14 (4.9%) minor and one (0.4%) major wound complication, 15 (5.3%) minor and one (0.4%) major general complication, and four (1.4%) re-ruptures.

Complications / Achilles Tendon Rupture Management	Non-Surgical Management	Percutaneous Repair: Immobilization	Percutaneous Repair [1]: Early Mobilization	Open Surgery [2]: Immobilization	Open Surgery [2]: Early Mobilization
N	645	247	122	3718	283
Minor Wound	–	12 (4.9%)	8 (6.6%)	457 (12.3%)	14 (4.9%)
Major Wound	–	–	4 (3.3%)	86 (2.3%)	1 (0.4%)
Minor General	55 (8.5%)	21 (8.5%)	18 (14.8%)	301 (8.1%)	15 (4.9%)
Major General	4 (0.6%)	2 (0.8%)	1 (0.8%)	29 (0.8%)	1 (0.4%)
Re-rupture	63 (9.8%)	9 (3.6%)	8 (6.6%)	82 (2.2%)	4 (1.4%)

Table 1. Overview of complications in a review by Wong and co-workers [43]
[1] At least four different percutaneous techniques were used
[2] The preferred method for early-diagnosed ruptures has been simple end-to-end suture, but collected data revealed that 41 different open techniques were used.

Wong and co-workers [43] found that, in general, the number of publications reporting Achilles tendon ruptures was increasing, and the trend for the number of reported complications was decreasing. Few studies used standardized subjective scoring to assess patient satisfaction and recovery after an Achilles tendon rupture.

In conclusion, the published studies show a trend towards earlier mobilization. Open repair followed by early mobilization does produce the best functional recovery, with an acceptable complication rate.

Bhandari and co-workers [4] (2002)

Bhandari and co-workers [4] published the results of a quantitative systematic review of only randomized and quasi-randomized trials to determine the effect of surgical versus non-surgical management of acute Achilles tendon ruptures on the rate of re-rupture. Computerized databases were searched to locate clinical studies and the results of this meta-analysis were compared with recommendations in the literature.

A pooled analysis of five studies with 421 patients revealed a non-significant difference in the proportion of patients who regained normal functionality after surgical or non-surgical management (71% versus 63%, respectively). Similarly, an analysis of six studies including 448 patients did not reveal any difference in the risk of spontaneous complaints (heel aches while walking, increased shoe size because of the widening of the Achilles tendon and ankle stiffness) at follow-up between surgical repair and non-surgically-treated groups (19% versus 25%, respectively).

Apart from this pooled analysis, Bhandari and co-workers [4] studied recommendations with regards to the management of Achilles tendon ruptures that were made in 22 review articles and textbooks. They found that 16 researchers strongly favoured surgery (72.7%); four were non-committal (18.2%), and two strongly favoured non-surgical therapy (9.1%).

According to Bhandari and co-workers [4], the most obvious limitation to surgical intervention is the increased risk of infection. In the current group of trials, there was a 4.7% incidence of infection after surgery and no infections after non-surgical management. Wound slough may occur at a rate of 0.85%, and sural nerve injury at a rate of 6% after surgical repair. Deep venous thrombosis was more common after the non-surgical management of Achilles tendon ruptures (1.5%).

Bhandari and co-workers [4] postulated that strong recommendations require a large, randomized trial comparing surgery and non-surgical therapy for acute Achilles tendon ruptures.

Kocher and co-workers [17] (2002)

Kocher and co-workers [17] performed an expected-value decision analysis to determine the optimal management strategy for the management of acute Achilles tendon rupture, whether surgical or non-surgical. Included were randomized controlled trials, cohort studies and case series; altogether, 25 studies reporting data on surgical management and ten studies reporting data concerning non-surgical management were evaluated.

Complications	Major	Moderate	Minor
	Re-rupture Second re-rupture Tendon lengthening Deep infection Chronic fistula DVT (pulmonary embolus)	Sural nerve injury Wound problems not requiring reoperation	Adhesion of the scar

Table 2. Complication categories in a review by Kocher and co-worker[17].

As in the review by Wong and co-workers [43], the severity of complications was divided into three groups (Table 2).

This systematic review revealed that the probability of re-rupture after non-surgical management was 12.1%, whereas the re-rupture rate after surgical repair was only 2.2%. However, the probability of a moderate (mainly wound) complication after surgical repair was 7.5% versus 0.3% after non-surgical management. As in the three previous reviews, this study also showed that surgical management was the optimal management strategy for acute Achilles tendon rupture. Results in terms of return to work and the rate of return to the previous level of sports participation were summarized, but no conclusions were drawn.

Like Bhandari and co-workers [4], Kocher and co-workers [17] described the fact that variations in specific management regimens existed within the two treatment arms [2]. Furthermore, they did not study percutaneous repair since the data were insufficient.

In conclusion, Kocher and co-workers advocated a model of shared decision-making in which the physician and the patient were jointly involved in the medical decision-making process.

Lynch [20] (2003)

Lynch [20] performed a comprehensive literature search to retrieve relevant English language articles, comparing surgical and non-surgical management. Lynch identified five prospective randomized controlled trials between 1966 and 2002.

The assessed outcomes included not only re-rupture rates and complications, but also plantar flexion strength and the time to return to work and to return to sports. A definition of the goals of management in acute Achilles tendon ruptures put forward by McComis and co-workers [24] was used: to restore tendon length and tension, to optimize ultimate strength and function, to reduce the time needed for rehabilitation, and to facilitate an early return to work and pre-injury levels of activity [24].

Lynch [20] also found that there is a lack of a universal, consistent protocols for subjective and objective evaluation following treatment, which renders the comparison of results difficult. In their opinion, surgical management is preferable to non-surgical management because it produces better functional outcomes.

As with the previous four reviewers, Lynch [20] found that the incidence of re-ruptures following non-surgical management was significantly higher than was the case after surgical management; only five patients need to be treated surgically to prevent one re-rupture.

The incidence of minor complications following surgical management is substantial, but these do not appear to affect functional outcomes. The return to sport at one year, the reduction in active plantar flexion, increased dorsi-flexion, isokinetic strength and endurance testing all revealed no significant differences.

Post-operatively early functional mobilization is more acceptable to patients than plaster cast immobilization, and generally results in improved functional outcomes, such as increased ROM and earlier returns to pre-injury levels of activity. This is probably because early motion helps to align the collagen fibres, thereby improving tensile strength and gliding ability.

Lynch [20] concluded that non-surgical management should be reserved for patients who refuse or who are unfit for surgical repair. In the end, patients should be involved in their management preferences.

Khan and co-workers [16] (2005)

Khan and co-workers performed a meta-analysis to identify the evidence from randomized controlled trials on the effectiveness of different interventions in the management of acute Achilles tendon ruptures. The researchers searched multiple databases and the reference lists of articles, and contacted the authors of the various studies. 12 trials involving 800 patients were included. The primary outcomes were complications of management and re-rupture. Other outcomes, such as the level of sports activity, patient satisfaction and length of hospital stay, were not included because they lacked the quantity and uniformity to support rigorous meta-analysis. Five comparisons were made.

Open surgical versus non-surgical management

This comparison concerns four trials comparing open surgical with non-surgical management, which included a total of 356 patients. There was a lower risk of re-rupture in the surgically-managed patients (3.5% versus 12.6% in the non-surgically-treated patients), with a higher risk of other complications including infection, adhesions and disturbed skin sensibility (34.1% versus 2.7%).

Post-operative splinting: cast immobilization versus cast immobilization followed by functional bracing

This comparison was studied in five studies. Re-rupture rates were reported in five studies, however, without a significant difference. In addition, five studies commented on the complications of management. The pooled rate of re-rupture was 5.0% (7/150) in the cast immobilization group and 2.3% (3/133) in the functional brace group. The pooled incidence of complications other than re-rupture was 50/140 (35.7%) in the cast immobilized group and 26/133 (19.5%) in the functional brace group.

Open surgical versus percutaneous repair

Two studies included 94 patients. The re-rupture rate in open surgery was 4.3% and 2.1% using a percutaneous technique. Complication rates other than re-rupture in open surgery were 26.1% compared with 8.3% in percutaneous repair. The pooled rate of reported complications (excluding re-rupture) was 26.1% in the open surgical group and 8.3% in the percutaneous group. The pooled rate of infection was 19.6% in the open surgical group and 0% in the percutaneous group.

Post-operative splinting: cast alone versus cast splinting followed by functional bracing

Data from 273 patients were available in five studies. The re-rupture rate in cast immobilization was 5.0% versus 2.3% for functional bracing. Other complications in the cast immobilization group rated 35.7% compared with 19.5% in the functional brace group (adhesions, altered sensibility, keloid or scar hypertrophy).

Comparing different non-surgical management regimens (cast versus functional bracing)

Only two studies were identified, evaluating 90 patients. Because of the small number of patients involved, no definitive conclusions could be drawn with regards to different non-surgical management regimes. The researchers could draw only limited conclusions from these two studies due to the small sample sizes, the difference in regimens and the minimal reporting of outcomes. The re-rupture rate in the brace group was 2.4%, compared with 12.2% in the cast immobilization group.

This meta-analysis concluded that non-surgically-managed patients have a more than three-times higher risk of re-rupture; however, they have a minimal risk of other complications, whereas one-third of surgically-treated patients sustained a complication.

There was a tendency towards a lower grade of complication – including infections – in the percutaneously-treated patients.

Post-operative management favours the outcome of functional bracing instead of a cast alone. Different regimens of post-operative splinting in a cast followed by a functional brace reduce the overall complication rate.

Khan and Smith[15] (2010)

Khan and Smith[15] published an update of the evidence for surgical treatment that was formerly presented in a review that covered all interventions for acute Achilles tendon rupture[16]. The aim of this study was to evaluate the relative effects of surgical versus non-surgical and different surgical interventions. Therefore, 12 (quasi-) randomized trials comparing surgical versus non-surgical and different surgical techniques were included. Re-rupture and complication rates, as well as long-term function, were the primary outcome measures.

Open surgical repair versus non-surgical treatment

In six studies, open surgery was compared with non-surgical treatment, involving 536 patients. The pooled results showed a higher rupture rate in the non-surgical group (12%) compared with the surgically-treated group (5%). The risk of overall wound infections was higher after surgery (Risk Ratio 4.89), whereas the pooled results of all reported complications other than re-rupture showed no significant differences.

Open versus percutaneous surgical repair

A comparison of open and percutaneous repair was considered in four studies. One of these studies reported three ruptures, of which two occurred in the open surgery group. The other three studies did not report any re-rupture. Infection occurred only in the open surgery group (18%). There were no differences in the incidence of other complications.

Different techniques

One study compared a two-strand versus a six-strand surgical technique and found no differences in the re-rupture rate, other complications or function on the long-term. Augmented versus simple surgical repair was compared in two studies, with no significant differences.

In conclusion, there is evidence that open surgery reduces the risk of re-rupture compared with non–surgical treatment; however, there is a significantly higher risk of other complications. Furthermore, there is inadequate evidence to allow any comment on different surgical techniques or the use of more complex reconstruction.

McMahon and co-workers [25] (2011)

McMahon and co-workers [25] performed a meta-analysis of randomized controlled trials to compare the clinical outcome of open and minimally-invasive surgery. Six studies, including 277 patients, comparing these two techniques were included. The primary outcome was the re-rupture rate. Additionally, the incidence of infections, nerve injuries, deep vein thrombosis, adhesions, pain, range of motion, the AOFAS score, and patient subjective outcomes, were all analysed.

No difference in the re-rupture rate between open and minimally-invasive surgery was detected. Although there was a small difference, a greater risk of developing a superficial wound infection was found. Patients were nearly three-times more likely to report a good or excellent outcome following minimally-invasive surgery in comparison with an open approach (odds ratio: 2.99). All other outcome measures were similar in both groups.

This meta-analysis was based on a relatively small population sample. Hence, more well-designed randomized controlled trials are required to perform an adequate evaluation of the outcomes of both procedures.

Zhao and co-workers [44] (2011)

Zhao and co-workers [44] published a meta-analysis of surgical versus non-surgical treatment to determine their effects on re-rupture and other complication rates. They identified eight randomized controlled trials, comparing surgical with non-surgical management, with 20 patients or more in each treatment group and at least one year follow-up. Complications were divided into three categories according to the classification given by Lo and co-workers [19]: major, moderate and minor. In addition, the time to return to work and the ability to return to previous sports activity level rates, a decreased range of motion rate (according to the method of Cetti and co-workers [6]) and other functional outcome measures were all analysed.

The re-rupture rate was 4.4% in the patients treated with open surgery versus 10.9% in the non-surgically-treated group, with a risk ratio of 0.4 in favour of the surgical treatment. In terms of complications, no differences in major complication rates were detected. However, moderate and minor complications were significantly more common in the surgically-treated group. The time to return to work was reported in two studies, and was shorter after surgical treatment. Other outcome measures did not show any significant differences.

In conclusion, surgical treatment appears to reduce the risk of re-rupture compared with non-surgical treatment. However, the risk of moderate and minor complications is increased. Zhao and co-workers [44] recommend surgical treatment in young and active patients without medical complications. For those aged patients and those with lower sporting requirements, non-surgical management may be the most optimal treatment.

Jiang and co-workers [11] (2012)

Jiang and co-workers [11] performed a meta-analysis of the surgical versus non-surgical treatment for acute Achilles tendon rupture. Ten randomized controlled studies, with a total of 894 patients, were included. The outcome measures consisted of the re-rupture rate, complications other than re-ruptures, the number of patients recovering to a pre-injury sports level, and sick leave.

The re-rupture rates for surgical and non-surgical treatments were 4.3% and 9.7%, respectively (risk ratio: 0.44). Nonetheless, the incidence of other complications was higher in the surgically-treated group. A complication rate of 26.6% was reported after surgery, whereas in the non-surgical group the complication rate was 7.2% (risk ratio: 4.07). No differences were found in the number of patients that returned to their pre-injury level of sports. The mean time for sick leave was shorter following surgical treatment.

The results of this meta-analysis confirm that surgical treatment can reduce the re-rupture rate, whereas non-surgical treatment might have a lower risk of other complications. Jiang and co-workers concluded that there was insufficient evidence regarding the difference in functional recovery and, therefore, that it is difficult to determine which treatment option is superior to the other.

Wilkins and Bisson [41] (2012)

Wilkins and Bisson [41] identified seven randomized controlled trials on the surgical versus non-surgical treatment of Achilles tendon ruptures that met their inclusion criteria. Studies comparing open surgical repair with non-surgical treatment, with adequate randomization and reporting on re-rupture rates, were included. Besides re-rupture rates, other complications (deep infections, scar complaints, etc.) and the time to return to work were used as secondary outcome measures.

The re-rupture rate was 3.6% in the surgically-treated group compared with 8.8% in the non-surgically-treated group; there was an odds ratio of 0.4 in favour of surgical treatment. Six of the seven studies included reported a higher re-rupture rate in the non-surgically-treated patients; however, in only one study was this difference statistically significant [21]. Of the other complications, the rate of deep infections, scar complaints, and sural nerve disturbances were significantly higher in the surgically-treated group. No differences were found in terms of deep vein thrombosis or return to work.

This systematic review showed that open surgical repair reduced the re-rupture rate in comparison with non-surgical management. Several other complications, avoided with non-surgical treatment, occurred more frequently when surgical repair was performed.

Soroceanu and co-workers [37] (2012)

Soroceanu and co-workers [37] performed a meta-analysis of randomized trials on the surgical versus non-surgical treatment of acute Achilles tendon ruptures. A literature search yielded 615 studies, of which ten randomized controlled trials were included. All the studies compared surgical repair with non-surgical treatment. Surgical repair included either open or minimally-invasive techniques; both casting and splinting were described as non-surgical treatment. There were no restrictions on the basis of weight-bearing status or the early range of motion after surgery. The primary outcome measure was the re-rupture rate. Other complications, such as strength, range of motion, time to return to work, calf circumference and functional outcomes, were used as secondary outcome measures.

In terms of the re-rupture rate, the pooled results showed a significant risk difference of 5.5%, corresponding with a risk ratio of 0.4 in favour of surgical repair. However, there was a significant heterogeneity in the included studies. Using a meta-regression, the use of functional rehabilitation was a significant cause of heterogeneity. Hence, a stratified analysis of the re-rupture rates according to functional rehabilitation was performed, showing no differences between surgical and non-surgical treatments when a functional rehabilitation protocol with the early range of motion was used. However, a prolonged immobilization protocol resulted in an absolute risk reduction of 8.8%. The risk of complications other than re-rupture was 15.8% higher in the surgically-treated group, resulting in a risk ratio of 3.9 in favour of non-surgical treatment. The time to return to work was reported in four studies. The pooled data showed surgically-treated patients returning to work 19 days sooner. In terms of the other outcome measures, no clinically-relevant differences were found.

In a sub-analysis of four studies using functional rehabilitation, non-surgical treatment was shown to be a reasonable treatment option; the re-rupture rates were similar and the risk of other complications was lower in the non-surgically-treated group.

Van der Eng and co-workers [40] (2013)

Van der Eng and co-workers [40] performed a systematic review of randomized controlled trials comparing surgical and non-surgical treatment. The aim of this review was to compare the re-rupture rates of surgical treatment followed by early weight-bearing and non-surgical treatment with early weight-bearing. Only studies published between 2001 and 2012 were included, resulting in seven eligible studies. Of the 576 patients involved, 290 were surgically treated and 286 were treated non-surgically. In one study, a minimally-invasive approach was employed, whereas in five studies open surgery occurred. Non-surgical treatment might consist of casting, bracing, orthosis and taping. Early weight-bearing was defined as weight-bearing initiated within the first four weeks following injury. Of the seven studies included, four used an early weight-bearing rehabilitation protocol. The secondary outcomes were minor and major complications.

In the four studies where early weight-bearing was employed, a re-rupture rate of 4% was reported in the surgically-treated group versus 12% in the non-surgically-treated group; however, this difference was not significant. The analysis of the three delayed weight-bearing studies, as well as all the included studies, showed no differences in the re-rupture rates. Moreover, in terms of complication rates no significant differences were detected.

Concerning the similar re-rupture rate in the surgical and non-surgical groups, the researchers concluded that none of the treatments were superior to the other.

Systematic Review → / RCT ↓	Lo[19] (1997)	Wong[43] (2002)	Bhandari[4] (2002)	Kocher[17] (2002)	Lynch[20] (2003)	Khan[16] (2005)	Khan[15] (2010)	McMahon[25] (2010)	Zhao[44] (2011)	Jiang[11] (2012)	Wilkins[41] (2012)	Soroceanu[37] (2012)	Van der Eng[40] (2013)
Coombs[7] (1981)	2,3	2,3	•	2,3	2,3	2,3	2,3	2,3	2,3	2,3	2,3	2,3	1c
Nistor[31] (1981)	•	•	•	•	•	•	•	1b	•	•	•	•	1c
Mortensen and co-workers[28] (1992)	x	•	1a,1d,2	x	1d,2	1d,2	•	1b,1d,2	1a,1d,2	1a,1d,2	1a,1d,2	1a,1d,2	1c
Saleh and co-workers[34] (1992)	?	•	1a	?	•	•	1a	1b	1a	1a	1a	1a	1c
Cetti and co-workers[6] (1993)	•	•	•	•	•	•	•	1b	•	•	•	•	1c
Cetti and co-workers[5] (1994)	x	?	1a, 5	•	?	•	1a	1b	1a	1a	1a	1a	1c
Thermann and co-workers[38] (1995)	4	?	•	4	4	3	3	1b	3	4	3	•	1c
Schroeder and co-workers[35] (1997)		2,3	2,3	2,3	2,3	•	•	•	2,3	•	2,3	•	1c
Mortensen and co-workers[27] 1999)		?	1a	x	•	•	1a	1b	1a	1a	1a	1a	1c
Majewski and co-workers[23] (2000)			•	4	4	3	3	•	3	4	3	•	1c
Möller and co-workers[21] (2001)			•	•	•	•	•	1b	•	•	•	•	•
Lim and co-workers[18] (2001)						•	•	•	1a	1a	1a	1a	1a
Petersen and co-workers[33] (2002)						•	1a	1b	1a	1a	1a	1a	1a
Kerkhoffs and co-workers[14] (2002)						•	1a	1b	1a	1a	1a	1a	1a
Maffulli and co-workers[22] (2003)						•	1a	1b	1a	1a	1a	1a	1a
Kangas and co-workers[12] (2003)						•	1a	1b	1a	1a	1a	1a	1a
Costa and co-workers[8] (2006)							1a	1b	1a	•	1a	1a	•
Twaddle and Poon[39] (2007)							•	1b	•	•	•	•	•
Aktas and co-workers[2] (2007)							•	1b	1a	1a	1a	1a	1a
Gigante and co-workers[10] (2008)							•	•	1a	1a	1a	1a	1a
Metz and co-workers[26] (2008)							•	1b	•	•	•	•	•
Aktas and Kocaoglu[1] (2009)							•	•	1a	1a	1a	1a	1a
Pajala and co-workers[32] (2009)							•	1b	1a	1a	1a	1a	1a
Valencia and Alcala[3] (2009)								•	1a	1a	1a	1a	1a
Nilsson-Hellander and co-workers[29] (2010)									•	•	•	•	•
Willits and co-workers[42] (2010)									•	•	•	•	•
Keating and Will[13] (2011)									•	•	?	?	•
Total	4	4	6	6	5	12	12	6	8	10	7	10	7

Table 3. Overview included studies

•	Included
X	Included, though not as a randomized controlled trial
?	Excluded for an unknown reason
1a	Study did not meet the inclusion criteria: surgical vs. non-surgical
1b	Study did not meet the inclusion criteria: conventional surgery vs. minimally-invasive surgery
1c	Study did not meet the inclusion criteria: only studies after 2000
1d	Study did not meet the inclusion criteria: other outcome measures
2	Only an abstract available / insufficient data reported
3	Inadequate randomization / inadequately concealed allocation
4	Excluded due to language restrictions
5	Duplicate study

Discussion

Between 1997 and 2013, 12 systematic reviews on the treatment of acute Achilles tendon ruptures have been published. These reviews comprise 26 different randomized controlled trials published between 1981 and 2011, and one unpublished study (Table 3). Of these randomized controlled trials, some were quasi-randomized and some did not describe the method of randomization. The methodological quality of the 13 systematic reviews is assessed using the AMSTAR checklist [36]. The AMSTAR checklist is an 11 item questionnaire used to measure the methodological quality of systematic reviews. The scores of the systematic reviews ranged from 2/11 to 10/11 points, indicating a wide variety of methodological quality (Table 4).

Study	Study Design		Methodological Quality	Re-rupture Rate	Other Complications	Return to Sport	Range of Motion	Other (satisfaction, strength, mean sick leave, etc.)
Lo [19] (1997)	Systematic Review	Surgical vs. Non-surgical	4/11	•	•	–	–	–
Wong [43] (2002)	Systematic Review	Surgical vs. Non-surgical	5/11	•	•	–	–	–
Bhandari [4] (2002)	Meta-analysis	Surgical vs. Non-surgical	8/11	•	•	–	–	–
Kocher [17] (2002)	Systematic Review	Surgical vs. Non-surgical	3/11	•	•	–	–	–
Lynch [20] (2003)	Systematic Review	Surgical vs. Non-surgical	2/11	•	•	•	–	–
Khan [16] (2005)	Meta-analysis	Surgical and Non-surgical	7/11	•	•	–	–	–
Khan [15] (2010)	Meta-analysis	Surgical Treatment	10/11	•	•	•	•	•
McMahon [25] (2010)	Meta-analysis	Open vs. Minimally-invasive	9/11	•	•	–	•	•
Zhao [44] (2011)	Meta-analysis	Surgical vs. Non-surgical	6/11	•	•	•	•	•
Jiang [11] (2012)	Meta-analysis	Surgical vs. Non-surgical	7/11	•	•	•	–	•
Wilkins [41] (2012)	Meta-analysis	Surgical vs. Non-surgical	4/11	•	•	–	–	•
Soroceanu [37] (2012)	Meta-analysis	Surgical vs. Non-surgical	4/11	•	•	–	•	•
Van der Eng [40] (2013)	Meta-analysis	Surgical vs. Non-surgical	5/11	•	•	-	•	•

Table 4. Overview of methodological quality and outcome measures.

Apart from the above-mentioned 27 randomized controlled trials, several cohort studies and case series have been published. Four reviews mixed the outcomes of randomized controlled trials with case series and cohort studies, which makes them more susceptible to bias. Lo and co-workers[19] included 15 case series and four randomized trials. Wong and co-workers[43] included 125 studies, of which 83 were retrospective, 20 were prospective and 18 were retrospective comparative studies. Only four were randomized controlled trials (Table 3). Kocher and co-workers[17] included 35 studies according to the inclusion criteria described by Lo and co-workers. Lynch[20] also included non-randomized trials; 16 studies were included, of which five were randomized trials (Table 4), six were comparative studies and five were reviews. Khan and co-workers[16] included quasi-randomized and randomized studies, as well as studies that stated that they were randomized but which did not, however, describe the method of randomization (Table 3).

Some of the reviewed studies that also included non-randomized trials or case series generated more detailed results because data on larger numbers of patients and more diverse outcome measures were available for analysis. Wong and co-workers[43], for example, included 125 studies and they were therefore able to describe complications in more detail.

Despite the inclusion of non-randomized trials and, therefore, a larger amount of studies in some reviews, there were no significant contradictions in the outcomes of those reviews that included data from non-randomized trials and those reviews that did not. Because of probable bias, the results from the reviews including non-randomized studies are hard to interpret and valid conclusions are difficult to draw.

We investigated the reviews with regard to the argumentation to include one randomized trial and exclude the other. The study by Coombs[7] was only reported as a conference abstract. Probably, most researchers excluded this study due to the inadequate reporting of the data and the fact that the randomization was not described. The studies by Mortensen and co-workers[28] and Schroeder and co-workers[35] were not included in several reviews, because only an abstract was available. The studies by Thermann and co-workers[38] and Majewski and co-workers[23] were written in German and were excluded in some reviews due to language restrictions [11, 17, 19, 20]. In addition, the randomization in these studies was not adequately stated, which was the reason for their exclusion in other reviews [15, 16, 41, 44] (Table 3).

Both Lo and co-workers[19] and Kocher and co-workers[17] classified two trials as being case series, while these trials should have been classified as being randomized trials [5, 27, 28]. In addition, Kocher and co-workers[17] erroneously included a case series published by Nistor in 1976 on the non-surgical management of acute Achilles tendon ruptures as a randomized study (Table 3).

Bhandari and co-workers[4] stated that Cetti and co-workers[5] (1994) was a duplicate publication of data from Cetti and co-workers[6] (1993), and therefore excluded the second study [5]. However, Cetti and co-workers [6] (1993) compares surgical with non-surgical management in a group of patients included from October 1982 to May 1984, whereas Cetti and co-workers [5] (1994) compared post-operative management in a rigid cast with post-operative management in a mobile cast in a group of patients included from September 1985 to November 1986. The groups are clearly different, and it is unlikely that the data were duplicated (Table 3).

Six reviews excluded studies for unknown reasons. Lo and co-workers [19] excluded Saleh and co-workers [34]; Wong and co-workers [43] excluded Cetti and co-workers [5] (1994), Thermann and co-workers [38] and Mortensen and co-workers [27] (1999); Kocher and co-workers [17] excluded Saleh and co-workers [34]; and Lynch [20] excluded Cetti and co-workers [5] (1994). Wilkins and Bisson [41] and Soroceanu and co-workers [37] both did not include the study by Keating and Will [13] for unknown reasons; however, Wilkins and Bisson did not report the date of their literature search and, therefore, we are not certain whether the study of Keating and Will [13] was available at that time. Van der Eng and co-workers [40] only included studies published between 2001 and 2012 (Table 3).

In conclusion, there are important differences between the reviews in terms of the inclusion and exclusion of studies. Some reviewers erroneously included non-randomized trials and some excluded adequately randomized trials. Despite these flaws, there were no significant contradictions in the outcomes of the reviews.

In terms of the outcome measures, all the studies reported on the re-rupture rate and major and minor complications as well. From the patients' point of view, other important parameters include the satisfaction rate and the ability to return to pre-injury levels of physical activity (i.e., work and sport). Several recent randomized controlled studies reported outcome measures such as length of hospital stay, the time to return to work, the time to return to sport, levels of sports activity, calf circumference or muscle hypotrophy, tendon elongation, power/strength-testing, range of motion, pain and patient satisfaction (Table 3). However, these outcome measures should be evaluated more extensively in future studies.

It is concluded that subjective outcome scores, as used by Möller and co-workers [21] are of great use in assessing patients' outcomes and making recommendations based on patients' needs and complaints following an Achilles tendon rupture. Moreover, the subjective scoring system the Achilles tendon total rupture score (ATRS), developed by Nilsson-Hellander and co-workers [30], has been designed as a patient-reported instrument for measuring the outcome after the surgical and non-surgical management of a total Achilles tendon rupture [30].

Most researchers prefer post-operative functional bracing with early weight-bearing instead of long-term cast immobilization [9,42]. There is currently a tendency to start weight-bearing directly after surgical reconstruction. A recent systematic review by Soroceanu and co-workers [37] supports this post-operative protocol. Where rehabilitation with early range of motion was employed, the re-rupture rates were equal for surgically- and non-surgically-treated groups, whereas the absolute risk reduction was 8.8% in the surgical group [37]. These results should, however, be interpreted with caution as they are based on the sub-analysis of only a few included studies. Additionally, these findings were supported by another recent systematic review by van der Eng and co-workers [40]. They found no differences in the re-rupture rates between surgical treatment followed by early weight-bearing and non-surgical treatment with early weight-bearing.

Conclusion

In conclusion, no definitive treatment recommendations can be made based on the available literature. All the reviewers suggest that management should be adjusted to the patient's needs, that non-surgical management leads to higher re-rupture rates and that surgical management leads to higher complication rates other than re-rupture. Most modern researchers prefer post-operative functional bracing instead of long-term cast immobilization.

The criteria for the inclusion or exclusion of randomized controlled trials are clearly stated, but often studies that might have been suitable for analysis were not retrieved or else were excluded for unknown reasons. This inconsistency creates substantial room for bias. Some of the older reviews also included non-randomized studies, which make the outcomes more prone to bias and generates less reliable results.

The ATRS and the Foot and Ankle Outcome Score are valid subjective scoring systems and are recommended for use in the assessment of patients with acute Achilles tendon ruptures.

References

1. Aktas S, Kocaoglu B. Open versus minimal invasive repair with Achillon device. Foot Ankle Int. 2009; 30(5): 391-397.
2. Aktas S, Kocaoglu B, Nalbantoglu U, Seyhan M, Guven O. End-to-end versus augmented repair in the treatment of acute Achilles tendon ruptures. J Foot Ankle Surg. 2007; 46(5): 336-340.
3. Avilla VJ, Guillon AM. Repair of acute Achilles tendon rupture. Comparative study of two surgical techniques. Acta Ortop Mex. 2009; 23(3): 125.
4. Bhandari M, Guyatt GH, Siddiqui F. Treatment of acute Achilles tendon ruptures: a systematic overview and metaanalysis. Clin Orthop Relat Res. 2002; (400): 190-200.
5. Cetti R, Henriksen LO, Jacobsen KS. A new treatment of ruptured Achilles tendons. A prospective randomized study. Clin Orthop Relat Res. 1994; 308: 155-165.
6. Cetti R, Christensen SE, Ejsted R, Jensen NM, Jorgensen U. Operative versus nonoperative treatment of Achilles tendon rupture A prospective randomized study and review of the literature. Am J Sports Med. 1993; 21(6): 791-799.
7. Coombs RRH. Prospective trial of conservative and surgical treatment of Achilles tendon rupture. J Bone Joint Surg Br. 1981; 63: 288.
8. Costa ML, MacMillan K, Halliday D. Randomised controlled trials of immediate weight-bearing mobilisation for rupture of the tendo Achillis. J Bone Joint Surg Br. 2006; 88(1): 69-77.
9. Garrick JG. Does accelerated functional rehabilitation after surgery improve outcomes in patients with acute Achilles tendon ruptures? Clin J Sport Med 2012; 22(4): 379-380.
10. Gigante A, Moschini A, Verdenelli A, Del TM, Ulisse S, de PL. Open versus percutaneous repair in the treatment of acute Achilles tendon rupture: a randomized prospective study. Knee Surg Sports Traumatol Arthrosc. 2008; 16(2): 204-209.
11. Jiang N, Wang B, Chen A, Dong F, Yu B. Operative versus nonoperative treatment for acute Achilles tendon rupture: a meta-analysis based on current evidence. Int Orthop. 2012; 36(4): 765-773.
12. Kangas J, Pajala A, Siira P, Hamalainen M, Leppilahti J. Early functional treatment versus early immobilization in tension of the musculotendinous unit after Achilles rupture repair: a prospective, randomized, clinical study. J Trauma. 2003; 54(6): 1171-1180.
13. Keating JF, Will EM. Operative versus non-operative treatment of acute rupture of tendo Achillis: a prospective randomised evaluation of functional outcome. J Bone Joint Surg Br. 2011; 93(8): 1071-1078.
14. Kerkhoffs GM, Struijs PA, Raaymakers EL, Marti RK. Functional treatment after surgical repair of acute Achilles tendon rupture: wrap vs. walking cast. Arch Orthop Trauma Surg. 2002; 122(2): 102-105.
15. Khan RJ, Carey Smith RL. Surgical interventions for treating acute Achilles tendon ruptures. Cochrane Database Syst Rev. 2010; (9): CD003674.
16. Khan RJ, Fick D, Keogh A, Crawford J, Brammar T, Parker M. Treatment of acute Achilles tendon ruptures. A meta-analysis of randomized, controlled trials. J Bone Joint Surg Am. 2005; 87(10): 2202-2210.
17. Kocher MS, Bishop J, Marshall R, Briggs KK, Hawkins RJ. Operative versus nonoperative management of acute Achilles tendon rupture: expected-value decision analysis. Am J Sports Med. 2002; 30(6): 783-790.
18. Lim J, Dalai R, Waseem M. Percutaneous vs. open repair of the ruptured Achilles tendon: a prospective randomized controlled study. Foot Ankle Int. 2001; 22(7): 559-568.
19. Lo IK, Kirkley A, Nonweiler B, Kumbhare DA. Operative versus nonoperative treatment of acute Achilles tendon ruptures: a quantitative review. Clin J Sport Med. 1997; 7(3): 207-211.
20. Lynch RM. Achilles tendon rupture: surgical versus non-surgical treatment. Accid Emerg Nurs. 2004; 12(3): 149-158.
21. Möller M, Movin T, Granhed H, Lind K, Faxen E, Karlsson J. Acute rupture of tendo Achillis a prospective, randomised study of comparison between surgical and non-surgical treatment. J Bone Joint Surg Br. 2001; 83(6): 843-848.
22. Maffulli N, Tallon C, Wong J, Lim KP, Bleakney R. Early weightbearing and ankle mobilization after open repair of acute midsubstance tears of the Achilles tendon. Am J Sports Med. 2003; 31(5): 692-700.
23. Majewski M, Rickert M, Steinbruck K. Achilles tendon rupture. A prospective study assessing various treatment possibilities. Orthopade. 2000; 29(7): 670-676.
24. McComis GP, Nawoczenski DA, DeHaven KE. Functional bracing for rupture of the Achilles tendon. Clinical results and analysis of ground-reaction forces and temporal data. J Bone Joint Surg Am. 1997; 79(12): 1799-1808.
25. McMahon SE, Smith TO, Hing CB. A meta-analysis of randomised controlled trials comparing conventional to minimally invasive approaches for repair of an Achilles tendon rupture. Foot Ankle Surg. 2011; 17(4): 211-217.
26. Metz R, Verleisdonk EJM, Geert J-MG. Acute Achilles tendon rupture minimally invasive surgery versus nonoperative treatment with immediate full weightbearing: a randomized controlled trial. Am J Sports Med. 2008; 36(9): 1688-1694.

27. Mortensen HM, Skov O, Jensen PE. Early motion of the ankle after operative treatment of a rupture of the Achilles tendon. A prospective, randomized clinical and radiographic study. J Bone Joint Surg Am. 1999; 81(7): 983-990.

28. Mortensen NH, Saether J, Steinke MS, Staehr H, Mikkelsen SS. Separation of tendon ends after Achilles tendon repair: a prospective, randomized, multicenter study. Orthopedics. 1992; 15(8): 899-903.

29. Nilsson-Helander K, Silbernagel KG, Thomee R. Acute Achilles tendon rupture: a randomized, controlled study comparing surgical and nonsurgical treatments using validated outcome measures. Am J Sports Med. 2010; 38(11): 2186-2193.

30. Nilsson-Helander K, Thomeé R, Grävare-Silbernagel K . The Achilles tendon total rupture score (ATRS) development and validation. Am J Sports Med. 2007; 35(3): 421-426.

31. Nistor L. Surgical and non-surgical treatment of Achilles tendon rupture. J Bone Joint Surg Am. 1981; 63: 394-399.

32. Pajala A, Kangas J, Siira P, Ohtonen P, Leppilahti J. Augmented compared with nonaugmented surgical repair of a fresh total Achilles tendon rupture. A prospective randomized study. J Bone Joint Surg Am. 2009; 91(5): 1092-1100.

33. Petersen OF, Nielsen MB, Jensen KH, Solgaard S. Randomized comparison of CAM walker and light-weight plaster cast in the treatment of first-time Achilles tendon rupture. Ugeskr Laeger. 2002; 164(33): 3852-3855.

34. Saleh M, Marshall PD, Senior R, MacFarlane A. The Sheffield splint for controlled early mobilisation after rupture of the calcaneal tendon. A prospective, randomised comparison with plaster treatment. J Bone Joint Surg Br. 1992; 74(2): 206-209.

35. Schroeder D, Lehmann M, Steinbrueck K. Treatment of acute Achilles tendon ruptures: open vs. percutaneous repair vs. conservative treatment. A prospective randomized study. Orthop Trans. 1997; 21: 1228.

36. Shea BJ, Grimshaw JM, Wells GA. Development of AMSTAR: a measurement tool to assess the methodological quality of systematic reviews. BMC Med Res Methodol. 2007; 7(1): 10.

37. Soroceanu A, Sidhwa F, Aarabi S, Kaufman A, Glazebrook M. Surgical versus nonsurgical treatment of acute Achilles tendon rupture. A meta-analysis of randomized trials. J Bone Joint Surg Am. 2012; 94(23): 2136-2143.

38. Thermann H, Zwipp H, Tscherne H. Functional treatment concept of acute rupture of the Achilles tendon. 2 years results of a prospective randomized study. Der Unfallchirurg. 1995; 98(1): 21.

39. Twaddle BC, Poon P. Early motion for Achilles tendon ruptures: is surgery important? A randomized, prospective study. Am J Sports Med. 2007; 35(12): 2033-2038.

40. van der Eng DM, Schepers T, Schep NW, Goslings JC. Rerupture rate after early weightbearing in operative versus conservative treatment of Achilles tendon ruptures: a meta-analysis. Foot Ankle Surg. 2013.

41. Wilkins R, Bisson LJ. Operative versus nonoperative management of acute Achilles tendon ruptures: a quantitative systematic review of randomized controlled trials. Am J Sports Med. 2012; 40(9): 2154-2160.

42. Willits K, Amendola A, Bryant D. Operative versus nonoperative treatment of acute Achilles tendon ruptures: a multicenter randomized trial using accelerated functional rehabilitation. J Bone Joint Surg Am. 2010; 92(17): 2767-2775.

43. Wong J, Barrass V, Maffulli N. Quantitative review of operative and nonoperative management of achilles tendon ruptures. Am J Sports Med. 2002; 30(4): 565-575.

44. Zhao HM, Yu GR, Yang YF, Zhou JQ, Aubeeluck A. Outcomes and complications of operative versus non-operative treatment of acute Achilles tendon rupture: a meta-analysis. Chin Med J. 2011; 124(23): 4050-4055.

"Anyone can hide. Facing up to things, working through them, that's what makes you strong."

Sarah Dessen

Chapter 26

Thromboprophylaxis and Wound Complications in Achilles Tendon Surgery

James D.F. Calder, Erica Arverud, Katarina Nilsson-Helander, Paul W. Ackermann, C. Niek van Dijk

Take Home Message

- *The incidence of symptomatic venous thromboembolism in foot and ankle surgery is similar to the risk of complications from chemical thromboprophylaxis, and routine use may therefore not be justified. The identification of those patients at greatest risk of developing venous thromboembolism may help to justify the cost and risk of giving thromboprophylaxis.*

- *Prevention is mandatory to reduce the complication rate. The use of pre-operative antibiotics and the avoidance of swelling that may endanger healing due to increased tension is of greatest importance.*

Introduction

The risk of venous thromboembolism (VTE) for patients undergoing orthopaedic surgery and lower limb immobilization following trauma is well documented [67], with death from a pulmonary embolus (PE) as a devastating potential consequence, yet debate surrounds the optimal method for the prevention of VTE and the risk-benefit analysis of such prophylaxis. The reported rate of deep vein thrombosis (DVT) is 44% after elective hip arthroplasty, 37% after hip fracture surgery, and 27% after elective knee arthroplasty, and

351

chemoprophylaxis following such procedures is now widely practiced. However, the risk of VTE following foot and ankle surgery appears low and the need for the routine use of such prophylaxis in patients undergoing foot and ankle surgery is not so clear due to the poor quality of the literature specifically dealing with the issue [26, 37, 60, 62]. The problems lie in identifying which patients and specific conditions are particularly at risk, and which method is most effective in preventing VTE while minimizing the risk, cost and inconvenience to the patient. This current concepts review critically analyses the available literature on the risks of developing VTE following foot and ankle surgery, which patients and conditions are particularly at risk, and the optimal methods available to reduce the incidence of VTE.

The Risk of Venous Thromboembolism

There are several problems when trying to assess the risk of VTE in foot and ankle surgery. Most of the larger studies have concentrated on investigating the incidence of VTE in patients undergoing hip and knee surgery, and very few well-conducted studies are available specifically examining the risk to patients with foot and ankle conditions. The majority of the larger studies also collect data prospectively yet review them retrospectively and rely upon identifying symptomatic VTE representing to the hospital or from follow-up questionnaires. As a result, there is undoubtedly under-reporting of the incidence of VTE in these studies.

Large, national database studies have given some insight into the incidence specifically of foot and ankle conditions. Jameson and co-workers investigated VTE and mortality within 90 days following surgery for ankle fractures, first metatarsal osteotomies, hindfoot fusions and total ankle replacements over a 43 month period using the English NHS database [26]. The respective incidence of DVT and PE following 45,949 ankle fractures was 0.12 and 0.17%; 0.01 and 0.02% following 33,626 first metatarsal osteotomies; and 0.03 and 0.11% after 7,033 hindfoot fusions. The incidence of PE following 1,633 total ankle replacements was 0.06% with no DVTs being reported. They concluded that the routine use of chemoprophylaxis agents such as low molecular weight heparin (LMWH) is not justified. They did, however, identify specific groups with a higher risk of VTE - those patients with ankle fracture who are >50 years old or who have a Charlson score ≥2. They comment that the National Institute for Health and Clinical Excellence (NICE) produces evidence-based guidelines on the appropriate treatment of patients in the NHS in England and Wales. NICE recently revised its guidelines for thromboprophylaxis, acknowledging the lack of robust evidence to support the routine use of chemoprophylaxis in orthopaedic patients though recommending that LMWH should be considered if limited mobility was expected post-operatively, if the patient is to be immobilized in a cast, or else if they undergo lower limb surgery lasting longer than 60 minutes. The length of treatment was not determined. Jameson and co-workers calculated that if the NICE guidelines were followed, this would cost £10.5 million over the study period whereas the cost for only giving chemoprophylaxis for the high risk groups they had identified would be £4.3 million [25].

Shibuya and co-workers reported the risk of VTE in 75,664 patients with isolated foot and ankle trauma from the National Data Trauma Bank (NDTB) [56]. There were the expected inherent flaws in this retrospective analysis of such a large cohort due to loss of data, but the authors openly reported how the data sets were analysed. The overall incidence of DVT and PE was 0.28 and 0.21% respectively. Increasing age was a risk factor for developing DVT, and a calculated 10 year difference in age would increase the risk of DVT by 20%. Obesity was also a significant risk factor increasing the likelihood of DVT and PE by a factor of 2.4 and 3 respectively. The authors concluded, therefore, that the routine use of chemoprophylaxis for the prevention of VTE in foot and ankle trauma patients was not warranted; however, patients should be assessed for risk on an individual basis.

Further studies have shown similarly low rates of VTE in patients undergoing foot and ankle procedures. Griffiths and co-workers, in a retrospective chart review of 2,654 patients, reported overall incidences of 0.27% DVT and 0.15% PE. 27 patients were lost to follow-up and if these were included in figures for the "worst-case scenario", then the rate of VTE was 1.43% [21]. The largest prospective multicentre study of 2,733 patients undergoing foot and ankle surgery was conducted by Mizel and co-workers, who reported a similarly low rate of VTE with an incidence of 0.22% DVT and 0.15% PE [36]. 50% of their patients underwent forefoot surgery, with 21.6% undergoing ankle surgery. They found that significant risk factors for VTE included non-weight-bearing status and immobilization. All these papers concluded that the routine use of thromboprophylaxis is not necessary but should be considered in higher risk patients.

Soohoo and co-workers reviewed the California discharge database, identifying 57,183 patients undergoing open reduction and internal fixation for ankle fractures. The readmission rate for PE was 0.34% [60]. This study is flawed by the fact that it reported only patients who were readmitted, ignoring patients who were admitted elsewhere, and the use of thromboprophylaxis was not documented (all were in-patients and, therefore, more likely to receive chemoprophylaxis). They subsequently looked at the same database for PE following the fixation of metatarsal fractures and found a rate of 0.27% in 1,477 patients (once again, this had the same study limitations). Phillips and co-workers in a prospective randomized study of the management of ankle fractures reported one non-fatal PE (0.7%) in a series of 138 patients [48]. Wukich and Waters reported an incidence of 0.4% DVT and 0.3% PE in 1,000 consecutive patients undergoing foot and ankle surgery during an 18 month period [65]. One confounding variable that may well have altered the true incidence of VTE is that patients who were admitted received thromboprophylaxis and 10% of their patients received LMWH for 15 days after discharge – interestingly, two of the seven patients who developed VTE were in this group.

Hanslow and co-workers reported a 4% incidence of clinically symptomatic VTE in a retrospective review of 602 patients undergoing foot and ankle surgery [22]. In this Level IV study, the risk factors for developing VTE included rheumatoid arthritis, recent air travel, previous history of VTE and immobilization. They deemed that 31% of their patients had a high risk to develop VTE, and these were therefore given chemical prophylaxis - interestingly the multivariate analysis demonstrated chemoprophylaxis as a risk factor for developing VTE.

When foot surgery is investigated by itself, similar low rates of VTE have been recorded. Felcher and co-workers retrospectively reviewed 7,264 patients undergoing podiatric surgery and identified the risk of VTE as 0.3% [12]. Previous history of VTE, use of the oral contraceptive pill (OCP) or hormone replacement therapy (HRT) and obesity were all independent risk factors. Slaybaugh and co-workers also performed a retrospective study on 1,822 patients undergoing podiatric surgery [58]. They reported rates of symptomatic DVT and PE of 0.5% and 0.1% respectively. Simon and co-workers in a prospective study investigating the effect of thigh tourniquet on the incidence of DVT after forefoot surgery in 71 patients, found no cases of thrombosis based on the results of I-labelled fibrinogen, Doppler ultrasound and phlebography [57]. Rink-Brune, in a retrospective review of 106 patients of the Lapidus procedure for the correction of hallux valgus, found only one DVT (0.9%) [51]. Wukich and co-workers reported a DVT in one patient undergoing opening wedge osteotomy for the treatment of primus varus in a series of 18 procedures (5.6%) [66]. Radl and co-workers found that 4% of patients showed venous thrombosis in a single centre, prospective, phlebographically-controlled study that quantified the rate of venous thrombosis in 100 patients who underwent Chevron osteotomy for the correction of hallux valgus deformity [49]. This Level II study concluded that the patients were at low risk of venous thrombosis after surgical treatment for hallux valgus. However, there was a significant correlation of VTE with increasing age with all four patients, with the VTE group having a mean age of 61.7 years compared with 48.4 years for the non-VTE group. They concluded that prophylaxis should be considered in patients over 60 years.

There is a concern that there may be a significant degree of under-reporting of VTE with such retrospective studies, and some smaller-sized but more controlled studies have demonstrated a higher rate of VTE. Solis and Saxby performed duplex ultrasound on the calves of 201 patients on their first post-operative visit following a foot and ankle operation [59]. Their incidence of below-knee DVT was 3.5% and at repeat ultrasound there was no progression of the DVT proximally. They suggested that the risks for DVT were hindfoot surgery and immobilization, tourniquet time and increasing age. They felt that the low incidence meant that routine prophylaxis is not required. Riou and co-workers investigated the incidence of VTE following immobilization for isolated non-surgical lower limb trauma. They performed compression ultrasound examination on 2,761 patients and found a symptomatic DVT rate of 1%, but following ultrasound the overall rate of DVT rose to 6.4%, suggesting that a significant number of patients remain asymptomatic [52]. Whether this is actually important and clinically significant is unknown, as the rate of proximal DVT - with which there is a greater risk of PE - was only 0.2%. Those over 50 years, rigid immobilization, a high injury severity score and non-weight bearing status were once again deemed to be the high risk groups for VTE.

Overall, the risk of VTE in patients undergoing foot and ankle surgery is much lower than that for hip and knee surgery. Reviewing the available data above, it appears that the risk of symptomatic DVT is approximately 0.5% and PE 0.2%. The true risk of DVT is certainly higher, but the clinical relevance of this is uncertain. Therefore, consideration should be given to identifying particular groups in whom chemoprophylaxis should be targeted.

Risk groups and factors for developing venous thromboembolism

One area of foot and ankle surgery exhibiting a higher risk of VTE concerns those with acute Achilles tendon rupture (ATR). Lapidus and co-workers performed colour duplex sonography (CDS) on 105 consecutive patients treated with acute Achilles tendon rupture [32]. They demonstrated a DVT rate of 35%. Nilsson-Helander and co-workers in a prospective series of 100 patients with acute Achilles tendon rupture, found a DVT in 32 of 95 patients (33.7%) who underwent CDS at eight weeks [40]. Five of these were proximal DVTs and there were three PEs. There was no difference in the risk for DVT in those treated surgically or non-surgically, and this view was further supported in a meta-analysis by Jiang and co-workers [26]. Lapidus and co-workers moreover, performed a prospective randomized trial with LMWH chemoprophylaxis on 91 acute Achilles tendon rupture patients and found no difference in DVT rates in the dalteparin 34% and placebo group 36% [32]. Similarly, Lapidus and co-workers found no effect of LMWH prophylaxis in a prospective randomized trial on 272 patients undergoing ankle fracture surgery, DVT rates being 21% in the dalteparin and 28% in the placebo group [31]. Jorgensen and co-workers studied the use of thromboprophylaxis for lower limb immobilization in 205 patients. Of the 41 patients with Achilles tendon rupture, eight (19.5%) had DVT [27]. Patel and co-workers, however, in a recent retrospective database analysis of 1,172 patients with Achilles tendon rupture, reported overall rates for DVT and PE 0.43 and 0.34%, respectively [44]. Concerns regarding the under-reporting of VTE in such studies have been previously discussed and another, smaller database review from New Zealand by Healy and co-workers reported a VTE rate of 6.3% in 208 patients with Achilles tendon rupture treated with immobilization [23]. They concluded that the incidence of VTE (which included three patients with PE) is similar to that following hip and knee surgery and, therefore, chemo-thromboprophylaxis should be considered. Saragas and co-workers likewise recommended chemoprophylaxis following operative repair of acute Achilles tendon rupture, when they reported a 5.7% incidence of DVT and one near-fatal PE (1.1%) [54]. Ingvar and co-workers, in a further chart review of 196 patients with Achilles tendon rupture, found that 3.6% had a DVT, and Persson and co-workers reported an incidence of 6.8% of symptomatic DVT following the repair of Achilles tendon rupture in a database of 800 patients [24, 47]. Interestingly, data from their screening programme showed that 45% of those with asymptomatic DVT had received LMWH chemoprophylaxis. Few studies have reported incidence in chronic Achilles tendon surgery, but Schon and co-workers in a prospective study of flexor hallucis longus tendon transfer for chronic Achilles tendinosis reported two DVTs in 46 patients (4.3%) [55].

Other authors have looked at the specific risk of those patients being treated for ankle fractures. Pelet and co-workers, in a retrospective chart review of 2,478 patients undergoing surgery for ankle fractures, found the incidence of ultrasound-confirmed symptomatic DVT was 2.7% and 0.3% for PE [46]. They concluded that thromboprophylaxis did not alter the occurrence of VTE. Although patients with risk factors for VTE such as obesity, smoking, increased age, HRT, OCP, neoplasia and previous history of VTE, had an increased rate of VTE (3.6%), this was not additionally affected by the use of thromboprophylaxis. Patil and co-workers performed a prospective study of the non-surgical management of stable ankle fractures treated in a below-knee cast [45]. Although no patients were symptomatic on the removal of the cast, ultrasound examination of 100 patients found a DVT in 5% in the absence of thromboprophylaxis. In view of the apparent low risk of DVT after ankle fractures, the authors recommended against routine thromboprophylaxis.

From the summary of papers given above, it would appear that patients undergoing surgery of the foot and ankle or with ankle fractures are at overall low risk of VTE. Those with acute Achilles tendon rupture may be at increased risk of symptomatic DVT, presumably due to immobilization in an equinus position. Specific patient-related factors increasing the individual's risk of VTE have been well-documented in the literature and the following factors specific to foot and ankle conditions should be considered [42] (Table 1):

Factor	Study
Age	≥40 years Shibuya [56] ≥50 years Wukich [66], Patel [44] ≥60 years Soohoo [61]
Obesity	Wukich [66], Brag [5], Shibuya [56], Patel [44], Pelet [46], Felcher [12]
Reduced weight-bearing status	Wukich [66], Hanslow [22], Brag [5], Riou [52]
Past history of VTE	Brag [5], Hanslow [22], Patel [44], Pelet [46], Felcher [12]
Immobilization	Solis [59], Hanslow [22], Riou [52]
Smoking	Edmonds [8], Pelet [46], Syed [62]
Oral contraception and hormone replacement therapy	Pelet [46], Felcher [12]
Air travel	Hanslow [22]
Rheumatoid arthritis	Hanslow [22]

Table 1. Specific patient-related factors increasing the individual's risk of VTE.

Methods of thromboprophylaxis

Various methods of thromboprophylaxis have been advocated, including aspirin, compression stockings and intermittent mechanical compression devices, inferior vena cava filters and both fractionated and unfractionated heparin [14]. To our knowledge, there are no randomized trials investigating the effects of coumarin derivatives in the prevention of VTE following lower limb immobilization. Pelet and co-workers, in their chart review of 2,478 patients, had 5.65% taking warfarin, but they could not demonstrate any modification in the rate of VTE [46]. Although the Pulmonary Embolism Prevention (PEP) Trial Collaborative Group demonstrated a 28% reduction in DVT in those patients taking aspirin following hip surgery, such results have not been demonstrated in foot and ankle disorders [1]. Gehling and co-workers conducted a small trial of aspirin versus LMWH, demonstrating equal effectiveness in preventing DVT following lower limb immobilization [18]. Griffiths and co-workers, in a retrospective case series, compared the VTE rate in 1,078 patients taking aspirin with 1,576 patients with no prophylaxis following foot and ankle surgery [21]. No protective effect against VTE could be demonstrated by using aspirin.

New oral anticoagulants may allow for the easier application of thromboprophylaxis - direct thrombin inhibitors (Dabigastran) and Xa inhibitors (Rivaroxaban) have been shown to be effective in the prevention of VTE in hip surgery, but they are only currently licensed for use following elective hip and knee arthroplasty [9, 10].

Mechanical devices such as venous calf and foot pumps, which apply intermittent pneumatic compression (IPC), have been shown to be effective in reducing VTE following lower limb surgery [2]. Knee length compression stockings have been shown to be as effective as thigh length stockings in an analysis of 14 randomized studies investigating VTE rates including 1,568 patients [53]. Thigh length stockings may also be difficult to apply and, if measured improperly, can act more as a tourniquet than as a graduated compression stocking [4, 5]. Recent studies demonstrate better DVT prophylaxis and fewer side effects with IPC compared to compression stockings. Venous compression by IPC alone or in combination with stockings has proven more effective than stockings alone in the prevention of both DVT and PE [3, 13, 36]. A meta-analysis of 16 studies including 3,887 post-operative and post-trauma patients suggests that the use of IPC yields results similar to heparin administration, but with the advantage of eliminating bleeding risks [6, 7]. IPC, moreover, seems to exhibit specific circulatory advantages as compared to LMWH when it comes to foot and ankle surgery, since distal circulation is impaired during post-operative immobilization. Moreover a recent review by Arverud and co-workers demonstrated that IPC in conjunction with DVT prevention also reduces pre- and post-operative oedema, leading to shortened hospital stays, improved joint mobility and pain relief, as well as having a possible effect on fractures and soft tissue repair [2].

The majority of papers have investigated the use of LMWH. A 2009 Cochrane review of six RCTs by Testroote and co-workers included 1,490 patients and reported an incidence of VTE ranging from 4.3% to 40% in patients immobilized in a plaster cast or brace for at least one week following leg injury who received no prophylaxis or placebo [63]. The incidence was significantly lower in those who received LMWH (event rates ranging from 0% to 37%; odds ratio 0.49). They concluded that the use of LMWH in outpatients significantly reduces VTE when immobilization of the lower leg is required. Ettema and co-workers, in a meta-analysis of six RTCs including 1,456 patients, concluded that the mean VTE rate was reduced from 17.1% to 9.6% with the use of LMWH [11]. Two studies compared the rates of DVT following lower leg immobilization using LMWH versus no treatment. Kujath and co-workers, in 253 patients, found a rate of 16.5% compared to 4.8% in the prophylaxis group, and Kock and co-workers found 4.3% versus 0% in the prophylaxis group (p<0.006) [29, 30]. Both studies could be criticized for not including controls or assessor blinding. Jorgensen and co-workers performed a RCT on 205 patients with lower limb immobilization and reported a DVT rate of 10% in the treatment group but 17% in the control group [27]. They could not, however, demonstrate a significant difference, possibly indicating a type II error as 12% had to stop injecting because of complications (bruising, haematoma, etc.) and nearly 1/3 of their initial 300 patients failed to complete the study.

Other studies have questioned the benefit of LMWH. Goel and co-workers, in a RCT of patients undergoing treatment with open reduction and internal fixation (ORIF) for isolated lower limb fractures, used either LMWH or saline control for 14 days within 48 hours of injury [20]. In 238 patients, the overall incidence of DVT was 11% and no significant differences were demonstrated between the two groups. However, funding ceased for this trial and therefore the 438 patients required according to the power calculation could not be recruited. Lapidus and co-workers in a placebo-controlled double-blind RCT of 272 patients undergoing LMWH therapy following ankle fracture reported that the overall incidence of phlebography-verified VTE was 21% in the LMWH group and 28% in the placebo group [31]. They concluded that although these patients seemed at high risk of VTE, most were asymptomatic and the routine use of LMWH was not recommended. Likewise, Riou and co-workers in their series of 2,761 patients with lower limb injuries treated non-surgically in a cast and assessed with ultrasound reported an overall rate 6.4% VTE, but could not prove the benefit of the routine use of LMWH, suggested instead a risk assessment approach [52]. Pelet and co-workers, in their chart review of 2,478 ankle fractures, could not demonstrate any influence on the VTE rate by the use of chemoprophylaxis [46]. Selby and co-workers, in a multicentre RCT of LMWH or placebo following the fixation of fractures distal to the knee, could not demonstrate a significant difference between the groups . Interestingly, they only chose to use ultrasound screening for proximal DVT, as they felt this to be more clinically important [54]. In consideration of when Achilles tendon rupture is specifically looked at, Lapidus and co-workers also performed a placebo-controlled RCT in 105 patients undergoing surgical repair. They could not identify any significant benefit of the use of LMWH in the 91 patients available for endpoint analysis (34% LMWH, 36% placebo) [30].

The effectiveness of LMWH in VTE prevention may be influenced by the timing of its commencement and the duration of it use. Zufferey and co-workers, in a meta-analysis of 13 RCTs, suggested that starting LMWH prophylaxis pre-operatively is associated with a reduced risk of asymptomatic DVT following major orthopaedic surgery [67]. Raskob and co-workers, in a methodological review of papers, concluded that pre-operative initiation is not required for good efficiency and that six hours post-operatively was the optimal timing for the commencement of LMWH (initiation <6 hours increases the risk of bleeding without improved efficacy and initiation at 12-24 hours post-operatively is less effective) [50].

Overall, the incidence of symptomatic DVT after foot and ankle surgery is about 0.5%, with an incidence of PE of about 0.2%, and the majority of authors conclude that the routine use of chemoprophylaxis after foot and ankle surgery or immobilization is not warranted [28]. Patients should be assessed regarding risk factors, such as age over 60 years, obesity, previous history of DVT, OCP/HRT and - possibly - those patients with an acute Achilles tendon rupture may need to be considered in a higher risk category. The combination of compression stockings and mechanical intermittent pneumatic compression while in hospital have evidence to support its use, but those with risk factors may benefit from protection with an oral factor Xa inhibitor or LMWH started at six hours following surgery and continued until mobile or else out of cast immobilization.

Complications of thromboprophylaxis

LMWH following foot and ankle surgery has complications associated with its use. The risk of bleeding following major orthopaedic surgery is reported as 1-2% [15], and has been reported as 0.3-1% specifically following surgery to the lower leg, requiring immobilization [33, 63]. Retroperitoneal bleeding occurred in one patient in the study by Lassen and co-workers, and Jorgensen and co-workers reported on 18 patients who stopped LMWH because of pain at the injection site, four with haematomas [27, 33]. They also reported an increased rate of wound infection in the LMWH group. Kock and co-workers also reported haematoma formation in four patients receiving LMWH thromboprophylaxis [29]. Ettema and co-workers, however, reported no increased risk of bleeding complications despite a reduction in the incidence of DVT following LMWH chemoprophylaxis after foot and ankle surgery [11]. Heparin-induced thrombocytopenia (HIT) is a potentially life-threatening adverse effect of heparin. It is more common in post-operative patients than medical patients, and occurs more often after unfractionated heparin (UH) than LMWH. Girolami and Girolami reported a 6.5% rate of HIT in patients using UH after orthopaedic surgery, while Martel and co-workers reported a rate of 2.6% compared to 0.2% following LMWH [19, 34].

Wound Complications

Several different types of wound complications are described in the literature. They can be roughly divided into major or minor complications. Movin and co-workers presented three categories: (1) General-, (2) Wound complications and (3) Re-ruptures [38].

In most randomized studies where surgical and non-surgical treatments are compared, the outcomes are presented as a comparison between re-ruptures and the number of wound infections.

Wound complications are one reason for selecting non-surgical treatment. Although wound complications do not usually lead to long-term problems, they can be troublesome for some patients. An infection can, in some patients, lead to devastating consequences, resulting in a poor outcome. According to Pajala and co-workers the incidence of deep infection as well as re-rupture has increased, with a prevalence of 2.2% [43].

Olsson and co-workers recently presented the results of a randomized controlled study comparing surgical and non-surgical treatment. In this study, including 100 patients, six patients in the surgical group sustained superficial infections, all of them healed with antibiotics. Willits and co-workers presented 2010, in a study an infection rate of one deep and four superficial infections out of 72 patients [64]. Furthermore, Metz and co-workers reported a high risk of skin-related complications in the non-surgical group related to the brace. Skin-related complications included, in most cases, minor superficial infections. As the definition of superficial and deep infection is lacking in most studies, it is difficult to compare the results from the different studies.

As a rule, most wounds heal with the addition of antibiotics and the avoidance of swelling [41, 64]. Patients with deep infections were significantly older, received corticosteroid medication more often, had sustained the tendon injury during everyday activities more frequently, and had a longer delay before treatment than those patients with simple re-ruptures.

Besides wound infections, patients may complain about scarring, decreased sensibility and aesthetic appearance. There are even patients who complain of impaired ankle function due to the scar [39].

Prevention is mandatory to reduce the complication rate. The use of pre-operative antibiotics and the avoidance of swelling that may endanger healing due to increased tension is of greatest importance. Negative wound pressure techniques could be used parallel to other treatments to reduce such tension.

Summary

The risk of asymptomatic VTE following foot and ankle surgery is lower than that in hip and knee surgery. Although some studies have recommended routine thromboprophylaxis [29, 30], these were based on the prevention of asymptomatic or distal DVTs. The incidence of symptomatic VTE is only approximately 0.5%, with the incidence of PE about 0.2% [12, 33, 35, 48, 52, 58, 61, 66]; most authors have therefore concluded that the routine administration of thromboprophylaxis after foot and ankle surgery or lower limb immobilization is not justified [12, 31, 32, 35, 45, 58, 61, 66]. When considering an intervention such as VTE prophylaxis that is intended for prevention as opposed to treatment, the risks and benefits must be carefully weighed. The efficacy of thromboprophylaxis has been established for hip and knee surgery, and mechanical methods are safe. In patients who are at high risk of VTE, the benefits of chemical thromboprophylaxis will generally outweigh the risks. However, in patients who are at a low risk of VTE, the risk/ benefit ratio may not be obvious. Complications such as bleeding and HIT, although infrequent, are increasingly recognized as being associated with adverse outcomes, increased cost and, potentially, an inability to resume therapy with needed anticoagulants. Therefore, an accurate and careful evaluation of a patient's thrombotic risk is essential to avoid the unnecessary or potentially harmful administration of medication. Patient risk factors such as age, obesity, previous history of VTE or cancer, OCP/HRT, and perhaps smoking, appear to be important, as do surgical factors such as immobilization, weight-bearing status and possibly air-travel. Achilles tendon rupture, whether treated surgically or non-surgically, also appears to be a specific risk factor. In high risk patients, it appears that starting chemical prophylaxis six hours post-operatively is appropriate, but there is no consensus on how long treatment should continue - most reports are for either until discharge from hospital or for approximately two weeks after surgery if the limb is immobilized.

There is very little agreement around the world in the various guidelines on the prevention of VTE, and most are based on hip and knee surgery. Struijk-Mulder compared 11 guidelines on thromboprophylaxis from nine countries [62]. Only the German and French guidelines recommend the use of chemical agents following the immobilization of lower extremities, while the Cardiovascular Disease Educational and Research Trust advises LMWH if risk factors are present. The American College of Chest Physicians (ACCP) publishes its recommendations regarding thromboprophylaxis every two to three years. The ACCP recommended that for patients with an isolated fracture of the lower extremity (including an ankle fracture), no thromboprophylaxis should be routinely given as it is uncertain whether thromboprophylaxis reduces clinically significant DVT or whether it is cost-effective [16, 17].

In conclusion, the incidence of symptomatic VTE in foot and ankle surgery is similar to the risk of complications from chemical thromboprophylaxis, and routine use may therefore not be justified. The identification of those patients at greatest risk of developing VTE may help to justify the cost and risk of giving thromboprophylaxis.

References

1. Pulmonary Embolism Prevention (PEP) Trial Collaborative Group Prevention of pulmonary embolism and deep vein thrombosis with low dose aspirin: pulmonary embolism prevention (PEP) trial. Lancet . 2000;355(9319 SRC - GoogleScholar):1715-1720.

2. Arverud E, Azevedo J, Labruto F, Ackermann P. Adjuvant compression therapy in orthopaedic surgery-an evidence-based review. European Orthopaedics and Traumatology 2013;4(1 SRC - GoogleScholar):49-57.

3. Asano H, Matsubara M, Suzuki K, Morita S, Shinomiya K. Prevention of pulmonary embolism by a foot sole pump. The Journal of bone and joint surgery British volume 2001;83(8):1130-1132.

4. Benko T, Cooke EA, McNally MA. Graduated compression stockings: knee length or thigh length. Clin Orthop 2001;383 SRC - GoogleScholar:197-203.

5. Brag A, Henninger H, Hintermann B, J. Risk factors for symptomatic deep-vein thrombosis in patients after total ankle replacement who received routine chemical thromboprophylaxis. Joint Surg Br 93B 2011;921-927.

6. Byrne B. Deep vein thrombosis prophylaxis: the effectiveness and implications of using below-knee or thigh-length graduated compression stockings. Journal of vascular nursing : official publication of the Society for Peripheral Vascular Nursing 2002;20(2):53-59.

7. Caprini JA. Stockings or no stockings: that is the question. Annals of surgery 2010;251(3):397-398.

8. Edmonds MJR, Crichton TJH, Runciman WB, Pradhan M. Evidence-based risk factors for postoperative deep vein thrombosis. ANZ journal of surgery 2004;74(12):1082-1097.

9. Eriksson BI, Borris LC, Friedman RJ et al. Rivaroxaban versus enoxaparin for thromboprophylaxis after hip arthroplasty. The New England journal of medicine 2008;358(26):2765-2775.

10. Eriksson BI, Dahl OE, Rosencher N et al. Dabigatran etexilate versus enoxaparin for prevention of venous thromboembolism after total hip replacement: a randomised, double-blind, non-inferiority trial. Lancet 2007;370(9591):949-956.

11. Ettema HB, Kollen BJ, Verheyen CCPM, B++ller HR. Prevention of venous thromboembolism in patients with immobilization of the lower extremities: a meta-analysis of randomized controlled trials. Journal of thrombosis and haemostasis : JTH 2008;6(7):1093-1098.

12. Felcher AH, Mularski RA, Mosen DM, Kimes TM, DeLoughery TG, Laxson SE. Incidence and risk factors for venous thromboembolic disease in podiatric surgery. Chest 2009;135(4):917-922.

13. Fordyce MJ, Ling RS. A venous foot pump reduces thrombosis after total hip replacement. The Journal of bone and joint surgery British volume 1992;74(1):45-49.

14. Forsythe RM, Peitzman AB, DeCato T et al. Early lower extremity fracture fixation and the risk of early pulmonary embolus: filter before fixation? The Journal of trauma 2011;70(6):1381-1388.

15. Francis CW. Prevention of VTE in patients having major orthopedic surgery. Journal of thrombosis and thrombolysis 2013;35(3):359-367.

16. Geerts WH, Heit JA, Clagett GP et al. Prevention of venous thromboembolism. Chest 2001;119(1 Suppl):132S-175S.

17. Geerts WH, Bergqvist D, Pineo GF et al. Prevention of venous thromboembolism: American College of Chest Physicians Evidence-Based Clinical Practice Guidelines (8th Edition). Chest 2008;133(6 Suppl):381S-453S.

18. Gehling H, Giannadakis K, Lefering R, Hessmann M, Achenbach S, Gotzen L. [Prospective randomized pilot study of ambulatory prevention of thromboembolism. 2 times 500 mg aspirin (ASS) vs. clivarin 1750 (NMH)]. Der Unfallchirurg 1998;101(1):42-49.

19. Girolami B, Girolami A. Heparin-induced thrombocytopenia: a review. Seminars in thrombosis and hemostasis 2006;32(8):803-809.

20. Goel DP, Buckley R, deVries G, Abelseth G, Ni A, Gray R. Prophylaxis of deep-vein thrombosis in fractures below the knee: a prospective randomised controlled trial. The Journal of bone and joint surgery British volume 2009;91(3):388-394.

21. Griffiths JT, Matthews L, Pearce CJ, Calder JDF. Incidence of venous thromboembolism in elective foot and ankle surgery with and without aspirin prophylaxis. Journal of Bone & Joint Surgery, British Volume 2012;94(2):210-214.

22. Hanslow SS, Grujic L, Slater HK, Chen D. Thromboembolic disease after foot and ankle surgery. Foot & ankle international / American Orthopaedic Foot and Ankle Society [and] Swiss Foot and Ankle Society 2006;27(9):693-695.

23. Healy B, Beasley R, Weatherall M. Venous thromboembolism following prolonged cast immobilisation for injury to the tendo Achillis. The Journal of bone and joint surgery British volume 2010;92(5):646-650.

24. Ingvar J, T+ñgil M, Eneroth M. Nonoperative treatment of Achilles tendon rupture: 196 consecutive patients with a 7% re-rupture rate. Acta orthopaedica 2005;76(4):597-601.

25. Jameson SS, Augustine A, James P et al. Venous thromboembolic events following foot and ankle surgery in the English National Health Service. The Journal of bone and joint surgery British volume 2011;93(4):490-497.

26. Jiang N, Wang B, Chen A, Dong F, Yu B. Operative versus nonoperative treatment for acute Achilles tendon rupture: a meta-analysis based on current evidence. International orthopaedics 2012;36(4):765-773.

27. Jorgensen PS, Warming T, Hansen K et al. Vibeke Wille-Jorgensen molecular weight heparin (Innohep) as thromboprophylaxis in outpatients with a plaster cast: a venographic controlled study. Thromb Res 2002;105:477-480.

28. Kadous A, Abdelgawad AA, Kanlic E. Deep venous thrombosis and pulmonary embolism after surgical treatment of ankle fractures: a case report and review of literature. The Journal of foot and ankle surgery : official publication of the American College of Foot and Ankle Surgeons 2012;51(4):457-463.

29. Kock HJ, Schmit-Neuerburg KP, Hanke J, Rudofsky G, Hirche H. Thromboprophylaxis with low-molecular-weight heparin in outpatients with plaster-cast immobilisation of the leg. Lancet 1995;346(8973):459-461.

30. Kujath P, Spannagel U, Habscheid W. Incidence and prophylaxis of deep venous thrombosis in outpatients with injury of the lower limb. Haemostasis 1993;23 Suppl 1:20-26.

31. Lapidus LJ, Ponzer S, Elvin A et al. Prolonged thromboprophylaxis with Dalteparin during immobilization after ankle fracture surgery: a randomized placebo-controlled, double-blind study. Acta orthopaedica 2007;78(4):528-535.

32. Lapidus LJ, Rosfors S, Ponzer S et al. Prolonged thromboprophylaxis with dalteparin after surgical treatment of achilles tendon rupture: a randomized, placebo-controlled study. Journal of orthopaedic trauma 2007;21(1):52-57.

33. Lassen MR, Borris LC, Nakov RL. Use of the low-molecular-weight heparin reviparin to prevent deep-vein thrombosis after leg injury requiring immobilization. The New England journal of medicine 2002;347(10):726-730.

34. Martel N, Lee J, Wells PS. Risk for heparin-induced thrombocytopenia with unfractionated and low-molecular-weight heparin thromboprophylaxis: a meta-analysis. Blood 2005;106(8):2710-2715.

35. Mayle RE, DiGiovanni CW, Lin SS, Tabrizi P, Chou LB. Current concepts review: venous thromboembolic disease in foot and ankle surgery. Foot & ankle international / American Orthopaedic Foot and Ankle Society [and] Swiss Foot and Ankle Society 2007;28(11):1207-1216.

36. Mizel MS, Temple HT, Michelson JD et al. Thromboembolism after foot and ankle surgery. A multicenter study. Clinical orthopaedics and related research 1998;(348):180-185.

37. Morris RJ, Woodcock JP. Evidence-based compression: prevention of stasis and deep vein thrombosis. Annals of surgery 2004;239(2):162-171.

38. Movin T, Ryberg A, McBride DJ, Maffulli N. Acute rupture of the Achilles tendon. Foot and ankle clinics 2005;10(2):331-356.

39. Nilsson-Helander K, Silbernagel KG, Thomée R et al. Acute achilles tendon rupture: a randomized, controlled study comparing surgical and nonsurgical treatments using validated outcome measures. The American journal of sports medicine 2010;38(11):2186-2193.

40. Nilsson-Helander K, Thurin A, Karlsson J, Eriksson BI. High incidence of deep venous thrombosis after Achilles tendon rupture: a prospective study. Knee surgery, sports traumatology, arthroscopy : official journal of the ESSKA 2009;17(10):1234-1238.

41. Olsson N, Silbernagel KG, Eriksson BI et al. Stable surgical repair with accelerated rehabilitation versus nonsurgical treatment for acute achilles tendon ruptures: a randomized controlled study. The American journal of sports medicine 2013;41(12):2867-2876.

42. Paiement GD, Mendelsohn C. The risk of venous thromboembolism in the orthopedic patient: epidemiological and physiological data. Orthopedics 1997;20 Suppl:7-9.

43. Pajala A, Kangas J, Ohtonen P, Leppilahti J. Rerupture and deep infection following treatment of total Achilles tendon rupture. The Journal of bone and joint surgery American volume 2002;84-A(11):2016-2021.

44. Patel A, Ogawa B, Charlton T, Thordarson D. Incidence of deep vein thrombosis and pulmonary embolism after Achilles tendon rupture. Clinical orthopaedics and related research 2012;470(1):270-274.

45. Patil S, Gandhi J, Curzon I, Hui ACW. Incidence of deep-vein thrombosis in patients with fractures of the ankle treated in a plaster cast. The Journal of bone and joint surgery British volume 2007;89(10):1340-1343.

46. Pelet S, Roger ME, Belzile EL, Bouchard M. The incidence of thromboembolic events in surgically treated ankle fracture. The Journal of bone and joint surgery American volume 2012;94(6):502-506.

47. Persson LM, Lapidus LJ, L+ñrfars G, Rosfors S. Deep venous thrombosis after surgery for Achilles tendon rupture: a provoked transient event with minor long-term sequelae. Journal of thrombosis and haemostasis : JTH 2011;9(8):1493-1499.

48. Phillips WA, Schwartz HS, Keller CS et al. A prospective, randomized study of the management of severe ankle fractures. The Journal of bone and joint surgery American volume 1985;67(1):67-78.
49. Radl R, Kastner N, Aigner C, Portugaller H, Schreyer H, Windhager R. Venous thrombosis after hallux valgus surgery. The Journal of bone and joint surgery American volume 2003;85-A(7):1204-1208.
50. Raskob GE, Hirsh J. Controversies in timing of the first dose of anticoagulant prophylaxis against venous thromboembolism after major orthopedic surgery. Chest 2003;124(6 Suppl):379S-385S.
51. Rink-Brune O, A, J. Lapidus Arthrodesis for Management of Hallux ValgusГÇöReview of 106 Cases. Ankle Surg 2004;43(5 SRC - GoogleScholar):290-295.
52. Riou B, Rothmann C, Lecoules N et al. Incidence and risk factors for venous thromboembolism in patients with nonsurgical isolated lower limb injuries. The American journal of emergency medicine 2007;25(5):502-508.
53. Sajid MS, Tai NRM, Goli G, Morris RW, Baker DM, Hamilton G. Knee versus thigh length graduated compression stockings for prevention of deep venous thrombosis: a systematic review. European journal of vascular and endovascular surgery : the official journal of the European Society for Vascular Surgery 2006;32(6):730-736.
54. Saragas NP, Ferrao PNF. The incidence of venous thromboembolism in patients undergoing surgery for acute Achilles tendon ruptures. Foot and ankle surgery : official journal of the European Society of Foot and Ankle Surgeons 2011;17(4):263-265.
55. Schon LC, Shores JL, Faro FD, Vora AM, Camire LM, Guyton GP. Flexor hallucis longus tendon transfer in treatment of Achilles tendinosis. The Journal of bone and joint surgery American volume 2013;95(1):54-60.
56. Shibuya N, Frost CH, Campbell JD, Davis ML, Jupiter DC. Incidence of acute deep vein thrombosis and pulmonary embolism in foot and ankle trauma: analysis of the National Trauma Data Bank. The Journal of foot and ankle surgery : official publication of the American College of Foot and Ankle Surgeons 2012;51(1):63-68.
57. Simon MA, Mass DP, Zarins CK, Bidani N, Gudas CJ, Metz CE. The effect of a thigh tourniquet on the incidence of deep venous thrombosis after operations on the fore part of the foot. The Journal of bone and joint surgery American volume 1982;64(2):188-191.
58. Slaybaugh RS, Beasley BD, Massa EG. Deep venous thrombosis risk assessment, incidence, and prophylaxis in foot and ankle surgery. Clinics in podiatric medicine and surgery 2003;20(2):269-289.
59. Solis G, Saxby T. Incidence of DVT following surgery of the foot and ankle. Foot & ankle international / American Orthopaedic Foot and Ankle Society [and] Swiss Foot and Ankle Society 2002;23(5):411-414.
60. Soohoo NF, Krenek L, Eagan MJ et al. Complication rates following open reduction and internal fixation of ankle fractures. Joint Surg Am 2009;91 SRC - GoogleScholar:1042-1049.
61. Soohoo NF, Farng E, Zingmond DS. Incidence of pulmonary embolism following surgical treatment of metatarsal fractures. Foot & ankle international / American Orthopaedic Foot and Ankle Society [and] Swiss Foot and Ankle Society 2010;31(7):600-603.
62. Syed FF, Beeching NJ. Lower-limb deep-vein thrombosis in a general hospital: risk factors, outcomes and the contribution of intravenous drug use. QJM : monthly journal of the Association of Physicians 2005;98(2):139-145.
63. Testroote M, Stigter W, de Visser DC, Janzing H. Low molecular weight heparin for prevention of venous thromboembolism in patients with lower-leg immobilization. The Cochrane database of systematic reviews 2008;(4):CD006681.
64. Willits K, Amendola A, Bryant D et al. Operative versus nonoperative treatment of acute Achilles tendon ruptures: a multicenter randomized trial using accelerated functional rehabilitation. The Journal of bone and joint surgery American volume 2010;92(17):2767-2775.
65. Wuckich D, Roussel A, Dial D, J. Correction of metatarsus primus varus with an opening wedge plate: a review of 18 procedures. Ankle Surg JulAug 2009;48(4 SRC - GoogleScholar):420-426.
66. Wukich DK, Waters DH. Thromboembolism following foot and ankle surgery: a case series and literature review. The Journal of foot and ankle surgery : official publication of the American College of Foot and Ankle Surgeons 2008;47(3):243-249.
67. Zufferey P, Laporte S, Quenet S et al. Mismetti low-molecular-weight heparin regimen in major orthopaedic surgery A meta-analysis of randomised trials. Downloaded from wwwthrombosisonlinecom DOI 1011600086:TH03-02.

*"Employ thy time well, if thou
meanest to get leisure."*

Benjamin Franklin

Chapter 27

Techniques of Reattachment and Reconstruction of the Achilles Tendon

Nicola Maffulli, Umile G. Longo, Angelo Del Buono,
Vincenzo Denaro

Take Home Message

- *Missed or chronic Achilles tendon ruptures may cause muscle hypotrophy and tendon retraction resulting in a defect that must be augmented with endogenous or exogenous tissue.*

- *The aim of Achilles tendon reconstruction is to restore plantar flexion power, restore normal range of movement of the ankle joint, and ensure durable and pliable soft tissue coverage.*

- *The surgical management of insertional Achilles tendinopathy includes Achilles tendon debridement, calcaneal osteotomy and retrocalcaneal bursa excision. When complete tendon detachment is required, reattachment procedures can be performed using either anchors or transosseous sutures.*

Reconstruction

Achilles tendon ruptures represent more than 40% of all tendon ruptures requiring surgical management [27, 28]. Around 20% of acute Achilles tendon ruptures are not diagnosed at the time of injury and become chronic, necessitating more complicated management than acute injuries [8, 13, 15]. The management of chronic ruptures of the Achilles tendon is usually different from that of an acute rupture, as the tendon-ends have normally retracted [5, 31, 32]. Reconstruction of chronic Achilles tendon rupture is challenging but critical for successful ambulation. Missed or chronic Achilles tendon ruptures may cause muscle hypotrophy and tendon retraction, resulting in a defect that must be augmented with endogenous or exogenous materials. The blood supply to this area is relatively poor, and the tendon-ends need to be freshened to allow healing. Due to the increased gap, primary repair is not generally possible [31]. The aim of Achilles tendon reconstruction is to restore plantar flexion power and restore normal ankle range of movement, and allow durable and pliable soft tissue coverage [2, 14, 21, 22, 25, 29, 43, 48, 53].

Several open surgical techniques using a single longitudinal incision for exposure have been described for the reconstruction of the Achilles tendon, including flap tissue turn-down using one [7, 26] or two flaps [1], local tendon transfer [10, 44, 54, 55] and autologous hamstring tendon harvesting [34]. Complications, such as wound breakdown and infection (9%) [49], are not infrequent, and they are probably related to the paucity of the soft tissue vascularity, and may require reconstructive surgical procedures to cover soft tissue defects [23]. Minimally invasive reconstruction of the Achilles tendon, in the presence of a large gap lesion, has been described using an ipsilateral free semitendinosus tendon graft or peroneus tendon to improve the overall function with a low rate of complications [33, 36, 38-41]. Long-term follow-up has shown good results for both techniques.

Reconstructive procedures can be also necessary in the case of chronic avulsion of the Achilles tendon, as the calcaneus can be totally denuded of tendon tissue, or else only a small tuft of frayed tissue may remain attached to the calcaneus and thus be inadequate to allow a direct repair. In these patients, if it is not possible to directly reattach the Achilles tendon, a tendon graft can be necessary and can be fixed in a minimally invasive fashion using a free semitendinosus tendon graft with interference screw fixation in the calcaneus through a Cincinnati incision [37]. Bibbo and co-workers [3] described a transcalcaneal suture technique for the repair of Achilles tendon sleeve avulsion through a longitudinal incision. This technique, to be used in patients who do not have a large tendon defect, allows the reinsertion of the tendon into the calcaneus. However, when a large tendon defect is present, the surgeon must consider a tendon graft to bridge the gap and produce a strong construct.

Peroneus brevis transfer

The patient is positioned prone. Three skin incisions are performed [5]: 1) the first incision is 5 cm long, made 2 cm proximal and just medial to the palpable end of the residual tendon; 2) the second incision is 3 cm long and is also longitudinal, but it is 2 cm distal and lateral to the distal end of the tendon rupture; 3) the third incision is a 2 cm long at the base of the fifth metatarsal.

The distal Achilles tendon stump is first mobilized to allow access to the base of the lateral aspect of the distal tendon close to its insertion. It should be possible to palpate the medial tubercle of the calcaneus. The ruptured tendon-end is then resected back to a macroscopically healthy tendon, and a locking suture is run along the free tendon edge to prevent the separation of the bundles. The proximal tendon is then mobilized from the proximal wound; any adhesions are divided and further soft tissue release anterior to the soleus and gastrocnemius allows for maximal excursion, minimizing the gap between the two tendon stumps. A locking suture is thereafter run along the free tendon edge to allow adequate exposure and to prevent separation of the bundles. The tendon of the peroneus brevis is harvested and a locking suture is applied to the tendon-end before release from the metatarsal base. The peroneus brevis tendon is identified at the base of the distal incision of the Achilles tendon following the incision of the deep fascia overlying the peroneal muscles compartment. The tendon of the peroneus brevis is then withdrawn through the distal wound. This may take significant force, as there may be tendinous vinculae between the two peroneal tendons distally. The muscular portion of the peroneus brevis is then mobilized proximally to allow for increased excursion of the tendon of the peroneus brevis. A longitudinal tenotomy parallel to the tendon fibres is made through both stumps of the tendon. With the ankle in maximal plantar flexion, a suture is used to suture the peroneus brevis to both sides of the distal stump. The peroneus brevis tendon is then passed beneath the intact skin bridge into the proximal incision, and passed from medial to lateral through a transverse tenotomy in the proximal stump. Finally, the tendon of the peroneus brevis is sutured back onto itself on the lateral side of the proximal incision. A previously prepared removable scotch cast support with Velcro straps is applied.

Post-operatively, patients are allowed to bear weight as comfort allows with the use of crutches. After two weeks, the back shell is removed and physiotherapy is commenced with the front shell in situ preventing dorsiflexion of the ankle, focusing on proprioception, plantar-flexion of the ankle, and inversion and eversion training. During this period of rehabilitation, the patient is permitted to bear weight as comfort allows with the front shell in situ. The front shell may finally be removed after 6 weeks. A heel raise after the removal of the cast is usually not recommended, and patients normally regain a plantigrade ankle over a couple of weeks.

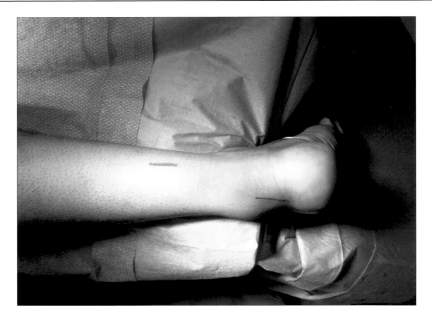

Figure 1. Picture showing the two landmarks where the two incisions are made. The proximal incision is 1 cm medial to the medial edge of the tendon and approximately 5 cm above the palpable defect. The distal incision is 2 cm below the defect, 1 cm lateral to the lateral edge of the tendon, extended to the postero-superior tuberosity of the calcaneus.

Ipsilateral free semitendinosus tendon graft transfer for chronic tears of the Achilles tendon

The patient is positioned prone [35]. Two skin incisions are made: 1) the first incision is 5 cm long, made 2 cm proximal and just medial to the palpable end of the residual tendon; 2) the second incision is 3 cm long and is also longitudinal but is 2 cm distal and in the midline over the distal end of the tendon rupture (Figure 1). The proximal and distal Achilles tendon stumps are mobilized, freeing them of all peritendinous adhesions. The ruptured tendon-end is then resected back to a macroscopically healthy tendon, and a locking suture is run along the free tendon edge to prevent the separation of the bundles. The proximal tendon is thereafter mobilized from the proximal wound, adhesions are divided, and further soft tissue release anterior to the soleus and gastrocnemius allows for maximal excursion, minimizing the gap between the two tendon stumps. A locking suture is run along the free tendon edge to allow adequate exposure and to prevent the separation of the bundles. After trying to reduce the gap of the ruptured Achilles tendon, and if the gap produced is greater than 6 cm despite maximal plantar flexion of the ankle and traction on the Achilles tendon stumps, the ipsilateral semitendinosus tendon is harvested.

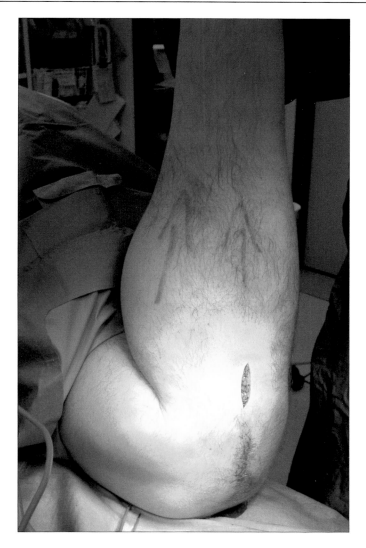

Figure 2. Longitudinal 3 cm long incision over the pes anserinus to harvest the semitendinosus tendon.

The semitendinosus tendon is harvested through a short, vertical, longitudinal incision over the pes anserinus (Figure 2). The semitendinosus tendon is passed through a small incision in the substance of the proximal stump of the Achilles tendon and is sutured to the Achilles tendon at the entry and exit points (Figure 3). The semitendinosus tendon is then passed beneath the intact skin bridge into the distal incision and passed from medial to lateral through a transverse tenotomy in the distal stump (Figure 4). With the ankle in maximal plantar flexion, the semitendinosus tendon is sutured to the Achilles tendon at entry and exit points. The repair is tensioned in maximal equinus. One end of the semitendinosus tendon is then passed again beneath the intact skin bridge into the proximal incision and passed from medial to lateral through a transverse tenotomy in the proximal stump. The other end of the semitendinosus tendon is then passed again from medial to lateral through a transverse tenotomy in the distal stump. The reconstruction may be further augmented if needed. A previously-prepared removable cast support is applied post-operatively.

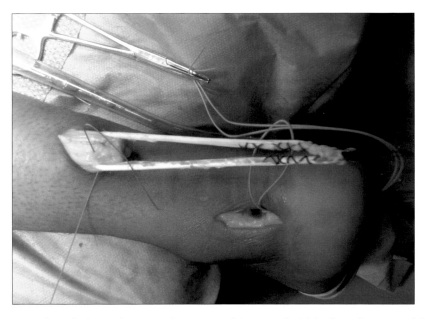

Figure 3. The tubularized semitendinosus graft is passed within the substance of the proximal stump of the Achilles tendon through a small incision. It will be secured to the Achilles tendon at both the entry and exit points.

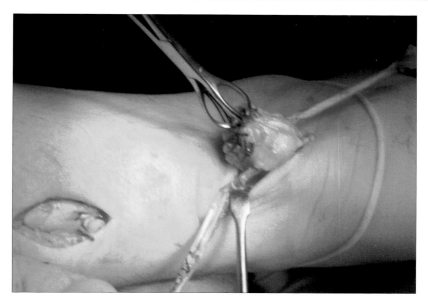

Figure 4. Medial-to-lateral passage of the semitendinosus tendon through a transverse tenotomy in the distal stump.

Less invasive semitendinosus reconstruction for chronic avulsion of the Achilles tendon

The patient is positioned prone. Two skin incisions are made: 1) the first incision is 5 cm, made 2 cm proximal and just medial to the palpable end of the residual tendon; 2) the second incision is a 5 to 7 cm semicircular Cincinnati skin incision [6], made over the area of the Achilles tendon insertion. After trying to reduce the gap of the ruptured Achilles tendon, and if the gap does not allow the tendon to reach the bone despite maximal plantar flexion of the ankle and traction on the Achilles tendon stump, the ipsilateral semitendinosus is harvested. The tendon is prepared in the usual fashion (Figure 5).

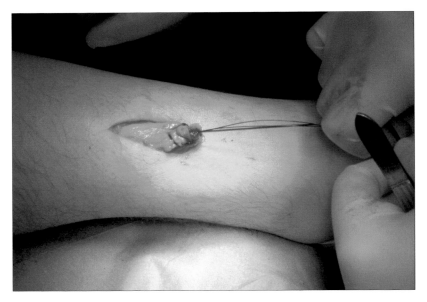

Figure 5. Appearance of the proximal stump after preparation.

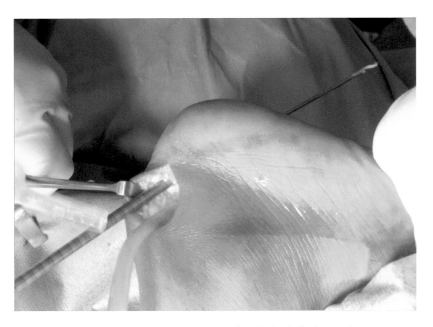

Figure 6. Reamer and K wire passage through a hole drilled into the calcaneus. As it is shown, this surgical step is made keeping the ankle in maximal plantar flexion.

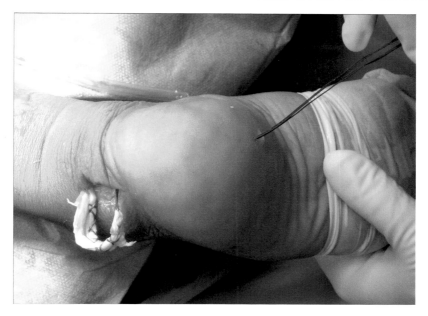

Figure 7. After osteotomy of the posterior tuberosity of the calcaneus, the semitendinosus graft is passed through the calcaneus.

A cannulated headed reamer corresponding to the graft's diameter is used to perforate the calcaneus to allow the passage of the double-looped semitendinosus tendon graft. A wire is then passed through the tunnel (Figure 6). The proximal tendon is then mobilized from the proximal wound, as described above. The semitendinosus tendon is passed through a small incision in the substance of the proximal stump of the Achilles tendon and is sutured to the Achilles tendon at the entry and exit points. The semitendinosus tendon is then passed beneath the intact skin bridge into the distal incision, and then through the calcaneus tunnel (Figure 7). With the ankle in maximal plantar flexion, the semitendinosus tendon is fixed using a bioabsorbable interference screw inserted over a guide wire into the calcaneus (Figure 8).

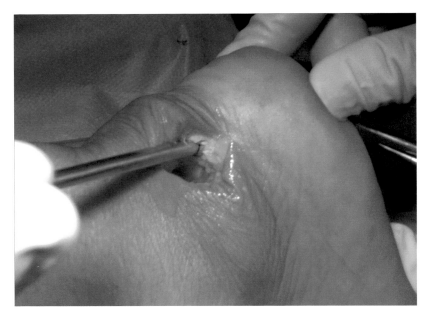

Figure 8. The system is finally secured by a bioabsorbable screw inserted into the previously drilled tunnel. The ankle is still plantar-flexed.

Reattachment

Insertional Achilles tendinopathy results in isolated pain at the Achilles tendon insertion site due to intratendinous degeneration. When non-surgical measures fail, surgical treatment may be necessary. Reattachment procedures with either anchors [42] or transosseous sutures [52] can be indicated in patients with insertional Achilles tendinopathy.

This condition can be difficult to manage. Bursectomy, excision of the distal paratenon, detachment of the tendon, removal of the calcific deposit, and the reinsertion of the Achilles tendon with bone anchors, have all been proved to be safe and effective [42].

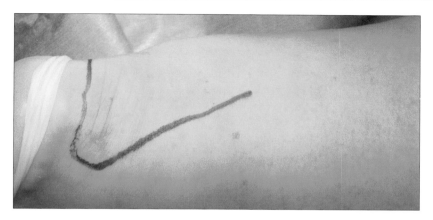

Figure 9. Mark of the incision performed for complete exposure of the tendon insertion and posterior tuberosity of the calcaneus.

Surgical technique

The procedure is performed as day-care surgery. The patient is prone, under general anaesthesia. A longitudinal incision is undertaken 1 cm medial to the medial border of the tendon, extended from the lower one third of the tendon up to 2 cm distal to the calcaneal insertion (Figure 9). The paratenon is dissected from the tendon and excised, taking care to preserve the anterior fat in Kager's triangle without injuring the mesotenon. When retrocalcaneal bursitis is present, the bursa is removed. Once the tendon has been exposed, the appearance of the tendon is checked. Between one and three longitudinal tenotomies are performed in the areas in which the tendon has lost its normal appearance or where softening or thickening are appreciable. Areas of degeneration are removed. The longitudinal tenotomise are left open. Once the site of calcific tendinopathy has been appreciated, it is defined proximally, medially and laterally with the tip of a syringe needle (Figure 10). At least one third of the Achilles tendon surrounding the area of calcific tendinopathy is detached or else - at times - a total disinsertion is made. The area of calcific tendinopathy is excised. The area of hyaline cartilage over the postero-superior tuberosity of the calcaneus may be macroscopically degenerated. In such an instance, this area is removed via osteotomy.

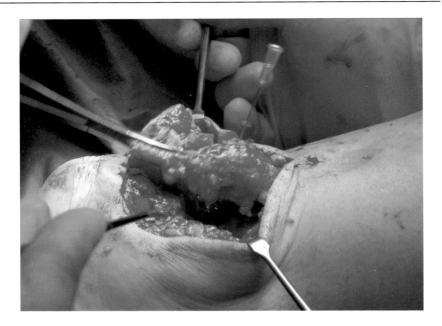

Figure 10. Definition of the ends of the calcific area.

The tendon is reinserted into the calcaneus using bone anchors (Mitek GII, Ethicon Ltd., Edinburgh, Scotland) (Figure 11). Two bone anchors are used when one third to 50% of the Achilles tendon is disinserted; three bone anchors are used when the disinsertion involves 50% to 75% of the Achilles tendon; four bone anchors are used when 75% or more of the tendon is detached; and five anchors are used when the Achilles tendon is totally disinserted. The Achilles tendon is then advanced from proximal to distal and reinserted into the calcaneus.

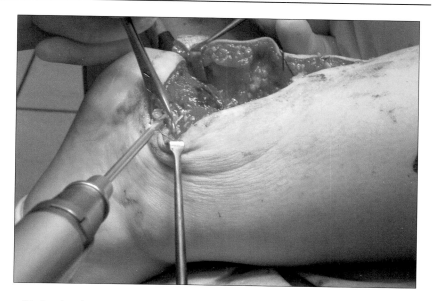

Figure 11. Anchor insertion into the calcaneal bone.

In a longitudinal study [23], 21 patients with recalcitrant calcific insertional Achilles tendinopathy underwent surgical removal of the calcific degeneration of the Achilles tendon and tendon reinsertion using bone anchors. After an average follow-up of four years, 16 patients reported good or excellent results; five patients had not returned to their pre-injury sporting activity. Only one patient had undergone a second operation. Based on a VISA-A assessment, all the patients fared markedly better compared to the baseline condition. The final average VISA was 88.1; the average pre-operative score was 62.4.

Alternative approach

Depending upon the extent of the detachment, place stiches utilizing the Bunnel suturing technique. Start suturing from the distal end of the tendon. For this technique, it is best to start and finish on the superficial side of the tendon. Select the anchor insertion site on the distal border of the tendon insertion site. Utilize knotless tensionable suture anchors (FOOTPRINT™ Ultra PK, Smith & Nephew, Andover, MA). For medial, central or lateral insertional tendinopathy, a partial detachment and a reinsertion of the detached portion of the tendon is performed. In case of calcification over the full width of the insertion, the complete tendon is detached and reinserted with three anchors.

Post-operative management

A synthetic below knee cast is applied keeping the ankle plantigrade. Patients are discharged on the day of surgery. They are recommended to walk on crutches [18] and are allowed to bear weight on the operated leg as tolerated, and they are also recommended to keep the leg elevated as much as possible for the first two post-operative weeks. The cast is removed after two weeks. At that stage, a synthetic anterior below the knee slab is applied with the ankle in a neutral position - patients are encouraged to bear weight on the operated limb and gradually progress to full weight-bearing, and isometric contractions of the gastrocnemius-soleus complex are started. Return to sport is allowed at 20 to 24 weeks from the index procedure.

Discussion

There are no evidence-based guidelines for choosing the type of operative management of chronic ruptures and avulsion of the Achilles tendon. Two classification systems have been proposed for chronic ruptures of the Achilles tendon [24, 45], both based on the length of the tendon defect. Under Kuwada's classification [24], a Type I lesion is a partial rupture and is managed with plaster cast immobilization. A Type II lesion is a complete rupture with a defect up to 3 cm: it is managed with end-to-end repair. A Type III lesion is a complete rupture with a defect of 3-6 cm. It is managed with a tendon graft, with or without augmentation with a synthetic graft. A Type IV lesion is a complete rupture with a defect more than 6 cm long after the debridement of the ends of the tendon to healthy tissue. A gastrocnemius recession, a free tendon graft and/ or a synthetic tendon graft are used for this type of lesion. Under Myerson's classification [45], a Type 1 defect is no more than 1-2 cm long. It is managed with end-to-end repair and a posterior compartment fasciotomy. Type 2 defects range between 2 and 5 cm. They are managed with V-Y lengthening, with or without a tendon transfer. A Type 3 defect is >5 cm and is bridged by the use of a tendon transfer, alone or in combination with a V-Y advancement. Neither of these two classifications systems is evidence-based, and there is no published evidence that these schemes - if followed - would provide a better functional result than any other management philosophy.

Several techniques have been used to perform the reconstruction of chronic Achilles tendon ruptures [56]. The entirety of the plantar flexor muscle plays a role in the push-off phase of walking [12] and, when its tendons are harvested for the Achilles tendon, reconstruction may result in a loss of push-off strength. This could be more invaliding in athletic and young people [12, 17]. The plantaris tendon has been used to reinforce the reconstruction [16, 30], but this tendon is thin and is not always present [30]. The tendon of the flexor hallucis longus and that of the peroneus brevis have also been used to reconstruct chronic ruptures of the Achilles tendon [34, 54]. The flexor hallucis longus plays an important role in foot biomechanics [19, 20] and it has been used for transfer through a single-incision technique. Its use has resulted in decreased flexion strength at the interphalangeal joint of the hallux, as demonstrated by decreased distal phalangeal pulp pressure, but the patients' function remains high [9, 50].

Transfer of the tendon of the peroneus brevis is safe but technically demanding. It affords good recovery, even in patients with a chronic rupture, and the plantar flexion strength of their ankle can be reduced [49]. Biomechanical studies have indicate that the tendons of the peroneus brevis and the flexor hallucis longus are comparable for the reconstruction of chronic Achilles tendon ruptures [51]. Advocates of the tendon of the flexor hallucis longus report that the flexor hallucis longus is the strongest muscle of the ankle after the gastrocnemius-soleus complex, and that it is an ankle flexor. Its transfer may therefore supply some strength to plantar flexion of the ankle. In this context, the force exerted by the flexor hallucis longus is probably one order of magnitude lower than that of the gastrocnemius-soleus complex, and that, following tendon transfer, normally the relevant muscles loses one grade of force. Hence, it is possible that the only real contribution of the flexor hallucis longus - or, for that matter, any other technique aiming to bridge the gap - is to provide much needed biological material connecting the two stumps of the chronically torn Achilles tendon, allowing the gastrocnemius-soleus complex to return to more normal function. In this respect, the strong free semitendinosus graft provides this connection, and acts as an autologous biological scaffold for the Achilles tendon. Obviously, less invasive semitendinosus reconstruction does not deprive the foot of motor strength and power, is safe, and - given the length of the semitendinosus tendon - can be used to bridge large gaps.

The semitendinosus tendon is routinely used - in isolation or together with the gracilis tendon - as a free graft in the reconstruction of the anterior cruciate ligament [57], as it is easy to harvest and its harvesting produces no long-term disability [11, 47].

Turndown flaps are a popular choice [4, 7], and variations of the technique have recently been reported [46]. However, these techniques require wide exposure. Also, it has recently been demonstrated that, in Achilles tendon ruptures, the areas proximal and distal to the rupture itself exhibit profound biochemical and gene expression changes, and cannot be considered 'healthy and normal' [18]. The use of tendon transfers would supply an area with profound histopathological abnormalities with healthy tissue which would favour healing.

Conclusions

Chronic ruptures and avulsions of the Achilles tendon are potentially debilitating. The choice of management is partly guided by the size of the tendon defect with the optimal management being surgical. There are many different techniques which can be used to repair or reconstruct the rupture. The comparison of different techniques is difficult, due to the studies involved being retrospective and, generally, small. Every patient is different, and can present with varied co-morbidity, varied time of presentation and different lengths of the Achilles tendon retraction gap. Management should be tailored to the individual concerned. Tissue engineering technology shows promise, but is currently in its infancy and its application in clinical studies is probably still far away. Further research and clinical trials are needed to evaluate its efficacy in humans.

References

1. Arner O, Lindholm A. Subcutaneous rupture of the Achilles tendon; a study of 92 cases. Acta Chir Scand Suppl. 1959;116(Supp 239):1-51.
2. Bevilacqua NJ. Treatment of the neglected Achilles tendon rupture. Clin Podiatr Med Surg. 2012;29(2):291-299, viii.
3. Bibbo C, Anderson RB, Davis WH, Agnone M. Repair of the Achilles tendon sleeve avulsion: quantitative and functional evaluation of a transcalcaneal suture technique. Foot Ankle Int. 2003;24(7):539-544.
4. Bosworth DM. Repair of defects in the tendo Achillis. J Bone Joint Surg Am. 1956;38-A(1):111-114.
5. Carmont MR, Maffulli N. Less invasive Achilles tendon reconstruction. BMC Musculoskelet Disord. 2007;8:100.
6. Carmont MR, Maffulli N. Management of insertional Achilles tendinopathy through a Cincinnati incision. BMC Musculoskelet Disord. 2007;8:82.
7. Christensen I. Rupture of the Achilles tendon; analysis of 57 cases. Acta Chir Scand. 1953;106(1):50-60.
8. Cienfuegos A, Holgado MI, Díaz del Río JM, González Herranz J, Lara Bullón J. Chronic Achilles rupture reconstructed with Achilles tendon allograft: a case report. J Foot Ankle Surg. 2013;52(1):95-98.
9. Coull R, Flavin R, Stephens MM. Flexor hallucis longus tendon transfer: evaluation of postoperative morbidity. Foot Ankle Int. 2003;24(12):931-934.
10. Dekker M, Bender J. Results of surgical treatment of rupture of the Achilles tendon with use of the plantaris tendon. Arch Chir Neerl. 1977;29(1):39-46.
11. Ferretti A, Conteduca F, Morelli F, Masi V. Regeneration of the semitendinosus tendon after its use in anterior cruciate ligament reconstruction: a histologic study of three cases. Am J Sports Med. 2002;30(2):204-207.
12. Ferris L, Sharkey NA, Smith TS, Matthews DK. Influence of extrinsic plantar flexors on forefoot loading during heel rise. Foot Ankle Int. 1995;16(8):464-473.
13. Flint JH, Wade AM, Giuliani J, Rue JP. Defining the Terms Acute and Chronic in Orthopaedic Sports Injuries: A Systematic Review. Am J Sports Med. 2013.
14. Giza E, Frizzell L, Farac R, Williams J, Kim S. Augmented tendon Achilles repair using a tissue reinforcement scaffold: a biomechanical study. Foot Ankle Int. 2011;32(5):S545-549.
15. Hadi M, Young J, Cooper L, Costa M, Maffulli N. Surgical management of chronic ruptures of the Achilles tendon remains unclear: a systematic review of the management options. Br Med Bull. 2013.
16. Incavo SJ, Alvarez RG, Trevino SG. Occurrence of the plantaris tendon in patients sustaining subcutaneous rupture of the Achilles tendon. Foot Ankle. 1987;8(2):110-111.
17. Jacob HA. Forces acting in the forefoot during normal gait - an estimate. Clin Biomech (Bristol, Avon). 2001;16(9):783-792.
18. Karousou E, Ronga M, Vigetti D, Passi A, Maffulli N. Collagens, proteoglycans, MMP-2, MMP-9 and TIMPs in human Achilles tendon rupture. Clin Orthop Relat Res. 2008;466(7):1577-1582.
19. Kirane YM, Michelson JD, Sharkey NA. Contribution of the flexor hallucis longus to loading of the first metatarsal and first metatarsophalangeal joint. Foot Ankle Int. 2008;29(4):367-377.
20. Kirane YM, Michelson JD, Sharkey NA. Evidence of isometric function of the flexor hallucis longus muscle in normal gait. J Biomech. 2008;41(9):1919-1928.
21. Kosaka T, Yamamoto K. Long-term effects of chronic Achilles tendon rupture treatment, using reconstruction with peroneus brevis transfer, on sports activities. West Indian Med J. 2011;60(6):628-635.
22. Kraemer R, Wuerfel W, Lorenzen J, Busche M, Vogt PM, Knobloch K. Analysis of hereditary and medical risk factors in Achilles tendinopathy and Achilles tendon ruptures: a matched pair analysis. Arch Orthop Trauma Surg. 2012;132(6):847-853.
23. Kumta SM, Maffulli N. Local flap coverage for soft tissue defects following open repair of Achilles tendon rupture. Acta Orthop Belg. 2003;69(1):59-66.
24. Kuwada GT. Classification of tendo Achillis rupture with consideration of surgical repair techniques. J Foot Surg. 1990;29(4):361-365.
25. Lapidus LJ, Ray BA, Hamberg P. Medial Achilles tendon island flap--a novel technique to treat reruptures and neglected ruptures of the Achilles tendon. Int Orthop. 2012;36(8):1629-1634.
26. Lee YS, Lin CC, Chen CN, Chen SH, Liao WY, Huang CR. Reconstruction for neglected Achilles tendon rupture: the modified Bosworth technique. Orthopedics. 2005;28(7):647-650.
27. Longo UG, Ronga M, Maffulli N. Achilles tendinopathy. Sports Med Arthrosc. 2009;17(2):112-126.
28. Longo UG, Ronga M, Maffulli N. Acute ruptures of the Achilles tendon. Sports Med Arthrosc. 2009;17(2):127-138.
29. Lui TH. Minimally invasive flexor hallucis longus transfer in management of acute Achilles tendon rupture associated with tendinosis: a case report. Foot Ankle Spec. 2012;5(2):111-114.
30. Lynn TA. Repair of the torn Achilles tendon, using the plantaris tendon as a reinforcing membrane. J Bone Joint Surg Am. 1966;48(2):268-272.

31. Maffulli N. Rupture of the Achilles tendon. J Bone Joint Surg Am. 1999;81(7):1019-1036.

32. Maffulli N, Ajis A, Longo UG, Denaro V. Chronic rupture of tendo Achillis. Foot Ankle Clin. 2007;12(4):583-596, vi.

33. Maffulli N, Del Buono A, Spiezia F, Maffulli GD, Longo UG, Denaro V. Less-Invasive Semitendinosus Tendon Graft Augmentation for the Reconstruction of Chronic Tears of the Achilles Tendon. Am J Sports Med. 2013.

34. Maffulli N, Leadbetter WB. Free gracilis tendon graft in neglected tears of the Achilles tendon. Clin J Sport Med. 2005;15(2):56-61.

35. Maffulli N, Longo UG, Gougoulias N, Denaro V. Ipsilateral free semitendinosus tendon graft transfer for reconstruction of chronic tears of the Achilles tendon. BMC Musculoskelet Disord. 2008;9:100.

36. Maffulli N, Longo UG, Hüfner T, Denaro V. [Surgical treatment for pain syndromes of the Achilles tendon]. Unfallchirurg. 2010;113(9):721-725.

37. Maffulli N, Longo UG, Spiezia F, Denaro V. Free hamstrings tendon transfer and interference screw fixation for less invasive reconstruction of chronic avulsions of the Achilles tendon. Knee Surg Sports Traumatol Arthrosc. 2010;18(2):269-273.

38. Maffulli N, Loppini M, Longo UG, Maffulli GD, Denaro V. Minimally Invasive Reconstruction of Chronic Achilles Tendon Ruptures Using the Ipsilateral Free Semitendinosus Tendon Graft and Interference Screw Fixation. Am J Sports Med. 2013.

39. Maffulli N, Spiezia F, Longo UG, Denaro V. Less-invasive reconstruction of chronic Achilles tendon ruptures using a peroneus brevis tendon transfer. Am J Sports Med. 2010;38(11):2304-2312.

40. Maffulli N, Spiezia F, Pintore E, et al. Peroneus brevis tendon transfer for reconstruction of chronic tears of the Achilles tendon: a long-term follow-up study. J Bone Joint Surg Am. 2012;94(10):901-905.

41. Maffulli N, Spiezia F, Testa V, Capasso G, Longo UG, Denaro V. Free gracilis tendon graft for reconstruction of chronic tears of the Achilles tendon. J Bone Joint Surg Am. 2012;94(10):906-910.

42. Maffulli N, Testa V, Capasso G, Sullo A. Calcific insertional Achilles tendinopathy: reattachment with bone anchors. Am J Sports Med. 2004;32(1):174-182.

43. Magnussen RA, Glisson RR, Moorman CT. Augmentation of Achilles tendon repair with extracellular matrix xenograft: a biomechanical analysis. Am J Sports Med. 2011;39(7):1522-1527.

44. McClelland D, Maffulli N. Neglected rupture of the Achilles tendon: reconstruction with peroneus brevis tendon transfer. Surgeon. 2004;2(4):209-213.

45. Myerson MS. Achilles tendon ruptures. Instr Course Lect. 1999;48:219-230.

46. Nilsson-Helander K, Sward L, Silbernagel KG, Thomee R, Eriksson BI, Karlsson J. A new surgical method to treat chronic ruptures and reruptures of the Achilles tendon. Knee Surg Sports Traumatol Arthrosc. 2008;16(6):614-620.

47. Papandrea P, Vulpiani MC, Ferretti A, Conteduca F. Regeneration of the semitendinosus tendon harvested for anterior cruciate ligament reconstruction. Evaluation using ultrasonography. Am J Sports Med. 2000;28(4):556-561.

48. Park YS, Sung KS. Surgical reconstruction of chronic Achilles tendon ruptures using various methods. Orthopedics. 2012;35(2):e213-218.

49. Pintore E, Barra V, Pintore R, Maffulli N. Peroneus brevis tendon transfer in neglected tears of the Achilles tendon. J Trauma. 2001;50(1):71-78.

50. Richardson DR, Willers J, Cohen BE, Davis WH, Jones CP, Anderson RB. Evaluation of the hallux morbidity of single-incision flexor hallucis longus tendon transfer. Foot Ankle Int. 2009;30(7):627-630.

51. Sebastian H, Datta B, Maffulli N, Neil M, Walsh WR. Mechanical properties of reconstructed Achilles tendon with transfer of peroneus brevis or flexor hallucis longus tendon. J Foot Ankle Surg. 2007;46(6):424-428.

52. Sundararajan PP. Transosseous fixation in insertional Achilles tendonitis. J Foot Ankle Surg. 2012;51(6):806-812.

53. Thompson J, Baravarian B. Acute and chronic Achilles tendon ruptures in athletes. Clin Podiatr Med Surg. 2011;28(1):117-135.

54. Wapner KL, Pavlock GS, Hecht PJ, Naselli F, Walther R. Repair of chronic Achilles tendon rupture with flexor hallucis longus tendon transfer. Foot Ankle. 1993;14(8):443-449.

55. Wilcox DK, Bohay DR, Anderson JG. Treatment of chronic Achilles tendon disorders with flexor hallucis longus tendon transfer/augmentation. Foot Ankle Int. 2000;21(12):1004-1010.

56. Wong J, Barrass V, Maffulli N. Quantitative review of operative and nonoperative management of Achilles tendon ruptures. Am J Sports Med. 2002;30(4):565-575.

57. Yasuda K, Tsujino J, Ohkoshi Y, Tanabe Y, Kaneda K. Graft site morbidity with autogenous semitendinosus and gracilis tendons. Am J Sports Med. 1995;23(6):706-714.

*"Exercise to stimulate,
not annihilate."*

Lee Haney

CHAPTER 28

ACTIVITY RESUMPTION AFTER ACHILLES TENDON DISORDERS

Ruben Zwiers, Maayke N. van Sterkenburg, C. Niek van Dijk

Take Home Message

• *Activity resumption should be adapted to the individual and to the treatment undertaken, and the patient's and surgeon's expectations should be aligned at the outset of treatment.*

• *Incomplete rehabilitation and too early a return to activity can lead to an increased risk of morbidity and chronic symptoms.*

Introduction

Achilles tendinopathy and Achilles tendon ruptures affect a person's ability to be physically active. From the patient's perspective, the time to return to previous activities, such as walking, stair climbing, work and return to normal sporting activities, are important outcome measures. Return to sport has become increasingly important as an outcome measure, as Achilles tendon problems are common in physically-active individuals. The average time to return to sport is dependent on the extent of the injury, the sports activity and the desired level of sporting involvement.

In this chapter, the various aspects that influence sports ability and the expected time for return to sport are discussed. Furthermore, the different levels of activity are described, and recommendations concerning the time before different activity levels can be resumed are discussed.

General considerations

Prior injury is one of the greatest risk factors for lower limb injury in athletes. Especially during the time after a recovery period, athletes are prone to a new injury [40]. A too early return to activity with incomplete recovery can impair athletic performance and lead to the development of chronic symptoms. Achilles tendinopathy is a condition well-known for its propensity of recurrence. It is not unusual for patients with Achilles tendinopathy to have pain for many years [1, 3, 52].

A recent epidemiological study on elite professional rugby union players showed that chronic or overuse conditions around the foot – in comparison with acute injuries – took on average more than twice as long to recover [46]. It was also found that the presentation of a recurrent overuse injury kept the player away from training and playing nearly four times longer than the first presentation of an overuse condition, highlighting the need to allow for complete recovery before return to contact sports.

When planning return to activities, it is important to identify and treat any risk factors that may have contributed to the development of the condition in the first place. The incidence of Achilles tendon disorders and other overuse injuries is rising as more people participate in recreational and competitive sports, and as the duration and intensity of training regimes increases [13, 17, 32, 61]. Training errors are one of the most common causes of Achilles tendon overuse injuries [50] and as such it is important to recognise and correct them as a part of the rehabilitation protocol.

Inadequate rehabilitation and sport resumption prior to full recovery are risks that might be minimized with appropriate guidance in the return to sport phase. A study by Hagglund and co-workers compared the re-injury rates of tendon injuries in soccer teams with and without assistance in grading the return to sports. They reported a re-injury rate of 44% in the teams with no assistance in grading the return, whereas in teams with a standardized progression programme that gradually increased loading during the return to sport phase, there were no recurrences following tendon injuries [12]. This indicates the importance of including a gradual and controlled progression in the rehabilitation programme for returning to full sports activity, giving the athlete sufficient time to recover and evaluate symptoms.

Since athletes do not continuously suffer from their Achilles tendon during sports activity, players may be tempted to return to activity prematurely. The evaluation of symptoms, such as stiffness, pain and swelling after training, especially the following day, is a crucial factor prior to determining the appropriate increase in training intensity [52, 53]. A well-designed and meticulously-planned programme for return to sport will help with the guidance in achieving a balance between adequate and healthy loading and overloading of the Achilles tendon.

Factors influencing return to sport

Return to preoperative activity levels depends on the recovery of different factors. In the case of Achilles tendon rupture, the tendon needs to be at least partially healed before it can be loaded. It is, however, not only the quality of the healed tendon that determines whether a patient can resume activities of daily living, such as walking and stair climbing, or return to sport. The range of motion (ROM), especially dorsiflexion, should be normal or near to normal, and depending on the level of activity, strength and proprioception have to be normalized as does the sport's specific demands. Pain and swelling are other factors that might influence a successful return to pre-injury activity levels. When returning to full resumption of sport, the sport-specific demands have to be taken into consideration.

Literature overview of sports resumption after Achilles tendon rupture

An overview is provided here of the best available evidence on sports resumption following different treatment regimens for an Achilles tendon rupture.

Non-surgical versus surgical treatment

A differentiation should be made between non-surgically and surgically-treated patients. Nistor and Möller and co-workers reported no differences in terms of the level of sporting activity in these two group [26, 41]. However, Cetti and co-workers described that, of 111 patients treated for an acute Achilles tendon rupture, 57% of the surgically-treated group and only 29% of the non-surgically-treated patients managed to reach the same level of sporting activity as before the injury 9. Thermann and co-workers found no differences in functional outcomes between surgical and functional non-surgical treatment in terms of the duration of rehabilitation [56].

A randomized controlled study by Keating and co-workers found return to previous levels of sports activity in 26 of 37 patients (70%) in the surgical group (using an open technique) and 25 of 39 (64%) in the non-surgical group. The mean time to return to full sporting activity was 34 weeks (14 to 52 weeks) in the surgical group and 35 weeks (17 to 52 weeks) in the non-surgical group [20].

Metz and co-workers compared minimally-invasive surgery with non-surgical treatment with immediate full weight-bearing. In the surgical group, 24 of 36 patients (67%) returned to their previous levels of sports within one year, versus 27 of 33 patients (82%) in the non-surgical treatment group. Seven patients (four in the surgical group and three in the non-surgical group) had reasons other than their Achilles tendon ruptures for not returning to or changing the

385

type of sport in question [38]. A recent meta-analysis by Jiang and co-workers concluded that there was no difference in sports resumption between surgical and non-surgical treatments [16].

It can be concluded that in most studies no significant differences in sports resumption are found between surgical and non-surgical treatment.

Post-operative casting versus functional bracing

Post-operatively, patients can be immobilized in a cast or they can be treated by means of functional bracing. Maffulli and co-workers [27] reviewed the available literature on the treatment of Achilles tendon ruptures. Post-operative functional bracing resulted in a four week shorter period for a return to normal walking compared with post-operative casting. Functional bracing allowed patients to resume sports four weeks earlier than cast immobilization. These researchers concluded that post-operative treatment avoiding rigid immobilization of the ankle must be considered for all athletes and well-motivated, reliable patients. At the fourth post-operative week, the ankle should dorsiflect to neutral in a synthetic slab in which plantar flexion is allowed. At six weeks, the slab should be removed and high-level athletes who comply with the post-operative protocol normally should be able to return to sports activities three months post-operatively.

Costa and co-workers [10] performed two independent, randomized controlled trials in order to assess the potential benefits of immediate weight-bearing mobilization after rupture of the Achilles tendon. The first trial compared post-operative casting with functional bracing. The majority of the patients in both groups had returned to their pre-injury state by six months after the injury.

Kangas and co-workers [18] performed a randomized, clinical study where they concluded that isokinetic calf muscle strength recovered better in the post-operative functional bracing group. In a second study, they investigated subjective outcome measures such as pain, stiffness and footwear restrictions, and saw similar results for both groups. Mortensen and co-workers [39] described a period of rehabilitation of seven and a half months in the cast group, compared with four months in the functional brace group. They also studied the time to reach the pre-injury level of activity, and concluded that the functional brace group needed six months for recovery compared with nine months in the cast group. Kerkhoffs and co-workers [21] reported a time to return to sports of 73 days (range 54-112) in a cast group and 57 days (49-70) for a functional brace group. Suchak and co-workers randomized patients in the two week post-operative period to either weight-bearing or non-weight-bearing groups for an additional four weeks. At six months, 67% of the patients managed with weight-bearing as tolerated, and 63% of those managed with non-weight-bearing returned to at least partial sports activity [55].

Functional non-surgical treatment versus plaster cast immobilization

Costa and co-workers[10] compared non-surgical treatment with immediate weight-bearing mobilization to plaster-cast immobilization. There was, however, no evidence of any treatment effect in terms of time to return to sports.

Percutaneous versus open surgical treatment

Lim and co-workers[24] compared a small group of active patients, who were treated with a percutaneous suture to open surgery, and noted that four out of nine of the open group reached their pre-injury level of sports activity compared with nine out of eleven in the percutaneous group. Lansdaal[22] found that in 163 patients treated with minimally-invasive surgery, the average time to return to full sports activity was 167 days.

Literature overview of sports resumption after mid-portion Achilles tendinopathy

Concerning mid-portion Achilles tendinopathy, rest from Achilles tendon loading activities is generally recommended early in the rehabilitation[2, 44, 47]. At the next rehabilitation stage, activities such as deep-water running and cycling are suggested as a complement. Resumption of activities such as running and jumping is generally recommended when the symptoms have subsided. Studies often have an intervention for a minimum of 12 weeks, and then report that return to sports is allowed. In studies on surgical treatment for Achilles tendinopathy, more specific guidelines can be found, with return to sports generally recommended between weeks 12 and 24 following surgery[3, 31].

Non-surgical treatment

A systematic review on non-surgical treatment for mid-portion Achilles tendinopathy by Magnussen and co-workers identified four randomized treatment studies reporting on return to sport or return to previous activity[35].

Roos and co-workers in a randomized controlled trial, compared three groups: eccentric exercise, night splint and a combination of both. Of the patients participating in sports prior to the onset of symptoms, in the eccentric group, five out of eight patients returned to their pre-injury activity level after 12 weeks. In the combined group, three out of eight patients returned, while in the splint group one out of 10 patients had returned to sports after 12 weeks[48]. In a prospective randomized study, Mafi and co-workers[34] found that eccentric exercises more efficient in terms of return to activity. At 12 weeks follow-up, 82% of the patients in the eccentric exercise group versus 36% of the concentric exercise group patients resumed previous activity. In addition, Silbernagel and co-workers reported that 55% of the patients in the eccentric exercise group to returned to initial activity levels, compared with 34% in the concentric group at one year follow-up. This difference was not statistically significant[53].

In addition, in terms of injection therapies, no significant differences in return to sport are reported. Brown and co-workers [8] found that 77% of the patients returned to sport in a group treated with Aprotinin injections versus 85% in the placebo group at one year of follow-up. A randomized controlled trial by de Vos and co-workers [11] showed no difference in return to sports activity between a group treated with platelet-rich plasma injections and a placebo (57 versus 58% at 12 weeks follow-up).

Surgical treatment

In terms of return to sport after open surgery for mid-portion Achilles tendinopathy, the outcome varies. In a study by Maffulli and co-workers [30] nine of 14 athletes with unilateral Achilles tendinopathy with central core lesions did not return to pre-injury levels of activity. Paavola and co-workers [45] found that 84% of patients returned to their pre-injury levels of physical activity. Maffulli and co-workers [33] reported 36 of 45 patients with excellent or good outcomes after open surgery, while the remaining patients could not return to normal activity levels. Bohu and co-workers [6] reported that 75.6% of patients returned to former levels of activity at 37.4 months of follow-up. The average time for resume to running was 6.7 months, and 11.1 months for a return to competitive sports.

Two more recent studies reported the results of patients treated by means of an endoscopic technique. Steenstra and van Dijk [54] reported that most of 20 patients were able to resume their sporting activities after four to eight weeks. Vega and co-workers [58] described eight patients treated using an endoscopic technique. All the patients were able to return to their previous sports activity without difficulty or posterior discomfort.

Literature overview of sports resumption after insertional Achilles tendinopathy

Although the epidemiological data is limited, existing studies show that symptomatic insertional tendinopathy is four-times less common than non-insertional tendinopathy [4, 45]. Patients with insertional Achilles tendinopathy tend to be older and less active than those with retrocalcaneal bursitis [60]. This will greatly affect the specific design and expectations of any programme.

Debridement and detachment/re-attachment

The post-operative regimen and return to activity after the detachment of the Achilles insertion depends on how much of the insertion has been detached. Avulsion of the Achilles after surgery is a major concern, but most reported incidents occurred after a slip or fall in the early post-operative period [59, 60].

McGarvey and co-workers presented a series of 22 patients treated with a posterior tendon-splitting approach. The surgical technique consisted of synovectomy, bursectomy and the excision of the calcaneal prominence where necessary [37]. Post-operative care for patients who underwent debridement alone consisted of two weeks in a weight-bearing equinus cast followed by a posterior shell for two weeks and then a shoe with a heel-lift for a further two weeks. Strengthening training started at six weeks post-operatively. Patients were encouraged to start running at three months. Where the surgery involved detachment and reattachment of the Achilles tendon, weight-bearing was not allowed until two weeks post-operatively. Range of motion training was started four weeks post-operatively, with strengthening after eight weeks. 20 out of 22 patients resumed normal activity at three months following surgery. Only 13 of the 22, however, were able to return to unlimited activities.

Saxena [49] performed a retrospective review of elite and non-elite track and field athletes after surgery for all types of chronic tendinopathy, and recorded the time to return to sport. Eleven patients underwent open excision of the calcaneal prominence with a mean return to activity after 15 weeks. Six athletes had insertional Achilles tendinopathy debridement with reattachment of the tendon using suture anchors and returned to activity after 12 weeks. There was a significant difference overall between the elite and non-elite group with respect to return to activity (7.9 ± 4.7 versus 15.0 ± 6.2 weeks), but Saxena acknowledged that this was likely to be biased by the fact that many of the elite runners had undergone soft tissue procedures.

Maffulli and co-workers [29] reported on 21 patients with calcific insertional Achilles tendinopathy who were treated surgically by the removal of the calcific deposit and the reinsertion of the tendon with one or more bone anchors, depending of the degree of disinsertion. Of the 21 patients in this study, 16 reported good or excellent outcomes. These patients had returned to their pre-injury levels of activity at an average of 24.5 weeks. The remaining five patients could not return to their previous levels of sports activity despite prolonged, supervised post-operative physiotherapy, with cryotherapy, massage, ultrasound, and pulsed magnetic and laser therapy.

In a recent study, the same group reported on 30 patients who underwent debridement and an osteotomy of the postero-superior corner of the calcaneus for insertional Achilles tendinopathy without calcific component. A weight-bearing cast for 2 weeks was applied and immediately after surgery weight-bearing as tolerated using crutches was allowed. Stationary cycling a swimming were recommended from the second week after removal of the cast. Patients were encouraged to gradually progress to full weight-bearing. Twenty-six patients returned to their pre-injury levels of activity at a mean of 32 weeks (24 to 38) after surgery. The remaining four patients did not return to their previous levels of sports activity, despite prolonged, supervised post-operative physiotherapy [28].

Surgical treatment for retrocalcaneal bursitis

Arthroscopic and minimally-invasive surgery aims to reduce the complications associated with open techniques and may allow for a faster return to sports and other activities [25]. One study reported on return to sport following the open resection of a calcaneal prominence [5]. Of the 22 patients, four returned to unrestricted sports activities, whereas 15 were able to participate in sports activities with limitations.

Since the introduction of a procedure to remove inflamed bursal tissue as well as the postero-superior part of the calcaneus using an endoscopic approach, several case series have been published. Van Dijk and co-workers [57] published the results of 21 such procedures in 20 patients in 2001. Patients were encouraged to perform active range of motion exercises and weight-bearing immediately after surgery. Nineteen out of 20 patients showed good to excellent results. Patients returned to work at an average of seven weeks and sports at an average of 12 weeks. The average time to full weight bearing was four weeks. Additionally, Scholten and van Dijk [51] presented the outcome of 39 endoscopic calcaneoplasty procedures in 36 patients. Of them, 30 had good or excellent results with sports resumption at an average of 11 weeks.

Ortman and co-workers [43] retrospectively assessed the return to activity after endoscopic decompression of the retrocalcaneal space. The average return to normal daily functioning was eight weeks. They divided their cohort into athletic and non-athletic groups, and reported that all athletes returned to their previous levels of activity at an average of 12 weeks. Other studies on this procedure did not report data for a return to sports activity [15, 23, 36].

Return to sport algorithms

Based on the current literature and expert opinion of the Achilles Tendon Study Group, return to sport algorithms for patients recovering from Achilles tendon rupture and mid-portion Achilles tendinopathies were compiled. Limited evidence is available on return to sport in relation to different conditions around the Achilles insertion. However, the return to sport algorithm described by Silbernagel and co-workers [52] can be employed in a rehabilitation protocol for insertional Achilles tendon-related problems.

Achilles tendon rupture

After Achilles tendon rupture, recovery and activity resumption can be divided into four levels of increasing intensity. The greater the physical demands, the higher the level and quality of recovery needed.

Level 1: Walking

The first phase of Achilles tendon rupture healing is a return to normal walking. This phase begins at day 0 and ends when the patient is able to walk normally again. The most important factor, which determines the return to normal walking, is the quality of tissue healing. As the tissue heals, the mechanical properties of the tendon improve, making it possible to increase the load. Patients can switch from unloaded to loaded activities as soon as it is tolerated. After removal of a cast or external support, the patients can switch from static to dynamic training. The next step is to proceed from concentric to eccentric muscle training and, when this is achieved, it should be followed by progression from open- to closed-chain exercises. Proprioception is taught in order to achieve active stability. An acceptable level of proprioception is reached when the time spent while standing on a single leg is either normal or near-normal. The range of motion should be near-normal by the end of phase 1. No passive stretching is allowed in this phase. Concerning strength, there should be no more than a 25% left/right difference, which can be measured by performing repeated one-leg heel-raises, comparing left to right [19]; toe walking should also be possible at this point. The ability to perform a single heel-rise appears to be related to functional outcomes and return to physical activity [42]. Pain and swelling must be absent within 48 hours after any increased activity.

When all these variables are similar to those of the unaffected limb, the patient can safely resume unrestricted normal walking without any external support.

Level 2: Running

The next level of activity is to resume running. This phase demands the recovery of speed, force and endurance. It begins when the patient is able to walk normally and ends when the patient can return to easy jogging. This is achieved by training technical skills, force and endurance, and improving the cardiovascular status as well. The goal of this programme is to enable controlled, sideward movement, and to regain a normal ROM. At the end of this phase, there should be a left/right difference in strength of less than 12%. Following increased activity, pain and swelling should be absent within 24 hours.

Level 3: Non-contact sports

The third level of activity is the return to non-contact sports. This involves further training of speed, force and endurance. This phase begins when easy jogging is possible and ends when the patient is able to return to non-contact sports. It consists of the further training of speed to allow running on even ground and sprinting. Muscle strength is equally trained.

At the end of this phase, rope jumping, turning and twisting should be possible, and endurance training is advanced. Muscle strength should be normal, and while some pain may occur after increased activity it should be absent after 24 hours.

Level 4: Contact sports

The highest level of activity is defined as the return to contact sports. This phase begins when non-contact sports are resumed and ends when patients can safely return to contact sports. The final training of speed, muscle strength and endurance should enable the patient to return to contact sports, which involves running on uneven ground, generating explosive force, changing direction and other sports-specific movements.

On the basis of the current literature already described and the expert opinion of the Achilles Tendon Study Group, the following timeline was proposed:

Level 1: Return to normal walking

The most important factor, which determines the return to normal loading, is the quality of tissue healing. In the case of cast immobilization after surgery, one can expect this phase to last for up to 12 weeks. At the end of this 12 week period, the patient should have progressed to unrestricted walking without external support. In the case of functional treatment after surgery, this period is expected to be reduced to eight weeks (Level III evidence) [27]. However, a functional perspective rather than a time perspective is of major importance when rehabilitation is advanced. Although its relation with normal gait patterns needs further research, the simple heel-rise test appears to be an important milestone in early rehabilitation [42].

Level 2: Return to running

The expert panel recommends this phase as taking a minimum of 4-6 weeks.

Level 3: Return to non-contact sports

This phase can be expected to take another 4-6 weeks (Level V evidence).

Level 4: Return to contact sports

If patients participate in contact sports, this typically needs another 4-6 weeks of rehabilitation (Level V evidence, Figure 1) (Table 1).

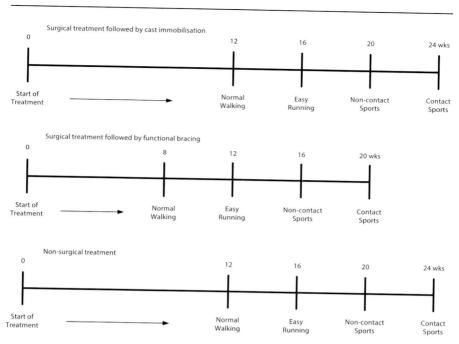

Figure 1. There is no evidence for a prolonged period of time before sports can be resumed in non-surgically-treated patients, but a significantly smaller number of patients are able to return to their previous levels of activity.

Phase	Goal	Duration	Training of	End Terms	Activity
Level 1	Return to normal loading	12 weeks ↑↓	Proprioception	Active Stability (negative Rhomberg-test by standing on one leg	Normal Walking
			ROM	Normal ROM No passive streching allowed	
			- Static to Dynamic - Excentric to Concentric - Open chain to Closed chain	Improved speed Force: <25% L/R-difference (measured by heel raise test)	
				Pain/swelling after increased activity should dissappear <48 hrs	
Level 2		4 weeks ↑↓	Technical skills	Controlled sideward movements Normal ROM	Running
			Force	Force: <12% L/R-difference	
			Endurance Cardiovascular status		
				Pain/swelling after increased activity should dissapear <24 hrs	
Level 3	Return to sport specific loading	4 weeks ↑↓	Speed	Running oneven ground Sprinting	Non-contact Sports
			Force	Normal force Rope jumping Turning/twisting Some pain after increased activity should dissapear < 24 hrs	
			Endurance		
Level 4		4 weeks ↑↓	Speed	Running oneven ground	Contact Sports
			Force	Explosive force Change of direction Sport specific movements	
			Endurance		

Table 1. In the case of functional bracing after operative treatment for acute Achilles tendon rupture, this phase can be shortened to eight weeks (algorithm adapted from van Sterkenburg and co-workers.

The expected times given to resume each of the activity levels represent averages. There are individual differences, for example, where one patient is quicker while another needs more time to reach the same rehabilitation goal. The most important signs to monitor as to whether a patient can speed up or else has to slow down in relation to the average time include pain and swelling after activity – especially increased pain the day after increased activity – and delayed tissue healing.

Mid-portion and insertional tendinopathy

We advise to use the return to sport algorithm introduced by Silbernagel and co-workers [52] as an important part of the rehabilitation protocol for both insertional and mid-portion Achilles tendon pathology.

Return to sport phase is a balancing act between a swift return to full activity and avoiding overloading and re-injury of the tendon. A gradual progression into each specific sports activity is recommended in the literature regardless of injury [12, 14, 52]. To be successful in guiding the athlete in the return to sports phase following Achilles tendinopathy, an algorithm is recommended where the load of the activity, the athletes perceived exertion with the activity, the symptoms and pain level, and recovery-days, are all incorporated in the decision-making. Step one is to find, for each athlete, specific activities that meet the requirements for each level (low, medium and high) based on the pain level and the perceived exertion [7]. The clinician's knowledge of how to progress the load on the Achilles tendon is of great importance, along with an understanding of the athlete's specific sports requirements. In Table 2, the requirements for each activity level are shown along with an example of the various activities for a long-distance runner.

Classification of Activities	Pain Level During Activity VAS	Pain Level After Activity (Next Day) VAS	Athletes Perceived Exertion (in regards to the Achilles Tendon) Borg Scale*	Recovery Days Needed Between Activities	The Individual Athletes Activity
Light	1-2	1-2	6-10	0 days (can be performed daily)	*Walking fast for 70 min*
Medium	2-3	3-4	11-14	2 days	*Jogging on flat surface for 40 minutes*
High	4-5	5-6	15-18	3 days	*Running 90% of desired speed for 30 minutes*

Table 2. Classification scheme of activities during return to sports (with an example of a long-distance runner).

Several activities can be added for each activity level. A specific training schedule for approximately two to three weeks is then planned for the athlete. Low level activities can be performed daily. For medium levels of activity, two days of recovery are needed, during which the athlete should not perform activities of the same or a higher level. High level activities need three days of recovery from medium and/or high level activities. When the athlete improves (i.e., when the pain level and the perceived exertion level decreases), a revised classification is performed. This is usually done every two to three weeks. A previous medium level of activity might then become low and a new activity can be added on the high activity list. The proposed return to sport algorithm has been developed based on the knowledge gained in a randomized study where some patients were allowed to continue tendon loading activities during the rehabilitation while using the pain-monitoring model [52].

In a clinical setting, the return to sports algorithm has been used for both recreational and elite athletes. Its advantage lies in using a well-structured plan with a gradual progression of loading the Achilles tendon and a gradual return to sports. Often, the athlete's coach or strength and conditioning coach is involved when activities and return to activities are discussed and decisions are taken. Further studies need to be performed on the effectiveness of the return to sports algorithm.

Conclusion

The period of time before sporting activities can be resumed depends on a combination of several factors. Besides the pathology and treatment, a motivated, compliant athlete can resume sports earlier than one who is not. Activity resumption should be adapted to the individual and to the treatment undertaken, and the patient's and surgeon's expectations should be aligned at the outset of treatment. Incomplete rehabilitation and too early return to activity can lead to recurrent symptoms with considerable morbidity.

References

1. Alfredson H. Chronic midportion Achilles tendinopathy: an update on research and treatment. Clin Sports Med. 2003; 22(4): 727-741.

2. Alfredson H, Ohberg L, Zeisig E, Lorentzon R. Treatment of midportion Achilles tendinosis: similar clinical results with US and CD-guided surgery outside the tendon and sclerosing polidocanol injections. Knee Surg Sports Traumatol Arthrosc. 2007; 15(12): 1504-1509.

3. Alfredson H, Pietila T, Jonsson P, Lorentzon R. Heavy-load eccentric calf muscle training for the treatment of chronic Achilles tendinosis. Am J Sports Med. 1998; 26(3): 360-366.

4. Astrom M, Rausing A. Chronic Achilles tendinopathy: A survey of surgical and histopathologic findings Mats. Clin Orthop Relat Res. 1995; 316: 151-164.

5. Biyani A, Jones DA. Results of excision of calcaneal prominence. Acta Orthop Belg. 1993; 59(1): 45-49.

6. Bohu Y, Lefevre N, Bauer T. Surgical treatment of Achilles tendinopathies in athletes. Multicenter retrospective series of open surgery and endoscopic techniques. Orthop Traumatol Surg Res. 2009; 95(8): 72-77.

7. Borg G. Borg's perceived exertion and pain scales. Human Kinetics; 1998.

8. Brown R, Orchard J, Kinchington M, Hooper A, Nalder G. Aprotinin in the management of Achilles tendinopathy: a randomised controlled trial. Br J Sports Med. 2006; 40(3): 275-279.

9. Cetti R, Christensen SE, Ejsted R, Jensen NM, Jorgensen U. Operative versus nonoperative treatment of Achilles tendon rupture A prospective randomized study and review of the literature. Am J Sports Med. 1993; 21(6): 791-799.

10. Costa ML, MacMillan K, Halliday D. Randomised controlled trials of immediate weight-bearing mobilisation for rupture of the tendo Achillis. J Bone Joint Surg Br. 2006; 88(1): 69-77.

11. de Vos RJ, Weir A, van Schie HT. Platelet-rich plasma injection for chronic Achilles tendinopathy: a randomized controlled trial. JAMA. 2010; 303(2): 144-149.

12. Hägglund M. Epidemiology and prevention of football injuries. 2007.

13. Houshian S, Tscherning T, Riegels-Nielsen P. The epidemiology of Achilles tendon rupture in a Danish county. Injury 1998; 29(9): 651-654.

14. Humble RN, Nugent LL. Achilles' tendonitis. An overview and reconditioning model. Clin Podiatr Med Surg. 2001; 18(2): 233.

15. Jerosch J, Schunck J, Sokkar SH. Endoscopic calcaneoplasty (ECP) as a surgical treatment of Haglund's syndrome. Knee Surg Sports Traumatol Arthrosc. 2007; 15(7): 927-934.

16. Jiang N, Wang B, Chen A, Dong F, Yu B. Operative versus nonoperative treatment for acute Achilles tendon rupture: a meta-analysis based on current evidence. Int Orthop. 2012; 36(4): 765-773.

17. Kader D, Saxena A, Movin T, Maffulli N. Achilles tendinopathy: some aspects of basic science and clinical management. Br J Sports Med. 2002; 36(4): 239-249.

18. Kangas J, Pajala A, Siira P, Hamalainen M, Leppilahti J. Early functional treatment versus early immobilization in tension of the musculotendinous unit after Achilles rupture repair: a prospective, randomized, clinical study. J Trauma. 2003; 54(6): 1171-1180.

19. Kannus P. Etiology and pathophysiology of chronic tendon disorders in sports. Scand J Med Sci Sports. 1997; 7(2): 78-85.

20. Keating JF, Will EM. Operative versus non-operative treatment of acute rupture of tendo Achillis: a prospective randomised evaluation of functional outcome. J Bone Joint Surg Br. 2011; 93(8): 1071-1078.

21. Kerkhoffs GM, Struijs PA, Raaymakers EL, Marti RK. Functional treatment after surgical repair of acute Achilles tendon rupture: wrap vs walking cast. Arch Orthop Trauma Surg. 2002; 122(2): 102-105.

22. Lansdaal JR, Goslings JC, Reichart M. The results of 163 Achilles tendon ruptures treated by a minimally invasive surgical technique and functional after treatment. Injury 2007; 38(7): 839-844.

23. Leitze Z, Sella EJ, Aversa JM. Endoscopic decompression of the retrocalcaneal space. J Bone Joint Surg Am. 2003; 85-A(8): 1488-1496.

24. Lim J, Dalai R, Waseem M. Percutaneous vs. open repair of the ruptured Achilles tendon; a prospective randomized controlled study. Foot Ankle Int. 2001; 22(7): 559-568.

25. Lohrer H, Arentz S. Die Impingementlaesion der distalen Achillessehne bei Bursitis subachillae und Haglund-Pseudoexostose-eine therapeutische Herausforderung. Sportverletzung-À Sportschaden. 2003; 17(04): 181-188.

26. Möller M, Movin T, Granhed H, Lind K, Faxen E, Karlsson J. Acute rupture of tendo Achillis a prospective, randomised study of comparison between surgical and non-surgical treatment. J Bone Joint Surg Br. 2001; 83(6): 843-848.

27. Maffulli N. Rupture of the Achilles tendon. J Bone Joint Surg Am. 1999; 81(7): 1019-1036.

28. Maffulli N, Del BA, Testa V, Capasso G, Oliva F, Denaro V. Safety and outcome of surgical debridement of insertional Achilles tendinopathy using a transverse (Cincinnati) incision. J Bone Joint Surg Br. 2011; 93(11): 1503-1507.

397

29. Maffulli N, Testa V, Capasso G, Sullo A. Calcific insertional Achilles tendinopathy: reattachment with bone anchors. Am J Sports Med. 2004; 32(1): 174-182.

30. Maffulli N, Binfield PM, Moore D, King JB. Surgical decompression of chronic central core lesions of the Achilles tendon. Am J Sports Med. 1999; 27(6): 747-752.

31. Maffulli N, Longo UG, Gougoulias N, Denaro V. Ipsilateral free semitendinosus tendon graft transfer for reconstruction of chronic tears of the Achilles tendon. BMC musculoskeletal disorders. 2008; 9(1): 100.

32. Maffulli N, Sharma P, Luscombe KL. Achilles tendinopathy: aetiology and management. JRSM. 2004; 97(10): 472-476.

33. Maffulli N, Testa V, Capasso G. Surgery for chronic Achilles tendinopathy yields worse results in nonathletic patients. Clin J Sport Med. 2006; 16(2): 123-128.

34. Mafi N, Lorentzon R, Alfredson H. Superior short-term results with eccentric calf muscle training compared to concentric training in a randomized prospective multicenter study on patients with chronic Achilles tendinosis. Knee Surg Sports Traumatol Arthrosc. 2001; 9(1): 42-47.

35. Magnussen RA, Dunn WR, Thomson AB. Nonoperative treatment of midportion Achilles tendinopathy: a systematic review. Clin J Sport Med. 2009; 19(1): 54-64.

36. Maquirriain J. Endoscopic Achilles tenodesis: a surgical alternative for chronic insertional tendinopathy. Knee Surg Sports Traumatol Arthrosc. 2007; 15(7): 940-943.

37. McGarvey WC, Palumbo RC, Baxter DE, Leibman BD. Insertional Achilles tendinosis: surgical treatment through a central tendon splitting approach. Foot Ankle Int. 2002; 23(1): 19-25.

38. Metz R, Verleisdonk EJM, Geert J-MG. Acute Achilles tendon rupture minimally invasive surgery versus nonoperative treatment with immediate full weightbearingGÇöA randomized controlled trial. Am J Sports Med 2008;36(9):1688-1694.

39. Mortensen HM, Skov O, Jensen PE. Early motion of the ankle after operative treatment of a rupture of the Achilles tendon. A prospective, randomized clinical and radiographic study. J Bone Joint Surg Am. 1999; 81(7): 983-990.

40. Murphy DF, Connolly DAJ, Beynnon BD. Risk factors for lower extremity injury: a review of the literature. Br J Sports Med. 2003; 37(1): 13-29.

41. Nistor LARS. Surgical and non-surgical treatment of Achilles tendon rupture. J Bone Joint Surg Am. 1981; 63: 394-399.

42. Olsson N, Karlsson J, Eriksson BI, Brorsson A, Lundberg M, Silbernagel KG. Ability to perform a single heel rise is significantly related to patient reported outcome after Achilles tendon rupture. Scand J Med Sci Sports. 2012.

43. Ortmann FW, McBryde AM. Endoscopic bony and soft-tissue decompression of the retrocalcaneal space for the treatment of Haglund deformity and retrocalcaneal bursitis. Foot Ankle Int. 2007; 28(2): 149-153.

44. Paavola M, Kannus P, Orava S, Pasanen M, Jarvinen M. Surgical treatment for chronic Achilles tendinopathy: a prospective seven month follow up study. Br J Sports Med. 2002; 36(3): 178-182.

45. Paavola M, Orava S, Leppilahti J, Kannus P, Jarvinen M. Chronic Achilles tendon overuse injury: complications after surgical treatment. An analysis of 432 consecutive patients. Am J Sports Med. 2000; 28(1): 77-82.

46. Pearce CJ, Brooks JH, Kemp S, Calder JD. The epidemiology of foot injuries in professional rugby union players. Foot Ankle Surg. 2011; 17(3): 113-118.

47. Rompe JD, Furia J, Maffulli N. Eccentric loading compared with shock wave treatment for chronic insertional Achilles tendinopathy. A randomized, controlled trial. J Bone Joint Surg Am. 2008; 90(1): 52-61.

48. Roos EM, Engstrom M, Lagerquist A, Soderberg B. Clinical improvement after 6 weeks of eccentric exercise in patients with mid-portion Achilles tendinopathy - a randomized trial with 1-year follow-up. Scand J Med Sci Sports. 2004; 14(5): 286-295.

49. Saxena A. Results of chronic Achilles tendinopathy surgery on elite and nonelite track athletes. Foot Ankle Int. 2003; 24(9): 712-720.

50. Schepsis AA, Jones H, Haas AL. Achilles tendon disorders in athletes. Am J Sports Med. 2002; 30(2): 287-305.

51. Scholten PE, van Dijk CN. Endoscopic calcaneoplasty. Foot Ankle Clin. 2006; 11(2): 439-46, viii.

52. Silbernagel KG, Thomee R, Eriksson BI, Karlsson J. Continued sports activity, using a pain-monitoring model, during rehabilitation in patients with Achilles tendinopathy: a randomized controlled study. Am J Sports Med. 2007; 35(6): 897-906.

53. Silbernagel KG, Thomee R, Thomee P, Karlsson J. Eccentric overload training for patients with chronic Achilles tendon pain - a randomised controlled study with reliability testing of the evaluation methods. Scand J Med Sci Sports. 2001; 11(4): 197-206.

54. Steenstra F, van Dijk CN. Achilles tendoscopy. Foot Ankle Clin. 2006; 11(2): 429-38, viii.

55. Suchak AA, Bostick GP, Beaupre LA, Durand DC, Jomha NM. The influence of early weight-bearing compared with non-weight-bearing after surgical repair of the Achilles tendon. J Bone Joint Surg Am 2008;90(9):1876-1883.

56. Thermann H, Zwipp H, Tscherne H. [Functional treatment concept of acute rupture of the Achilles tendon. 2 years results of a prospective randomized study]. Der Unfallchirurg 1995;98(1):21.

57. van Dijk CN, van Dyk GE, Scholten PE, Kort NP. Endoscopic calcaneoplasty. Am J Sports Med 2001;29(2):185-189.

58. Vega J, Cabestany JM, Golano P, Perez-Carro L. Endoscopic treatment for chronic Achilles tendinopathy. Foot Ankle Surg 2008;14(4):204-210.

59. Wagner E, Gould JS, Kneidel M, Fleisig GS, Fowler R. Technique and results of Achilles tendon detachment and reconstruction for insertional Achilles tendinosis. Foot Ankle Int 2006;27(9):677-684.

60. Watson AD, Anderson RB, Davis WH. Comparison of results of retrocalcaneal decompression for retrocalcaneal bursitis and insertional achilles tendinosis with calcific spur. Foot Ankle Int 2000;21(8):638-642.

61. Wilder RP, Sethi S. Overuse injuries: tendinopathies, stress fractures, compartment syndrome, and shin splints. Clin Sports Med 2004;23(1):55-81.

"Children are not just small adults."

Mercer Rang

Chapter 29

Achilles Tendon Problems in Children

Jeffrey R. Sawyer, Derek M. Kelly, William C. Warner, James H. Beaty

Take Home Message

- *In children, the Achilles tendon may require surgical lengthening to correct tightness or the contractures associated with congenital, developmental, neurological and post-traumatic disorders.*

- *While traumatic Achilles tendon injuries are rare in children, overuse injuries do occur in athletic adolescents.*

- *Both open and percutaneous lengthening techniques can be successful, but care must be taken to avoid over-lengthening.*

Introduction

Unlike in adults, Achilles problems in children rarely involve tendon rupture or tendinopathy. In children, tendons and ligaments are relatively strong compared to the physis, so trauma usually affects the weaker physis rather than the tendon. Tendon lacerations, while rare, are more common than tendon ruptures in this age group [12, 28, 33, 35, 39]. Injuries to the insertions of tendons onto bone are more frequent than injuries to the body of the tendon [23] and overuse injuries can occur in athletic adolescents. Problems can also exist with a variety of conditions in which the tendon is involved secondarily. Congenital, developmental and neurological disorders may all involve the Achilles tendon.

401

Traumatic injuries

Tendon laceration or rupture

Achilles tendon laceration or rupture is rare in children but may occur as part of severe trauma, such as from a lawn-mower or bicycle spoke injury [1, 2, 28, 40]. Vosburgh and co-workers [40] reported complete disruption of the Achilles tendon in four of six patients with posterior injuries caused by riding lawn mowers. They concluded that obtaining a clean wound for closure was more important than any consideration of early repair or transfer after Achilles tendon lacerations. Reconstructive surgery was done in only one of their four patients with a complete disruption and segmental loss of the Achilles tendon; the other three were able to ambulate independently when a 'physiological tendon' was permitted to develop by scar formation.

More recently, Parkar co-workers [33] described the 'regeneration' of the Achilles tendon in a ten year old boy who had sustained an open calcaneal fracture and laceration of the tendon when his foot was caught in the spokes of a moped. The tendon was repaired and the fracture was stabilized with Kirschner wires.

Development of an infection required debridement that resulted in a loss of a 5 cm segment of the distal Achilles tendon. Free skin-flap coverage was done to control the infection, with tendon reconstruction planned as a second stage; however, at six weeks following flap coverage he could stand on tip-toe and had active plantar flexion of his ankle, while at the two year follow-up he had normal ankle function. The authors suggested that, rather than auto-regeneration, this may have simply been an adaptive response by the scar tissue.

Rupture of the Achilles tendon in children usually occurs as an avulsion of the tendon from the calcaneus rather than in the mid-portion, as is common in adults [26]. Although relatively common in adults, this is rare in children. Tudisco and Bisicchia [39] described the reconstruction of a neglected traumatic Achilles tendon rupture in a seven year old girl with excellent functional results and noted two other reports of traumatic ruptures in young patients. One, in a 14 year old girl who was struck across the mid-tendon by a swinging door, was treated operatively [35]. The other was in a seven year old girl who fell on her plantar-flexed foot and was treated non-surgically [12]. Both had good functional outcomes.

Overuse injuries

Insertional and non-insertional Achilles tendinopathy have been reported in adolescent athletes [5, 20]. Factors that may predispose an individual to tendon problems include foot pronation, tightness of the plantar fascia and Achilles tendon, cavus foot deformity and obesity. Technique errors and improper equipment can also contribute to the development of Achilles tendon problems, but the most common underlying cause is overuse [5, 20]. Non-surgical treatment that includes rest, NSAIDs and brief immobilization of the foot and ankle usually is effective; surgery is not indicated.

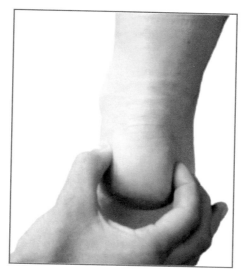

Figure 1. The 'squeeze test'. The application of gradual pressure over the medial and lateral sides of the calcaneal apophysitis elicit pain in patients with Sever's disease.

Sever's disease

Sever's disease is generally described as a traction apophysitis of the calcaneus, and has been attributed to chronic repetitive shear stress on the vertically-oriented apophysitis by the triceps surae and the plantar fascia. It is most common in athletic children between the ages of eight and 13 years. Heel pain is aggravated by activity, particularly running and jumping. Factors cited as contributing to the development of Sever's disease include overuse, foot pronation, a flat or high foot arch, leg length discrepancy and overweight or obesity [32]. Presenting symptoms can include limping, tenderness localized to the posterior heel at the insertion of the Achilles tendon, tightness of the Achilles tendon and decreased push-off strength. The diagnosis is generally a clinical one based on the patient's history of pain, with activity and a positive "squeeze test" (Fig. 1): pain is produced by medial and lateral compression of the heel where the calcaneal apophysitis attaches to the main body of the calcaneus. Although fragmentation and sclerosis of the calcaneal apophysitis on radiographs have been cited as indications of the condition (Fig. 2), studies have shown that there is little radiographic difference between the calcaneal apophysitis in children with and without Sever's disease. Some authors have suggested that obtaining radiographs in patients with a clinical diagnosis of Sever's disease is unnecessary [24]. Rachel and co-workers [34], however, recommended lateral radiographs in paediatric patients with heel pain so as to rule out other pathologies that may require more aggressive treatment (e.g., calcaneal stress fracture, bone cysts). Abnormal radiographs in 5% of their 96 patients led to changes in treatment plans because of the presence of a unicameral bone cyst, non-ossifying fibroma or stress fracture. Treatment is non-surgical and includes rest, activity modification and Achilles tendon-stretching. Shoe inserts, such as heel cups, pads or lifts, may also be beneficial. A brief period of immobilization in a brace or cast may be indicated for severe involvement or persistent symptoms, or else to ensure rest in non-compliant patients.

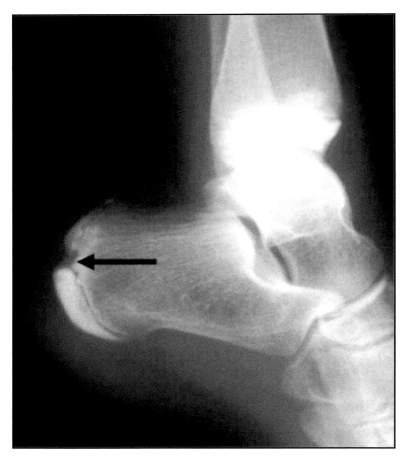

Figure 2. This lateral radiograph of the calcaneus shows fragmentation and sclerosis of the calcaneal apophysitis in a 13 year old long-distance runner with Sever's disease (from Frush TJ, Lindenfeld TN. Peri-epiphyseal and overuse injuries in adolescent athletes. Sports Health. 2009; 1: 201-211).

Progression of Sever's disease to calcaneal apophyseal avulsion fracture has been reported in four young athletes [25], two of whom required Achilles tendon repair for chronic injuries. The authors suggested that inadequate protection and continued repetitive trauma were responsible for this progression, and recommended more aggressive treatment of Sever's disease in athletes. Considering the frequency of Sever's disease, however, these fractures occur in only a very small subset of involved individuals.

Congenital and developmental disorders

Contracture of the Achilles tendon occurs as one of the components of a number of congenital, acquired and neuromuscular disorders, and tendon lengthening - or tenotomy - is an integral part of the surgical treatment of many foot deformities in these patients.

Flexible flatfoot

According to Mosca [29], flexible flatfoot is "common, often familial, rarely painful, and even more rarely disabling." In most children, the arch elevates spontaneously before the ages of eight to ten years, and flexible flatfoot is usually asymptomatic and requires no treatment. It is associated with a short Achilles tendon in approximately 25% of individuals with flat feet, and pain and functional disability are more frequent in these patients [15]. It is unclear whether the shortening of the Achilles tendon is a primary pathological feature or a secondary developmental deformity. Although a short Achilles tendon allows some mobility of the sub-talar joint, it limits ankle dorsiflexion. Mosca has described 'false' dorsiflexion, occurring when the dorsiflexion force is shifted to the sub-talar joint and which enables dorsiflexion of the calcaneus in relation to the talus; this often results in pain in the plantar-medial aspect of the mid-foot, and occasionally in the sinus tarsi area. Non-surgical treatment consists of stretching of the Achilles tendon in an attempt to convert the symptomatic flatfoot to an asymptomatic deformity. Stretching must be done with the forefoot in supination to avoid re-creating false dorsiflexion. Orthotics, generally, are not recommended because they do not correct the problem and can actually make symptoms worse. If operative treatment is indicated, Achilles tendon lengthening is usually combined with a joint-preserving osteotomy to correct the shape of the foot.

Idiopathic toe-walking

Toe-walking is common in children up to two or three years of age, but resolves in most children by school age. In older children, this abnormal gait pattern, in which a normal heel strike does not occur and most weight-bearing occurs through the forefoot, is considered pathological. In the absence of evidence of neurological, orthopaedic or psychiatric disease, the condition is considered to be idiopathic toe walking (ITW) [31]. Contractures and congenital shortness or tightness of the Achilles tendon have been identified in some children who are 'toe walkers', but this is not pathological as long as the foot remains flexible and the ankle can dorsiflex beyond neutral [37]. The condition becomes pathological once the contracture becomes fixed and the ankle is no longer completely flexible.

Non-surgical management of idiopathic toe walking may include physical therapy and braces, night splints or casting, to stretch the Achilles tendon and posterior calf musculature [14.] Chemodenervation of the gastrocnemius-soleus complex muscles with botulinum toxin, followed by serial casting, has also been reported to improve ankle range of motion [3, 13, 21]. The results of non-surgical treatment are mixed, with improvements in gait reported in 22% to 79% of patients [11, 14, 17]. The surgical management of idiopathic toe walking consists of lengthening the triceps surae muscle-tendon complex. The Silfverskiöld test (Fig. 3) is useful in determining the location of posterior muscle tightness that limits ankle dorsiflexion and where lengthening is needed. In general, lengthening of the Achilles tendon is indicated for patients with limited ankle dorsiflexion when the knee is flexed and extended (combined gastrocnemius and soleus tightness), and gastrocnemius lengthening is indicated for limited ankle dorsiflexion only when the knee is extended [38]. In two studies [16, 27,] Achilles tendon lengthening improved gait in 22 (88%) of 25 patients with idiopathic toe walking. Although complications are unusual after Achilles tendon lengthening, over- or under-correction is possible.

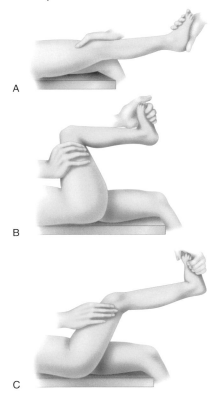

Figure 3. Silfverskiöld test for gastrocnemius tightness and contracture: A) With the knee extended, equinus is noted in the ankle; B) With the knee flexed, the ankle is easily dorsiflexed, indicating no soleus contracture; C) As the knee is extended, ankle dorsiflexion is resisted by tight gastrocnemius muscles. Improved ankle dorsiflexion with the knee flexed indicates the gastrocnemius muscles; equivalent ankle dorsiflexion with knee flexion and extension indicates Achilles tightness (from Sawyer JR. Cerebral palsy. In: Canale ST, Beaty JH, eds., Campbell's Operative Orthopaedics, 12th edition. Philadelphia: Elsevier. 2013; 1202-1254).

Congenital clubfoot

Abnormal shortening of the Achilles tendon is secondary to intrinsic foot deformity, and surgical release or lengthening is often necessary to correct the equinus in clubfoot. With the Ponseti method for clubfoot treatment, serial casting is used to correct all components of the deformity except equinus. Each cast holds the foot in the corrected position, allowing it to reshape gradually. Generally, five to six casts are required to correct the alignment of the foot and ankle fully. Before the application of the final cast, most infants require percutaneous Achilles tenotomy to gain adequate lengthening of the Achilles tendon and prevent a rocker bottom deformity.

Congenital vertical talus

The Achilles tendon is invariably contracted in children with congenital vertical talus, and the lengthening of the tendon is usually part of the surgical correction of congenital vertical talus. The exact surgery is determined by the age of the child and the severity of the deformity.

Neuromuscular disorders

Achilles tendon contracture, weakness or spasticity is common in children with neurological conditions, such as cerebral palsy, spina bifida, poliomyelitis and muscular dystrophy. In patients with cerebral palsy and spina bifida, the Achilles tendons are contracted and may require surgical lengthening [22]. In patients with poliomyelitis, certain muscles are paralysed and tendon transfer surgeries may be needed. The progression of muscular dystrophies may require both tendon transfer and tendon lengthening. Achilles tendon lengthening, however, must be appropriately-timed to avoid decreasing ambulatory ability by removing a compensatory mechanism. The plantarflexion contracture forces the knee into hyperextension, which helps overcome the weakness of the quadriceps muscles; after Achilles tendon lengthening, the plantigrade foot forces the use of the quadriceps muscles to stand and walk. If these muscles have become too weak, continued ambulation is not possible without braces. Other progressive neuropathies that may require the lengthening of the Achilles tendon include Charcot-Marie-Tooth disease and Friedreich ataxia.

Techniques for Achilles tendon lengthening

Achilles tendon lengthening can be done with open or percutaneous techniques [7,19]. If open Z-plasty lengthening is done in a walking child, care must be taken to suture the tendon in appropriate tension to prevent over-lengthening [8, 18, 36]. Vascular complications have been reported after percutaneous tenotomy in children with clubfoot deformities, possibly because of the vascular abnormalities known to be present in many of these children [4, 6, 9, 10, 30]. Dobbs and co-workers [9, 10] recommended Doppler examination of the peroneal artery if both the dorsalis pedis and posterior tibial pulses are not palpable; if the peroneal artery is found to be the only artery supplying the foot, they recommended open Achilles lengthening. Lengthening can also be done at the musculo-tendinous junction. This is often recommended for mild to moderate contractures, particularly if the Silverskiöld test indicates that the gastrocnemius is the primary contributor to the contracture.

Gastrocnemius-soleus lengthening (the Strayer procedure)

Through a posterior longitudinal incision over the middle of the calf (Fig. 4A), the aponeurosis of the gastrocnemius is exposed (Fig. 4B) and an inverted or transverse incision is made from lateral to medial through it (Fig. 4C). The raphae of the gastrocnemius-soleus and the plantaris tendon are released completely (Fig. 4D), then the ankle is brought into slight dorsiflexion to separate the ends of the tendon (Fig. 4E). A short-leg cast is applied and the patient is allowed to bear weight as tolerated. Knee extension is encouraged, and physical therapy to maintain ankle dorsiflexion is started at four weeks when the cast is removed. A maximal-dorsiflexion ankle-foot orthosis is worn at night for six months after surgery.

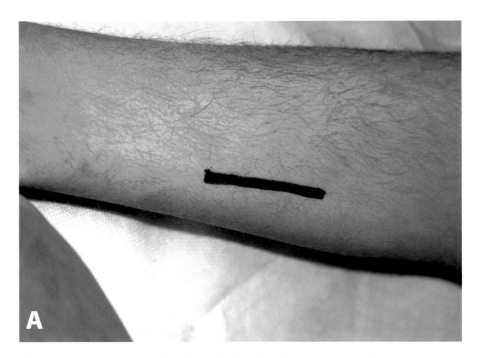

Figure 4. Gastrocnemius-soleus lengthening (the Strayer procedure): 4A. Incision.

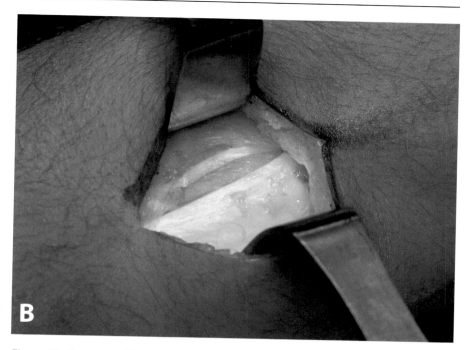

Figure 4B. Exposure of the gastrocnemius.

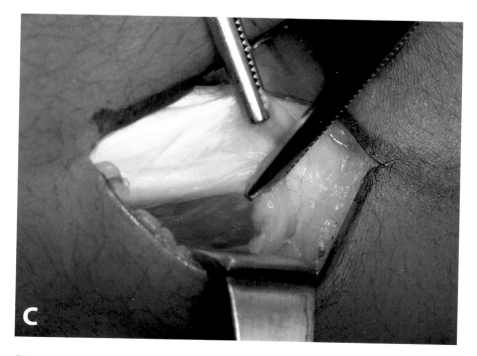

Figure 4C. Transverse incision.

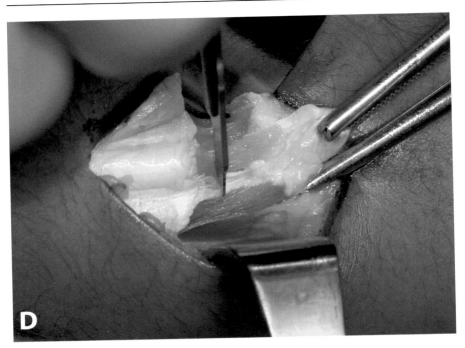

Figure 4D. Release of the gastrocnemius-soleus and plantaris tendons.

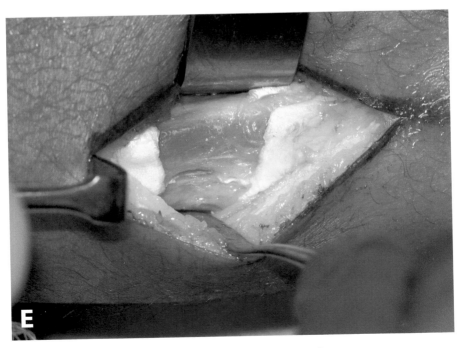

Figure 4E. Separation of the tendon-ends with ankle dorsiflexion.

410

Percutaneous Achilles tendon lengthening

With the patient prone and the leg prepared to the mid-thigh to include the toes, the knee is extended and the ankle is dorsiflexed to tense the Achilles tendon so that it is subcutaneous, easily outlined and away from the neurovascular structures anteriorly. Three partial tenotomies are made in the Achilles tendon (Fig. 5). The first medial cut is made just at the insertion of the tendon onto the calcaneus, through one half of the width of the tendon. The second tenotomy is made proximally and medially, just below the musculo-tendinous junction, and the third laterally through half the width of the tendon midway between the two medial cuts. If the heel is in varus, as it usually is, two incisions are made on the medial side of the heel, and on the lateral side if the heel is in valgus. The ankle is dorsiflexed to the desired angle. The incisions do not require closure, only a sterile dressing and a long leg cast with the knee in full extension.

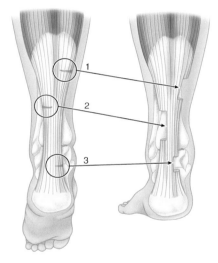

Figure 5. Percutaneous Achilles tendon lengthening (from Sawyer JR. Cerebral palsy. In: Canale ST, Beaty JH, eds., Campbell's Operative Orthopaedics, 12th edition. Philadelphia: Elsevier. 2013; 1202-1254).

Z-plasty lengthening of the Achilles tendon

A postero-medial incision is made midway between the Achilles tendon and the posterior aspect of the medial malleolus; the distal extent is at the superior border of the calcaneus and it continues proximally 4 to 5 cm (Fig. 6A). The Achilles tendon is exposed with sharp dissection directed posteriorly towards it, and the sheath is incised longitudinally for the length of the incision. Once the tendon is freed from the surrounding tissues, a longitudinal incision is made in the centre of the tendon from proximal to distal. The scalpel is turned medially or laterally distally to divide that half of the tendon transversely. For a varus deformity, the distal cut is made towards the medial side, and for a valgus deformity, it is made towards the lateral side. While the cut portion of the tendon is held with a forceps, the scalpel is brought to the proximal portion of the longitudinal incision in the tendon and is turned opposite the distal cut to divide that half of the tendon transversely to free the Achilles tendon completely. The plantaris tendon on the medial aspect of the Achilles tendon is divided transversely. Passive excursion of the triceps surae muscle is evaluated by using a Kocher clamp to pull the proximal stump of the tendon to its maximally-stretched length. The tendon is then allowed to retract halfway back to its resting length and is sutured to the distal tendon-end (Fig. 6B). Tension can be controlled by adjusting the position of the foot. The tendon repair is performed in a side-to-side fashion with heavy absorbable sutures, the wound is closed with absorbable or sub-cuticular sutures and skin strips, and a long-leg cast is applied.

Alternatively, the Z-plasty lengthening can be done in the coronal plane if equinus is the only deformity, with no varus or valgus component.

Ambulation is allowed as soon as the patient is comfortable. When the pain is gone (usually five to ten days), the cast is changed to a short leg cast, and walking is continued. Cast immobilization is continued for a total of six weeks. Bracing is used if the anterior tibial muscle is not strong or is not under volitional control. If there is no function in the anterior tibial muscle, full-time bracing is required. If the anterior tibial muscle functions only with withdrawal, full-time bracing is required for several months - and then at night only - to prevent the recurrence of Achilles tendon contracture.

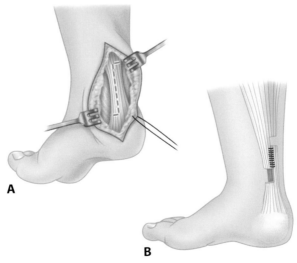

Figure 6. Z-plasty lengthening of the Achilles tendon: A) The longitudinal incision in the tendon is brought out proximally in one direction and distally in the opposite direction; B) The ends are sutured to repair the tendon (from Sawyer JR. Cerebral palsy. In: Canale ST, Beaty JH, eds., Campbell's Operative Orthopaedics, 12th edition. Philadelphia: Elsevier. 2013; 1202-1254).

Conclusion

Although not as frequent in children as in adults, problems with the Achilles tendon can cause pain and impair function. While traumatic Achilles tendon injuries are rare in children, overuse injuries do occur in athletic adolescents. In children, the Achilles tendon may require surgical lengthening to correct tightness or contractures associated with congenital, developmental, neurological and post-traumatic disorders. Both open and percutaneous lengthening techniques can be successful, but care must be taken to avoid over-lengthening.

References

1. Agarwal A, Pruthi M. Bicycle-spoke injuries of the foot in children. J Orthop Surg (Hong Kong). 2010; 18(3): 338-341.

2. Anger DM, Ledbetter BR, Stasikelis PJ, Calhoun JH. Injuries of the foot related to the use of lawn mowers. J Bone Joint Surg Am 1995; 77: 719-725.

3. Brunt D, Woo R, Kim HD, Kos MS, Senesac C, Li S. Effect of botulinum toxin type A on gait of children who are idiopathic toe-walkers. J Surg Orthop Adv. 2004; 13(3): 149-155.

4. Burghardt RD, Herzenberg JE, Ranade A. Pseudoaneurysm after Ponseti percutaneous Achilles tenotomy: a case report. J Pediatr Orthop. 2008; 28(3): 366-369.

5. Caine D, Cochrane B, Caine C, Zemper E. An epidemiologic investigation of injuries affecting young competitive female gymnasts. Am J Sports Med. 1989; 17: 811-820.

6. Changulani M, Garg N, Bruce CE. Neurovascular complications following percutaneous tendo Achillis tenotomy for congenital idiopathic clubfoot. Arch Orthop Trauma Surg. 2007; 127(6): 429-430.

7. Chen L, Greisberg J. Achilles lengthening procedures. Foot Ankle Clin. 2009; 14(4): 627-637.

8. Dalton GP, Wapner KL, Hecht PJ. Complications of Achilles and posterior tibial tendon surgeries. Clin Orthop Relat Res. 2001; 391: 133-139.

9. Dobbs MB, Gordon JE, Schoenecker PL. Absent posterior tibial artery associated with idiopathic clubfoot. A report of two cases. J Bone Joint Surg Am. 2994; 86(3): 599-602.

10. Dobbs MB, Gordon JEW, Walton T, Schoenecker PL. Bleeding complications following percutaneous tendo Achilles tenotomy in the treatment of clubfoot deformity. J Pediatr Orthop. 2004; 24(4): 353-357.

11. Eastwood DM, Menelaus MB, Dickens DR, Broughton NS, Cole WG. Idiopathic toe-walking: Does treatment alter the natural history? J Pediatr Orthop B. 2009; 9(1): 47-49.

12. Eidelman M, Nachtigal A, Katzman A, Bialik V. Acute rupture of Achilles tendon in a 7 year old girl. J Pediatr Orthop B. 2004; 13(1): 32-33.

13. Engström P, Gutierrez-Farewik EM, Bartonek A, Tedroff K, Oreffelt C, Haglund-Akerlind Y. Does botulinum toxin A improve the walking pattern in children with idiopathic toe-walking? J Child Orthop. 2010; 4(4): 301-308.

14. Fox A, Deakin S, Pettigrew G, Paton R. Serial casting in the treatment of idiopathic toe-walkers and review of the literature. Acta Orthop Belg. 2006; 72(6): 722-730.

15. Harris RI, Beath T. Hypermobile flat-foot with short tendo Achillis. J Bone Joint Surg Am. 1948; 30A(1): 116-140.

16. Hemo Y, Macdessi SJ, Pierce RA, Aiona MD, Sussman MD. Outcome of patients after Achilles tendon lengthening for treatment of idiopathic toe walking. J Pediatr Orthop. 2006; 26(3): 336-340.

17. Hirsch G, Wagner B. The natural history of idiopathic toe-walking: a long-term follow-up of fourteen conservatively treated children. Acta Paediatr. 2004; 93(2) 196-199

18. Hoefnagels EM, Waites MD, Belkoff SM, Swierstra BA. Percutaneous Achilles tendon lengthening: a cadaver-based study of failure of the triple hemisection technique. Acta Orthop. 2007; 78(6): 808-812.

19. Hoffman B, Nunley J. Achilles tendon torsion has no effect on percutaneous triple-cut tenotomy results. Foot Ankle Int. 2006; 27(11): 960-964.

20. Hogan KA, Gross RH. Overuse injuries in pediatric athletes. Orthop Clin North Am. 2003; 34(3): 405-415.

21. Jacks LK, Michels DM, Smith BP, Koman LA, Shilt J. Clinical usefulness of botulinum toxin in the lower extremity. Foot Ankle Clin. 2004; 9: 339-348.

22. Jaddue DA, Abbas MA, Sayed-Noor AS. Open versus percutaneous tendo Achilles lengthening in spastic cerebral palsy with equines deformity of the foot in children. J Surg Orthop Adv. 2010; 19(4): 196-199.

23. Järvinen TA, Kannus P, Maffulli N, Khan KM. Achilles tendon disorders: etiology and epidemiology. Foot Ankle Clin 2005; 10: 255-266.

24. Kose O. Do we really need radiographic assessment for the diagnosis of non-specific heel pain (calcaneal apophysitis) in children? Skeletal Radiol. 2010; 39(4): 359-361.

25. Lee KT, Young KW, Park YU, Park SY, Kim KC. Neglected Sever's disease as a cause of calcaneal apophyseal avulsion fracture: case report. Foot Ankle Int. 2010; 31(8): 725-728.

26. Lee SM, Huh SW, Chung JW, Kim DW, Kim YJ, Rhee SK. Avulsion fracture of the calcaneal tuberosity: classification and its characteristics. Clin Orthop Surg 2012; 4: 134-138.

27. McMulkin ML, Baird GO, Caskey PM, Ferguson RL. Comprehensive outcomes of surgically treated idiopathic toe walkers. J Pediatr Orthop. 2006; 26(5): 606-611.

28. Mine R, Fukui M, Nishimura G. Bicycle spoke injuries in the lower extremity. Plast Reconstr Surg. 2000; 106: 1501-1506.

29. Mosca VS. Flexible flatfoot in children and adolescents. J Child Orthop. 2010; 4: 107-121.

30. Mulier T, Molenaers G, Fabry G. A false aneurysm complicating a subcutaneous Achilles tendon lengthening. J Pediatr Orthop B. 1995; 4(1): 114-115.

31. Oetgen ME, Peden S. Idiopathic toe walking. J Am Acad Orthop Surg. 2012; 20(5): 292-300.

32. Ogden JA, Gane y TM, Hill JD, Jaakkola JI. Sever's injury: a stress fracture of the immature calcaneal metaphysis. J Pediatr Orthop. 2004; 24(5): 488-492.

33. Parkar AA, Taylor M, Patel N, Ramakrishnan V. Regeneration of tendo Achilles. J Bone Joint Surg Br 2010; 92: 885-887.

34. Rachel JN, Williams JB, Sawyer JR, Warner WC, Kelly DM. Is radiographic evaluation necessary in children with a clinical diagnosis of calcaneal apophysitis (Sever's disease)? J Pediatr Orthop. 2011; 31(5): 548-550.

35. Ralston EL, Schmidt ER Jr. Repair of the ruptured Achilles tendon. J Trauma 1971; 11: 15-21.

36. Salamon ML, Pinney SJ, Van Bergeyk A, Hazelwood S. Surgical anatomy and accuracy of percutaneous Achilles tendon lengthening. Foot Ankle Int. 2006; 27(6): 411-413.

37. Solan MC, Kohls-Gatzoulis J, Stephens MM. Idiopathic toe walking and contractures of the triceps surae. Foot Ankle Clin. 2010; 15(2): 297-307.

38. Stott NS, Walt SE, Lobb GA, Reynolds N, Nicol RO. Treatment for idiopathic toe-walking: results at skeletal maturity. J Pediatr Orthop. 2004; 24(1): 63-69.

39. Tudisco C, Bisicchia S. Reconstruction of a neglected Achilles tendon rupture in a young girl. J Orthopaed Traumatol. 2012; 13: 163-166.

40. Vosburgh CL, Gruel CRl, Herndon WA, Sullivan JA. Lawn mower injuries of the pediatric foot and ankle: observations on prevention and management. J Pediatr Orthop. 1995; 15: 504-509.

Chapter 30

Future Perspectives

Paul W. Ackermann

Take Home Message

- *First-line treatment for Achilles tendon pathology should exhibit non-invasive methods to promote tendon healing with focused exercise and biophysical procedures.*

- *Targeted minimally invasive surgical procedures should be considered in specific recalcitrant cases to initiate healing and alleviate pain.*

- *Biological augmentation techniques may in future promote tissue production.*

- *Biomaterial scaffolds could guide cell and new tissue ingrowth.*

- *Biomechanical loading techniques should help to enhance tissue remodelling.*

Introduction

Accurate diagnosis, standardized terminology and the thorough analysis of the underlying mechanisms involved in Achilles tendon disorders is a prerequisite to planning and administering correct management. The histopathological feature of tendinopathy can be characterized as a failed healing response displaying matrix disorganization, increased extracellular ground substance and separation between collagen fibres. In a failed healing response, one of the

417

following stages of the healing process may be deficient and necessitate exogenous stimulation: 1) induction, 2) production, 3) orchestration, 4) conduction and 5) modification (see chapter on healing and repair). Novel therapies can be applied as single treatments directed to promote a specific, failed stage of healing, or as combined therapies to enhance all stages of healing (e.g., after a surgical procedure).

In pain disorders, such as in tendinopathy, the focus of the therapy must address the pain-generating mechanism in a targeted manner. This requires knowledge and understanding of the underlying pathology. Novel findings demonstrate that the deficient healing response in tendinopathy is accompanied by the abnormal ingrowth of sensory nerves[3]. Sensory nerve-endings give rise to nociceptive signals on:

1. Mechanical activation (e.g., bone spur impingement);
2. High (low) temperature (one study assessed high temperature in racing horses);
3. Biochemical activation (e.g., autocrine/paracrine neuromediator activation).

This is why mechanical loading activity and biochemical activation cause nociception.

Novel procedures that may promote healing and target pain pathology are outlined:

Biophysical procedures and minimally invasive surgical approaches

In case of deficient healing, without bleeding and a lack of essential substances starting the repair process, it has been thought to induce a new trauma to re-start the healing process. Moreover, the Achilles tendon exhibits a delicate homeostasis dependent on successive increments in loading regimens for its cells and matrix to adapt and function normally[1].

Achilles tendon disorders should at first be treated with focused exercise and non-invasive techniques[3], and thus novel biophysical procedures, such as extracorporeal shockwave treatment (ESWT), low-intensity pulsed ultrasound (LIPUS) and low-level laser therapy (LLLT), to address pathology and initiate tendon and tendon-to-bone healing responses have emerged (see chapter 12). ESWT, LIPUS and LLLT all have positive experimental effects on tendon healing, and ESWT leads to the selective denervation of sensory unmyelinated nerve fibres without affecting larger motor neurons (see chapters 6 and 14). ESWT has shown encouraging clinical effects[12]. One clinically important aspect in administering focused eccentric exercise and biophysical therapy is that "overloading" sports activities may be avoided during the rehabilitation period. However, many parameters in terms of biophysical therapy remain unknown and diverging results from clinical studies may arise from unclear diagnosis, terminology and specifications of treatment. Future studies may offer more targeted protocols in terms of the timing and dosage of biophysical treatments.

Achilles tendon disorders that are resistant to non-invasive therapy and where an exact diagnosis can be made may open the possibility for a subsequent surgical procedure being performed using minimally invasive techniques. Such surgical procedures should at the same time target the pain-generating pathology. This can be performed, e.g., by the removal of bony spurs and the denervation of pathological nerve ingrowth into the Achilles tendon proper or into one of the bursae (retrocalcaneal, superficial calcaneal or subcalcaneal).

Thus, endoscopic or minimally invasive techniques have to be applied to sufficiently stimulate the healing response and address the pathology.

Biological augmentation techniques

Inhibition of pathological pathways

Novel treatments to improve tendon and tendon-to-bone healing may be directed towards the inhibition of pathological pathways, e.g., neuronal inflammation mediated by substance P (SP), mast cells and matrix metalloproteinases (MMPs) (Figure 1). Hence, the recent inhibition of MMP with doxycycline-improved tendon-to-bone healing in the rotator cuff [7]. Experimental studies verify that proteolytic metalloproteinases ADAM-12 (a disintegrin and metalloproteinase) and MMP-23 (matrix metalloproteinase) are significantly up-regulated in tendinopathy [8]. Metalloproteinases are released from, e.g., mast cells, which are activated by SP (Figure 1). Hence, approaches to mitigate tendinopathic processes could entail the inhibition of the above-mentioned pathways and molecules.

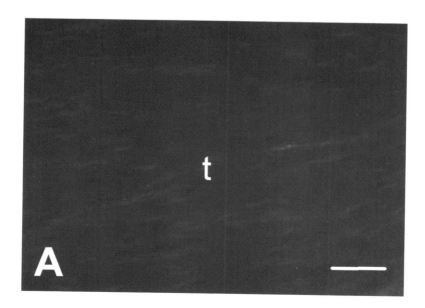

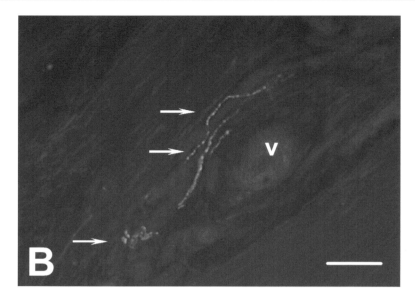

Figure 1. Achilles tendon of healthy control (A) and painful tendinopathy (B) after immunostaining for substance P (SP) and a picture taken with immunofluorescence microscopy. The arrows denote free nerve endings. The micrograph illustrates SP-positive nerve fibres in close vicinity to a proliferated vessel (B). v = blood vessel. Bar = 50 μm.

Improvement of growth factor delivery by autologous blood or platelet rich plasma (PRP)

Platelets are blood-derived cells that are activated after injury involving bleeding. Platelets release a wide variety of growth factors at the site of injury. Lately, in deficient healing conditions without bleeding such as Achilles tendon disorders, platelet rich plasma (PRP) injections have become a very popular treatment alternative [5]. A number of growth factors released by platelets, such as PDGF, VEGF, IGF-1, TGF-beta and FGF, promote repair in various soft tissue models. In addition, some (TGF-beta; BMP-2; IL-10) act as an anti-inflammatory on MMPs and cytokines. At this stage, the dose and treatment intervals of the cited growth factors working "exclusively" on tendon healing or – for instance – cartilage healing are unknown. Further research may induce more effective combinations than PRP as a "gunshot" treatment. Perhaps there will be a "tendon fraction" of growth factors in the future? Although in vitro and in vivo studies suggest a potential beneficial effect of the use of PRP in Achilles tendon pathology, the few well-conducted randomized controlled trials have shown limited evidence of clinical advantage (see chapter on PRP injections). Thus, at present, there are unknown variables (e.g., the delivery system, the local environment, receptor activation and tendon loading) which have to be mastered before growth factor delivery therapies (e.g., PRP) can become clinically effective.

Molecularly optimized mediator delivery

Normal tendon and tendon-to-bone repair involves infiltration into the wound area of tissue- and vascular-derived cells, which release a cascade of mediators (growth factors, cytokines, bone morphogenetic proteins and neuropeptides). These mediators have been supplemented in several experimental studies and have demonstrated promising results for the optimization of the repair process [2]. However, optimal delivery of growth factors has proven to be of limited clinical success. Molecular approaches, by which mesenchymal stem cells (MSCs) and genetically modified cells and gene therapy can synthesize and deliver the desired growth factors in a temporally and spatially orchestrated manner to the desired site, would be a powerful means to overcome the limitations of various delivery systems [4]. Hence, stem cells and genetically modified cells have produced the improved regeneration of tendon-to-bone insertion site [4]. The biological augmentation of Achilles re-attachment is an area where new techniques such as these may prove beneficial.

Biomaterial scaffolding

Novel biogenic or synthetic (e.g., bioresorbable polymers) scaffold grafts with biomimetic functionality will emerge to help the surgeon to cover tissue defects and promote cell and callus ingrowths. New grafts can also be used in a tissue-engineered manner to provide different properties to a tendon-to-bone insertion and to enhance stem cell and biological augmentation techniques.

If more than 2 cm of the tendon at its insertion is resected or 50% of the Achilles tendon is excised, then a grafting procedure should be considered. One of the greatest challenges to the clinician is to promote the biological fixation of the graft in different tissues (e.g., bone and tendon). Such fixation requires strategic biomimicry to be incorporated into the scaffold design to re-establish the critical structure-function relationship and to obtain a gradient of mechanical properties mimicking the four distinct layers of tendon-to-bone. Future biomaterial matrices will prove whether these principles can be incorporated into clinically effective products.

Biomechanical loading techniques

Mechanical loading promotes tendon repair, while excessive repetitive loading or immobilization are detrimental for tendon healing [11]. However, the exact timing, dosage and nature of loading during different healing phases and in various pathological conditions are not known. Hopefully, future treatments will give us better biomarkers to prescribe and administer biomechanical loading during healing and in pathological cases.

Mechanical loading of a healthy tendon results in the up-regulation of collagen expression and the increased synthesis of collagen protein, presumably regulated by the strain on the resident tenocytes. Exercise induces both formation and degradation of collagen, with a net loss during the first 36 hours after exercise but a net synthesis 36-72 hours post-exercise [11]. Thus, too frequent, intense loading may, over time, induce a net loss instead of the synthesis of collagen.

Immobilization, such as prolonged plaster casting, causes muscle hypotrophy and is detrimental to healing [1], as well as being potentially related to an increased mortality risk; recently, a high incidence of deep venous thrombosis has been reported after plaster cast immobilization for Achilles tendon ruptures. Moreover, in a rat model with plaster cast immobilization of the hind limb after Achilles tendon rupture, the ultimate tensile strength was reduced 80% and the mRNA expression of essential growth factors and matrix proteins was down-regulated at two weeks post-rupture compared to a freely mobilized group [13]. These results point to accelerated mobilization protocols.

Improved orthotic devices, which will allow earlier mobility, loading and improved circulation, may also be combined with novel methodologies of applying mechanical stimulation to the immobilized tendon. One method could be the application of external intermittent pneumatic compression (IPC) to the lower limbs (Figure 2) [6]. IPC, used clinically to prevent thrombosis and increase blood circulation [9], has experimentally proven positive effects on wound and fracture healing [10, 13] and improves tensile properties and collagen production in the healing of experimental Achilles tendon rupture [6, 13].

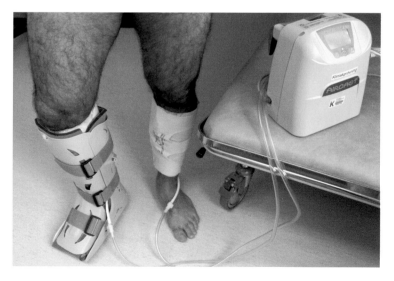

Figure 2. External intermittent pneumatic compression (IPC) applied to the lower limbs during immobilization. This is an experimental set-up currently assessed in prospective randomized clinical studies in order to decrease the risk of deep venous thrombosis and improve healing.

Whether IPC, new orthotics or novel biomarkers can improve tendon-to-bone repair and reverse the negative effects of immobilization in patients still needs further exploration.

Conclusion

There are several novel procedures to target the pathology of Achilles tendon problems. Minimally invasive, biophysical procedures, biological augmentation and biomaterial scaffolding techniques are increasingly being discussed. Each technique focuses on a different stage in the healing process. In addition, a new vision of current treatments, specifically in terms of loading and mobilization/immobilization after injury, may provide better results. Most treatment options are still experimental, and only a few preliminary clinical results have been published. Biological augmentation and biomaterial scaffolding techniques, both theoretically very promising, are still in their infancy. Supported by new studies, only the future can tell which novel treatment will provide the desired clinical results.

References

1. Ackermann PW. Neuronal regulation of tendon homoeostasis. International journal of experimental pathology. 2013;94(4):271-86.
2. Ackermann PW, Calder J, Aspenberg P. Healing and Repair Mechanism. In: van Diek CN, Karlsson J, Maffulli N, Thermann H, editors. Achilles Tendon Rupture: DJO Publications; 2008. pp. 17-26.
3. Ackermann PW, Renstrom P. Tendinopathy in sport. Sports Health. 2012;4(3):193-201.
4. Ackermann PW, Salo PT, Hart DA. Gene Therapy. In: Van Dijk N, Karlsson J, Maffulli N, editors. Achilles Tendinopathy Current Concept. London: DJO Publications 2010. pp. 165-75.
5. Andia I, Sanchez M, Maffulli N. Tendon healing and platelet-rich plasma therapies. Expert Opin Biol Ther. 2010;10(10):1415-26.
6. Arverud E, Azevedo J, Labruto F, Ackermann P. Adjuvant compression therapy in orthopaedic surgery - an evidence-based review. European Orthopaedics and Traumatology. 2013;4(1):49-57.
7. Bedi A, Fox AJ, Kovacevic D, Deng XH, Warren RF, Rodeo SA. Doxycycline-mediated inhibition of matrix metalloproteinases improves healing after rotator cuff repair. The American journal of sports medicine. 2010;38(2):308-17.
8. Jones GC, Corps AN, Pennington CJ, Clark IM, Edwards DR, Bradley MM, Expression profiling of metalloproteinases and tissue inhibitors of metalloproteinases in normal and degenerate human Achilles tendon. Arthritis and rheumatism. 2006;54(3):832-42.
9. Kakkos SK, Caprini JA, Geroulakos G, Nicolaides AN, Stansby GP, Reddy DJ. Combined intermittent pneumatic leg compression and pharmacological prophylaxis for prevention of venous thromboembolism in high-risk patients. Cochrane Database Syst Rev. 2008;(4):CD005258.
10. Khanna A, Gougoulias N, Maffulli N. Intermittent pneumatic compression in fracture and soft-tissue injuries healing. Br Med Bull. 2008;88(1):147-56.
11. Magnusson SP, Langberg H, Kjaer M. The pathogenesis of tendinopathy: balancing the response to loading. Nat Rev Rheumatol. 2010;6(5):262-8.
12. Rompe JD, Furia J, Maffulli N. Eccentric loading compared with shock wave treatment for chronic insertional Achilles tendinopathy. A randomized, controlled trial. The Journal of bone and joint surgery. 2008;90(1):52-61.
13. Schizas N, Li J, Andersson T, Fahlgren A, Aspenberg P, Ahmed M. Compression therapy promotes proliferative repair during rat Achilles tendon immobilization. J Orthop Res. 2010;28(7):852-8.